fourth edition

DIAGNOSIS AND EVALUATION IN SPEECH PATHOLOGY

WILLIAM O. HAYNES

Auburn University-Alabama

REBEKAH H. PINDZOLA

Auburn University-Alabama

LON L. EMERICK

Northern Arizona University-Flagstaff

PRENTICE HALL
Englewood Cliffs, New Jersey 07632

Library of Congress Cataloging-in-Publication Data

HAYNES, WILLIAM O.
    Diagnosis and evaluation in speech pathology / William O. Haynes,
Rebekah H. Pindzola, Lon L. Emerick. —4th ed.
        p. cm.
        Emerick's name appears first on the earlier edition.
        Includes bibliographical references and indexes.
        ISBN 0-13-210261-7
        1. Speech disorders—Diagnosis. 2. Speech disorders—Case
studies. I. Pindzola, Rebekah H. (Rebekah Hand) II. Emerick, Lon
L. III. Title.
        [DNLM: 1. Speech Disorders—diagnosis. WM 475 H424d]
RC423.H39 1992
616.85′5075—dc20
DNLM/DLC
for Library of Congress   91-21035
                                                                          CIP

Acquisitions Editor: Carol Wada
Copy Editor: Linda Pawelchak
Cover Designer: Carol Ceraldi
Prepress Buyer: Kelly Behr
Manufacturing Buyer: Mary Ann Gloriande

© 1992, 1986, 1979, 1973 by Prentice-Hall, Inc.
a Simon & Schuster Company
Englewood Cliffs, New Jersey 07632

Printed in the United States of America
10 9 8 7 6 5 4 3

ISBN 0-13-210261-7

Prentice-Hall International (UK) Limited, *London*
Prentice-Hall of Australia Pty. Limited, *Sydney*
Prentice-Hall Canada Inc., *Toronto*
Prentice-Hall Hispanoamericana, S.A., *Mexico*
Prentice-Hall of India Private Limited, *New Delhi*
Prentice-Hall of Japan, Inc., *Tokyo*
Simon & Schuster Asia Pte. Ltd., *Singapore*
Editora Prentice-Hall do Brasil, Ltda., *Rio de Janeiro*

CONTENTS

3

PSYCHOMETRIC CONSIDERATIONS IN DIAGNOSIS AND EVALUATION _____ 56

4

ASSESSMENT OF CHILDREN WITH LIMITED LANGUAGE _____ 80

5

ASSESSMENT OF SCHOOL-AGE AND ADOLESCENT LANGUAGE DISORDERS _____ 128

6

ASSESSMENT OF PHONOLOGICAL DISORDERS —————————— *154*

7

DISORDERS OF FLUENCY ————————————————— *198*

8

ASSESSMENT OF APHASIA AND ADULT LANGUAGE DISORDERS ——— *226*

12

ASSESSMENT OF RESONANCE IMBALANCE ─────────── *339*

13

THE DIAGNOSTIC REPORT ─────────────── *362*

appendix A

CHILD LANGUAGE ASSESSMENT
INTERVIEW PROTOCOL ─────────────── *373*

appendix B

EVALUATION CHECKLIST FOR
CARETAKER CHILD INTERACTION ─────────── *377*

appendix C

CODING SHEET FOR EARLY MULTIWORD ANALYSIS ──────── *379*

PREFACE

With this fourth edition of *Diagnosis and Evaluation in Speech Pathology*, we invite a new group of students and practitioners to consider the complex and fascinating arena of assessment in communication disorders. We are gratified that so many readers of the prior editions found in them the imprint of clinical relevance. This new edition embodies many changes. We have added chapters on assessment of resonance imbalance, evaluation of the laryngectomee, and psychometric considerations. The child language chapter has been split into two chapters—one on assessment of children with limited language and the other dealing with school-age and adolescent language disorders. The aphasia chapter has also been divided into two chapters—one on adult language disorders and the other on motor speech problems. These changes expand the length and scope of the text but are necessary in view of the proliferation of new research and changing trends in clinical practice.

In addition to the increased amount of information, we have also tried to cover both standardized as well as nonstandardized approaches to evaluation in all areas of communication disorders. Assessment is an ongoing process, so we need procedures to use in exploring client performance in a variety of contexts and for evaluating treatment progress. Standardized tests are not ideally suited for this purpose.

This edition has been designed as a resource for two groups. First, the text can act as an introduction to diagnosis and evaluation for students in training. We feel that it is important that students gain an early appreciation of diagnosis as a *process*, not just the administration of tests and scales. A diagnostician is much more than a neutral conduit through which test scores pass. Each case requires the clinician to think, solve problems, form hypotheses, gather data, and arrive at conclusions. Often, the diagnostic enterprise raises more questions than it answers, and then it becomes important to be a *clinician* rather than just a *technician*. Another emphasis for students is that assessment is done in the context of an interpersonal relationship. This edition reiterates our long-standing view that we diagnose *people,* not *problems.*

A second group that may find clinical relevance in this edition is made up of practitioners. These professionals are often asked to deal with a broad range of communication disorders and must constantly update and refine their skills in each area. It is difficult for students, professors, and practitioners to remain abreast of current views in assessment of even a single area in communication disorders. The task of keeping up-to-date in *all* areas sometimes seems impossible. Yet, it is just this impossibility with which practitioners in the 1990s must deal. A clinician who secures a position in a clinic, hospital, school system, or other facility will be expected to have diagnostic expertise across all communication disorder areas. The present text provides an overview of current thinking in diagnosis and evaluation. It can act as a sourcebook for new ideas and a guide to other relevant literature.

The authors would like to express appreciation to our students, clients, colleagues, and teachers who helped to mold our thinking about the assessment process. Also, we are especially indebted to the large number of scientists and practitioners who contributed the insights and applied clinical research cited in the present volume. We challenge students and colleagues to continue the refinement of our diagnostic procedures. Even though we have come a long way in our knowledge about assessment in communication disorders, many of our measurements are still in the early stages of their development. We must persist in our search for more efficient, predictive, and meaningful methods, for the best is yet to come!

William O. Haynes
Rebekah H. Pindzola
Lon L. Emerick

chapter

1

INTRODUCTION TO DIAGNOSIS AND EVALUATION:

Philosophical Issues and General Guidelines

Speech-language pathology is a wonderfully diverse profession that requires a practitioner to possess a wide range of skills, knowledge, and personal characteristics. A speech-language pathologist (SLP) works as a case selector, case evaluator, diagnostician, interviewer, parent counselor, teacher, coordinator, record keeper, consultant, researcher, and student. Because the boundaries between these various duties are not clearly defined and the clinician must move continuously from one area to another, it is inevitable that no one person can expect to be equally competent in all areas. The ultimate goal is to maximize one's strengths in all aspects to provide the best possible service to the communicatively handicapped individual.

Diagnosis is one of the most comprehensive and difficult tasks of the speech-language pathologist. The diagnosis of a client requires a synthesis of the entire field: knowledge of norms and testing techniques, skills in observation, ability to relate effectively and empathically, and a great deal of creative intuition. Furthermore, because speech is a function of the entire person, the diagnostician must try to scrutinize all aspects of behavior. We must try to remember that we are not simply working with speech sounds, fluency, vocal quality, or linguistic rules but rather with changing people in a dynamic environment. The experienced diagnostician does not look at objective scores of articulatory skill, point scales of vocal quality, or standard scores as ends in themselves, but rather as aspects of an individual's communication ability—we diagnose communicators, not communication. That revelation is a major factor in the transition from technician to professional clinician.

1

Because our diagnostic tools are imprecise and, largely in the experimental stages and communication disorders are by nature complex and perplexing, many of our diagnostic undertakings are incomplete and ambiguous. The lack of absolute and definitive answers to the various questions of diagnosis is often frustrating and demoralizing to the clinician. The ambiguous findings that sometimes culminate a diagnostic evaluation must be dealt with in a fashion that perpetuates the evaluative undertaking rather than closes the door on further probing. Diagnosis is a continuous and open-ended venture that results in answers or partial answers that themselves are open to revision with added information.

DIAGNOSIS AND EVALUATION DEFINED

Some clinicians, at first glance, may consider the words *diagnosis* and *evaluation* to be synonymous. It is our intent in this text to define *diagnosis* by referring to the classical Greek definition: distinguishing a person's problem from the large field of potential disabilities. The term *diagnosis* in the original Greek means to *distinguish.* The prefix *dia-* means *apart* and *-gnosis* translates as *to know.* In order to distinguish a person's particular problem from the many possibilities available, we must know the client thoroughly and how he/she responds in many conditions and performs a variety of tasks. *Evaluation* refers to the process of arriving at a diagnosis. Thus, informal probes, trial therapy tasks, and generalization data are part of evaluation. In the *American Heritage Dictionary* (1985), diagnosis is defined as "the act or process of identifying or determining the nature of a disease through examination." Our conception of diagnosis, then, includes a thorough understanding of the client's problem and not merely the application of a label. It is relatively simple to call a child language-impaired, but it is a more difficult matter to really understand how this child deals with linguistic symbols in a variety of tasks and situations. *This* is diagnosis in our view. We would also like to expand the notion of diagnosis to include distinguishing the nature of a person's problem at different points in time. Thus, diagnosis and evaluation are ongoing processes. We initially perform evaluation activities to arrive at an initial diagnosis, and we also examine the client repeatedly during the course of treatment. A client's diagnosis often changes over time. For example, a child may initially present with language delay and after a period of treatment be characterized as primarily a phonologically disordered youngster. A neurogenic patient may initially be referred to as aphasic but may experience further neurological damage and be rediagnosed as aphasic and dysarthric.

Another major thrust of this book is that diagnosis need not be confined to a two-hour block of time in a university setting or a 30-minute period in a medical facility. The extent of evaluation performed should be dictated by professional and not administrative criteria. The competent clinician will continue evaluation activities until the client's performance is as fully understood as is necessary to perform effective treatment.

We perform evaluation tasks with two major goals in mind. First, we evaluate to arrive at a good understanding or diagnosis of a client's problem. Sometimes these evaluation activities will be confined to an assessment period, and at other times they will be performed well into the beginning of treatment. We must often begin therapy with a client before arriving at a firm diagnosis. This is not optimal, but it is justified as long as we realize that (1) *any* treatment is experimental to a certain degree in the beginning, (2) most initial treatment goals will generally be "in the ball park" in terms of appropriateness (e.g., we probably would not engage in voice therapy for a stuttering client), and (3) just because we have begun treatment, we have not abandoned our efforts to define the parameters of the client's problem and arrive at a diagnosis. We can always "fine tune" a treatment program based on an increased understanding of a client's problem and capabilities.

A second major reason to perform evaluation activities is to monitor the client's progress in treatment and describe changes in the communication disturbance. In this use of evaluation activities, we are not necessarily trying to diagnose the problem, but to document treatment progress and determine possible changes in the course of treatment. In the chapters that deal with specific disorders, we will suggest evaluation tasks that are not in the formal test category but are often used for these purposes. Formal tests are primarily designed to categorize clients as exhibiting certain disorders, while evaluation tasks are used to gain insight into specific client abilities and gauge treatment progress. We will now discuss some of these purposes of diagnosis and evaluation in more detail.

DIAGNOSIS TO DETERMINE THE REALITY OF THE PROBLEM

One function of diagnosis is to determine whether the presenting communication pattern does indeed constitute a handicap. Before this is possible, however, it is necessary to have a clear idea of what constitutes a communication disorder. Van Riper's definition of a speech disorder is widely quoted: "Speech is abnormal when it deviates so far from the speech of other people that it calls attention to itself, interferes with communication, or causes the speaker or his listeners to be distressed" (Van Riper & Emerick, 1984, p. 34). Figure 1.1 depicts three components that must be considered in determining a communication disorder.

Figure 1.1   Components of a Definition of a Speech Disorder

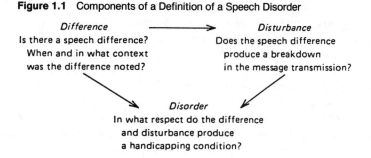

1. *Speech Difference:* This refers to whether or not the speech signal calls attention to itself and when this might occur. We can quantify the physical characteristics of the speech signal through recording, measurement, and observation. Speech spectrographs, pitch meters, and other instruments are available to help the diagnostician obtain an objective measure of the acoustic nature of the individual's speech. In other words, we must scrutinize the physical characteristics of the speech signal and judge its quality. But these data are of limited value unless it can be determined what *difference* a particular speech parameter makes.

The state of the art has not progressed in most areas of communication disorders to where we can simply take the quantified data, compare them with established numerical norms, and determine the correctness of the speech sample. Unfortunately, each diagnostician must develop a personal frame of reference. Vocal qualities are subject to individual impressions and even though a clinician may *know* that the voice is awry, evidence of the difference may often elude the sensors and algorithms of our high-tech instrumentation. In contrast, physicians are able to scrutinize data from a laboratory test and make an immediate diagnosis regarding the normalcy of an individual's blood count. This kind of reference information is not yet available to the SLP. The question of whether the presenting speech difference is different enough to be of concern thus becomes a matter of human judgment. This judgment involves filtering incoming data through the clinician's many synaptic junctions whose thresholds may have been worn thin by bias and experience. An inordinately critical or uncritical ear is a hazard with far-reaching implications.

What constitutes normal behavior? There are several definitions available, but we will discuss only two, representing the diverging philosophies with which each clinician must contend in establishing his/her own concept. The first theory we shall call the concept of *cultural norms.* The assumption is that there are behaviors that society considers aberrant in terms of group characteristics. According to this model, each bit of behavior can be judged against a real or theoretical standard, the nature of which is independent of the individual's personal idiosyncrasies. Thus, even a 70-year-old person with a hearing threshold of 30 dB in the high frequencies may be thought of as exhibiting a significant hearing loss.

The second theory we shall call the concept of *individual norms.* Advocates of this model assume that each individual has made a unique adjustment to life based on previous experiences, physical limitations, and the environment's reactions. Any judgment as to the normalcy of a bit of behavior must be contingent upon individual characteristics such as age, intelligence, and experience. Taken to the extreme, of course, this model would assert that each person is normal no matter what he/she does, since the behavior is the end product of all that plays upon the person; and to this extent the concept of individual norms loses meaning. But some case examples may help to clarify and give perspective. The audiologist who examines the hearing of the 70-year-old individual referred to earlier and obtains the typical presbycusic audiometric curve could make a case for the judgment that this person has "normal" hearing. According to personal norms, this is average or normal behavior for a person of 70; but according to cultural norms, the individual's hearing level is below the average for the total population. Follow-up procedures would be based, then, on the practical matter of getting a more efficient communication system for the individual and also on providing counseling so that the person will understand the nature of his/her hearing. Therefore, both cultural and personal norms play a part in diagnostic judgments and rehabilitative programs. A severely retarded 10-year-old with an unstimulable distortion of the /r/ phoneme may not be judged to have seriously defective speech; yet, an eight-year-old presenting a similar speech pattern, but a different intellectual potential, may be recommended for treatment. Such judgments have implications for case selection, and the clinician must reconcile the variances between the physical differences in the sounds involved and the individual variables in conjunction with what is normal for the population represented by the client. Each clinician must continually use both concepts of normalcy in diagnostic work.

There are all sorts of ways that a speech signal can call attention to itself and yet be perfectly appropriate. For example, Black English speakers may alter aspects of speech and language when their style shifts as they interact with members of one culture and then another. Although Standard English speakers may notice the differences in Black English, these variations certainly would not be viewed as evidence of a communication disorder. Another example might be when speakers alter their rate, loudness, and speech quality in order to tell a funny story or relate a particular experience in a dramatic way. Age is another variable. If the speaker is a child of two who exhibits many articulatory substitutions and omissions, does this difference constitute a problem? The answer can only lie in an examination of these errors against the context of normal two-year-old communication. Thus, a difference is not enough to constitute a communication disorder if the context suggests normality. This points out the importance of the SLP knowing contextual effects on communication and the contributions of age and the wide variety of cultural, ethnic, and geographical dialects on the speech signal.

2. *The Intelligibility of the Message:*   The second component of determining a communication disorder involves the perception of disturbance in the signal being transmitted. Is the signal distorted or is intelligibility affected? If the message transmission is adversely affected, there is a high probability of the existence of a problem. Many factors play a part in both the encoding and decoding processes, and the diagnostician must be capable of representing the standard for society when listening and making judgments. The essential judgment to be made involves how well the intentions of the speaker matched the perceptions of the listener and what factors affected this interaction. Are there attributes of the signal that distract the listener, thus altering the message? Is the signal indistinct, thus allowing only partial transmission of information? Is the signal distinct, but conveying a message other than that intended by the speaker? Is the signal distinct but conveying a message (albeit the one selected by the speaker) that is inappropriate for the context? We have, in the main, been content with clinical insight and intuitive estimates when we have judged the impact of speech differences upon intelligibility. Only a few research investigations have been concerned with this important problem (Yorkston & Beukelman, 1981).

The speech clinician is able to count the phoneme errors, quantify the number of repetitions or disfluencies per sentence, and establish various quotients of language ability, but as yet we are unable to assess the intelligibility of the transmitted message with any degree of reliability. In most cases the clinician resorts to scaling techniques (Black & Haggen, 1963; McCroskey & Mulligan, 1963) to mark the impact of the disorder on intelligibility, and we have little way to know the specific contributions of individual components of the speech signal or language used on overall signal distortion. Clearly, severe disfluency can interrupt a message; intermittent cessations of phonation and poor vocal qualities can distort transmission; inappropriate phoneme selection or production can lead to unintelligibility; and ambiguous vocabulary or sentence structure can lead to misinterpretations. Whatever the cause of the communication failure, we must document that it occurs. At present, however, we have no widely accepted system to use in this documentation for most areas of communication disorders.

3. *Handicapping Condition:* The final component in defining a disorder involves the determination of handicap in the life of the client. Emerick (1984) suggests:

> In the final analysis this third aspect justifies the existence of our profession. If the speech difference has no discernible impact on the child's behavior, and ultimately on his adjusting abilities and learning potential, there is little justification for concern on the part of the speech clinician. Although it is not feasible to compile a listing of all of the possible conditions under which a communication difference would become handicapping, it is generally agreed that communicative differences are considered handicapping when (1) the transmission and/or perception of messages is faulty; (2) the person is placed at an economic disadvantage; (3) the person is placed at a learning disadvantage; (4) the person is placed at a social disadvantage; (5) there is a negative impact upon the emotional growth of the person; or (6) the problem causes physical damage or endangers the health of the person.

There are numerous examples of famous people who are highly successful and seemingly content with their lives despite manifesting a communication disorder. Some famous personalities stutter all the way to the bank and have happy, fulfilling lives even though an SLP would have classified them as having a handicap. On the other hand, a minor deviation in a teacher or business executive may mean a significant handicap in terms of credibility and evaluation of job performance. If a person does not view his/her communication disorder as a handicap, it is difficult to justify clinical work or to motivate the client to improve communication skills.

DIAGNOSIS TO DETERMINE THE ETIOLOGY OF THE PROBLEM

Far too many clinicians view diagnosis as simply a labeling process; however, the actual labeling, or categorizing, is only a small part of the total assessment process. Classification systems within our profession are poor at best, and high-level abstractions (for example, stuttering) tend to emphasize the similarities within populations rather than the individual differences. The keen diagnostician looks upon classifications as communication conveniences to be viewed with suspicion. Of course, the convenience factor is important, and each clinician making a determination of the reality of the problem must be willing to label it. This must of necessity, however, follow an orderly description of the characteristics of the disorder so that it can be clear what route the diagnostician took in arriving at the final classification. A diagnosis that only describes the characteristics of the problem, without judging its type or class, is a dead end. The opposite path is also dangerous; the diagnostician who is willing to begin an evaluation by labeling the problem has reversed the orderly sequence of acquiring knowledge and often effectively closes his/her mind to factors that may later point away from the premature diagnosis.

The notion of *cause* has different meanings depending on its distance from the problem. As you look at a client in a diagnostic session, you search for reasons for the presenting behaviors. In fact, many of these reasons may be buried in the past and can only be revealed by painstaking effort. In many cases, cause and effect may be layered in complex patterns. Not only must we search through the client's past experience in order to uncover events that may help us alter current behaviors, but we must also guard against looking for causes in only one dimension of behavior. A child's brain damage, once identified, is probably not the only etiological factor, because communication is a complicated human function. Social, learning, motivational, and many other factors enter into the total process.

Classically, etiology has been defined in terms of predisposing, precipitating, and perpetuating factors. A classic example of predisposing factors is the apparent genetic predisposition to stutter. We know that stuttering tends to run in families; however, it could be that environmental factors cause it to surface. The wary diagnostician must watch for factors that occur with high regularity in association with certain communication disorders. Such data could ultimately be instrumental in uncovering some basic information regarding the nature of the disorder.

Precipitating factors are generally no longer operating and as such may or may not be identifiable. There is a philosophical question of whether we need to search for precipitating factors if they are not still operating, and the point is well taken. Each moment, however, a new set of precipitating factors is created that, acting as characteristics of the past, perpetuates behaviors of the present. Communication disorders are generally not static entities developed at a given point and perpetuated without modification through time; rather, they are ever-changing characteristics that are constantly influenced by intrinsic and extrinsic factors. A child with a language disorder may have begun to lag behind in linguistic development during a period of recurrent ear infections that occurred when language was being learned. If the otitis has long since disappeared and the language disorder remains, it is difficult for the diagnostician to observe or even pinpoint the true cause of the disability. Even if the child did have recurrent bouts with ear infections, it can never be truly substantiated that these infections actually precipitated or played a role in language delay. This is especially true since many children experience frequent ear infections and manage to develop language normally. In many cases the precipitating factors are clear, as in instances of stroke, vocal abuse, structural abnormalities, and certain congenital conditions.

The perpetuating factors are those variables currently at work on the individual. Almost without exception, habit strength is a prime perpetuating factor in many disorders since the client has made various compensations for the problem in terms of cognitive/linguistic strategies and motoric adjustments. Other factors are also crucial, however, and it is the diagnostician's task to uncover the environmental and physical factors that are reinforcing and thus perpetuating the disorder. A hearing loss may be precipitating and a perpetuating factor in a child's language delay. This child needs a thorough audiological evaluation and a prescription for amplification if indicated, or else the problem will perpetuate. A spouse who is noncommunicative with an aphasic patient and spends 100 percent of the time with this person is a participant in perpetuating the problem. Frequency of interaction needs to be increased and specific communicative strategies need to be emphasized if the aphasic patient is to communicate. We must always work to identify and, if possible, remove or reduce any factors that maintain a communication disorder.

DIAGNOSIS TO PROVIDE CLINICAL FOCUS

Although it is important to know the causes of the disorder, it is substantially more important to gain some insight into the possible ways to improve the client's communication. It is at this point that diagnosis and clinical management overlap. This is also where the importance of knowing a host of evaluation techniques becomes significant in the diagnostic enterprise. There is a series of questions that the diagnostician must ask:

1. What do I know about this condition?
   What are the usual etiologies?
   What are the usual effective treatment procedures?
   What is the typical prognosis?
2. What do I know about this person?
   What is the impact of the condition on the person?
   What are the person's strengths and weaknesses?
   How is this person like others I have worked with?
   How is this person different from others I have worked with?
3. What do I know about my own skills in treatment of this disorder and this type of person?
   How have I effectively approached similar problems?
   How have I effectively worked with similar people?
4. What do I know about the services of other professionals available for this person?
   What referrals need to be made?
   What consultations do I need to make?
5. What factors need to be removed, altered, or added to improve the prognosis?
   What inhibiting environmental factors exist?
   What organic factors need alteration?
   What can enhance the person's motivation?

If diagnosis is to be of utmost benefit, it must be goal-oriented. Many professionals have experienced the frustration of referring a child who they feel is autistic for an evaluation. When the report is received, the conclusion is that the child does indeed exhibit behaviors often seen in autistic children and the clinician's original suspicion is confirmed. Such a diagnostic report fails to provide the crucial final link, however, which is a series of recommendations for remedial procedures. Diagnosis is an empty exercise in test administration, data collection, and client evaluation if it fails to provide logical suggestions for treatment.

Most clinicians would like to believe that for each client there is a magic procedure that will work to improve communication. In almost every disorder area (fluency, voice, language, articulation), however, there are many procedures from which to select. Not only are there different types of treatments in terms of philosophy, entry level, and targets trained, but there are differences in the nature of the delivery system (e.g., highly structured, behavioral, client-directed, cognitive, etc.). Thus, the SLP is faced with a number of avenues from which to choose in terms of making treatment recommendations. Within the context of the diagnostic session(s), the well-trained and experienced clinician can make some clinical judgments regarding the types of treatment that may be of benefit to a particular client based on his/her performance on evaluation tasks. Sometimes the SLP can make these judgments in a general manner, using overall impressions from the diagnostic experience as a guide. On other occasions, some trial therapy can be performed in the context of evaluation tasks and actual data can be gathered to support one approach to treatment or another. This notion of using time in a diagnostic session to gain insight into performance on treatment tasks is known as *dynamic assessment* (Olswang et al., 1986; Wade & Haynes, 1989). We feel that dynamic assessment is an important part of any diagnostic venture because it is from these tasks that direction for treatment emerges. Wade and Haynes (1989) found that investing as little as 30 minutes of an evaluation in trial therapy demonstrated distinct performance differences in language-impaired children in the types of cues to which they responded. Almost every communication disorder area has a variety of variables to experiment with during a diagnostic session. We are of the opinion that treatment should be viewed rather like a single subject experimental design. No one really knows which type of treatment will be effective for a given client or which variables will have the most impact on performance. This is typically learned during the first stage of treatment as the clinician begins to fine tune the management program. However, the diagnostic session can easily be used to gain some insight into client tendencies and preferences. Aphasic clients may respond more favorably to certain combinations of cues in word retrieval. Stuttering clients may become more fluent using one particular technique than a second method. One client may express relief that the clinician is willing to talk about the psychological component of the problem during part of the diagnostic session, and this may suggest that this covert dimension should be a part of the treatment program. A language-impaired child may respond better to a structured task as opposed to a child-directed one, or vice versa. A voice case may be more able to alter vocal parameters using feedback from certain instrumentation rather than without this type of monitoring. A nonverbal child may show a marked tendency to learn a few gestures during a diagnostic session, as opposed to mastering vocal productions or words. We could continue with examples of ways the clinician can use a portion of the diagnostic session to learn about the client's response to certain treatment variables. Although the diagnostician should never make treatment recommendations based only on hunches, the judicious use of evaluation tasks in the assessment can suggest a reasonable starting point for treatment in many cases. Of course, these recommendations should be treated as working hypotheses and stated as such in the diagnostic report. The initial selection of a treatment option is in most cases only an educated guess and is always subject to change based on client performance. This is why we view evaluation as an ongoing process throughout the treatment experience.

DIAGNOSIS: SCIENCE AND ART

Diagnosis demands a unique blend of science and art (Silverman, 1984). The scientific method is applicable to our work as diagnosticians, both in guiding our procedures and in focusing our attitude of operation. The scientific method directs the diagnostician to observe all of the available factors, formulate testable hypotheses using clearly stated and answerable questions, test those hypotheses to determine their validity, and formulate conclusions based on the tested hypotheses. The method demands rigorous adherence to standardized procedures and has as its favorable characteristics objectivity, quantifiability, and structure. The scientific diagnostician tends to rely on tests, test data, and other procedures that lend themselves to quantification. As an attitude of operation, the scientific method implies that the diagnostician has not predetermined the test findings and that there is no bias in seeking the proof or disproof of hypotheses. The diagnostician sees hypotheses as something to be tested rather than something to be defended.

The self-fulfilling prophecy is a lethal but almost universal human characteristic; it must be counterbalanced by a scientific approach to testing. We are familiar with parents of language-impaired children who had traveled all over the country in search of a diagnostic explanation for the linguistic delay. Often these children are victims of the "fat folder syndrome" in which a case file has accrued over the years with reports from various authorities and clinics. Each report often reveals more about the examiner than the child as it cites facts in support of a theory of etiology congruent with the diagnostician's particular specialty. Finding what you want to find is not always in the realm of the scientific method. Diagnosticians often use their pet test instruments, as the famous quote goes, like the drunk uses the street lamp—more for support than illumination!

The strict adherence to fact that is demanded by the pure scientific method is often a bit confining. That, in part, may explain why we all practice the art of diagnosis at times. The artistic approach has several specific characteristics. The artist is less dependent on specific observations for the formation of hypotheses than on casual and nonstructured scrutiny. This type of clinician is perfectly willing to disregard formal test results or standard testing procedures in favor of what appears obvious on the basis of clinical experience and expertise. The hunch, or clinical intuition, plays a significant part in such evaluations. The diagnostician will contend that facts can be approached from several directions and that we are capable of assessing the same kinds of behaviors that are measured by formal tests. Such contentions are disconcerting to the test-bound person who has come to expect that the only valid way to gain information is through standardized procedures. One of the emphases in the present text is that these informal, nonstandardized evaluation procedures are valuable indeed in defining a client's problem and the potential response to treatment. In many ways, they may be more valid than standardized tests, as we will discuss in Chapter 3.

It is obvious that, in the extreme, there are weaknesses in both approaches. The scientist may tend to become so dependent on objective methods of measurement that there is a failure to see the client through the maze of percentiles and standard scores. The whole is greater than the sum of its parts, and every diagnostician must guard against simply measuring the isolated characteristics without getting a full picture of the individual. Do not build altars to any testing device; every objective instrument was once only a hunch in someone's mind. The art end of the science–art continuum is just as precarious, as the scientific end. The possibility of a diagnostician's projecting more than a modest amount of personal bias into the evaluation is greater when a less scientific approach is used. Clinical intuitions are often simply clinical biases, and it is very easy to make new evidence fit old categories. The diagnostician must find the proper mixture of each philosophy in establishing assessment procedures (Deutscher, 1983; Ringel, Trachtman, & Prutting, 1984).

THE DIAGNOSTICIAN AS A FACTOR

Ultimately, the most important diagnostic tool is the diagnostician. The clients we assess have seldom read the test manual, and the rigid structure of the testing situation may not be compatible with fluid and nonstructured styles of behavior. Tests are abstractions of behavior, and as such they represent only a fraction of the client's total repertoire of responses to the environment. What better measure of an individual's behavior than that behavior itself? Thus, the diagnostician becomes an important aspect of the evaluating situation in selecting measurements, interacting, responding, and assembling information.

What skills are necessary to develop in order to become an effective diagnostician? How do you develop them? There are no easy answers to these questions. Experience in the diagnostic process is an absolute necessity, but experience in terms of number of clients seen is not enough. Someone once said, "I've had 20 years of experience." The unfortunate thing, however, is that this person had the first year of experience repeated 19 times, which is altogether a different matter. The diagnostician must be able to gain from new experiences, and this demands *flexibility.* The stereotyped and stagnant diagnostician learns little from increased exposure to people and new situations, but those who use their experience as a pattern to be compared against, rather than as a mold into which all new experiences must fit, will continue to grow and learn. The diagnostician must be flexible enough within the testing situation to shift from predetermined plans to new modes of evaluation as the client presents unpredicted behaviors. The examiner who steadfastly plods through a series of tests even though a client is presenting some interesting new behavior or exhibiting valid instances of communication ability in nontest contexts will miss an important opportunity to gain insight into the problem. It is not atypical for beginning clinicians to panic in the face of an unexpected performance and become intransigent in their application of a series of formal tests because there is a certain degree of comfort in known processes. Continued experience in diagnosis may provide the flexibility needed to move freely to other avenues of information.

Practicing clinicians often eagerly accept new and novel techniques as they become available. As the profession moves into new, uncharted areas of concern, many new materials, tests, and techniques become available. New techniques must not be accepted or rejected carte blanche but rather must be scrutinized for their merit. We must learn to keep up with new developments by participating in an active continuing education program, both personal and professional. On the other hand, the beginning student must guard against the "recent article" syndrome to which we all fall prey upon occasion. Typically, the behavioral pattern goes something like this: You read an article that depicts a particular syndrome and explains the distinctive characteristics of a disorder; for a few weeks thereafter, every child you see appears to fall into the pattern described in the publication. Speech pathology witnessed a significant increase in the prevalence of "apraxia" in children following the publication of a series of articles on the topic. Although many of these cases may have been truly apraxic, others probably were fit into this category by frustrated, but thankful clinicians who had cases that perplexed them. The way to overcome the recent article syndrome, of course, is to be aware that it exists and to have a thorough understanding of the nature of human perception. With regard to new tests and measurements, techniques grossly foreign to experience tend to threaten and bewilder the inflexible clinician because they are perceived as attacks on trusted and time-proven methods. On the other hand, some clinicians get into the recent test syndrome and use the most popular test of the day simply because it is new. It is possible that training programs that emphasize formal testing, fixed therapy programs, and a focus on materials are more likely to produce an inflexible, nonevaluative clinician than those programs that emphasize theory, problem-solving ability, creativity, and descriptive assessment techniques.

A clinician must possess many important personal attributes. Rogers (1942) speaks of empathy, congruency, and unconditional positive regard as necessary characteristics of the clinician, and they most certainly apply to the diagnostic process as well. In many studies of clinical competence, both supervisors in speech-language pathology as well as adult clients perceive the interpersonal relationship to be a major factor in contributing to successful treatment

(Haynes & Oratio, 1978; Oratio, 1977). Generally these qualities must be nurtured through consistent effort and proper guidance in training programs through analysis by clinical supervisors and review of session videotapes by clinicians in training.

If the term *sensitivity* may be defined as a keenness of sense or a heightened awareness of incoming sensory data, then this term has meaning for the diagnostician. The clinician must be able to detect subtle physical, psychological, or interactional changes in a client's behavior, as these small changes may have significant meaning in the diagnostic process. For further reading in enhancing awareness skills, see the works of Johnson (1972) and others (Buscaglia, 1982; Emerick & Hood, 1975).

Insight into the meaning and clinical significance of behaviors must be developed from a thorough grounding in the basic processes requisite for communication. Each diagnostician must become so familiar with the normal process of language acquisition and normal communicative functioning that he/she has a built-in set of standards on which to base judgment. The insightful clinician is the knowledgeable professional who is capable of quickly comparing the client's behavior with the norm.

The development of an *evaluative attitude* is often a rather difficult task for the beginning clinician. We are, to a large extent, slaves to our experience; each clinician tends to bring a social attitude into the testing setting. Rather than looking upon the client's performance as having meaning for the evaluative process, we consult our own responses and formulate our own points of view in the give-and-take of the conversation. A critical, questioning attitude must be developed so that the clinician looks upon the behaviors in terms of their meaning rather than in terms of the response expected. Social interaction lends itself to superficiality, whereas the flow of the diagnostic interaction must, by design, lend itself to uncovering the meaning of the incorporated behavior. Effective diagnosticians tend to question the surface validity of behaviors and search for motivations, explanations, and interpretations that are not readily apparent.

Closely allied with the concept of the evaluative attitude is the idea of *persistent curiosity.* The diagnostician must develop an inquisitiveness that will make him/her persistent in searching for explanations. Answers are seldom apparent at first, and continuous effort is imperative. Training institutions often foster weakness in this area when they assign clients to students and expect therapy to get underway in a "reasonable" period of time. Additionally, they are so bound to the rigid university timetables that treatment is often discontinuous. In an attempt to give each student a variety of clinical experiences, they often tend to sever clinical undertakings with a client at each semester's end, knowing full well that the diagnostic or therapeutic process is not best served in this way. The student may not always understand that these have been decisions based on program convenience rather than client need and may develop the notion that diagnosis is a temporary therapy-initiating exercise to be completed in an hour or two. The curious and persistent clinician, however, continues to place the client in situations that will permit additional scrutiny. It would be ideal, albeit probably unworkable in training programs, for students to follow their clients over longer periods of time so they could see how diagnosis is an ongoing process and an integral part of treatment as the client changes.

Objectivity comes from practicing the art of controlled involvement. The diagnostician must cultivate objectivity because we are all subject to human errors. We must be warm, understanding, and accepting on the one hand and objective, evaluative, and detached on the other. Without some degree of balance between the two extremes, the diagnostician may so severely distort the interaction with the client that little information of value is obtained. Objectivity demands more than simply guarding against undue emotional involvement. To grow as a diagnostician, the examiner must be objective about his/her skills, knowledge, and personal characteristics, as well as taking an objective attitude toward the client.

Rapport may be defined as the establishment of a working relationship, based on mutual respect, trust, and confidence, that encourages optimum performance on the part of both client and clinician. Rapport is developed over a period of time and is not easily established in a single session or during a few minutes at the initiation of one diagnostic encounter. Rapport must not only be developed, it must be maintained, and this calls for continued effort. There is a growing literature in the area of formal tests that indicates that, especially with children, test performance varies with clinician familiarity (Fuchs et al., 1985). In essence, children tend to perform better if they have had an opportunity to become familiar with an examiner. Although the reasons for this are not totally clear, the concept of rapport is obviously involved.

Diagnosticians are people, too, and we often forget that they occasionally have "a bad day." They can experience the influence of pervasive personal problems and physical frailties that sometimes make them feel like they would rather have stayed at home in bed. The most knowledgeable and skillful diagnostician, however, may fail to achieve adequate results if he/she lacks the inquisitiveness necessary to encourage continuous effort and if there is no professional drive to serve each individual to the maximum potential. Each of us is subject to individual variations in daily behavior (physical problems, depression, stress, etc.) that can have a direct effect on performance; however, it is incumbent upon every professional to control those variations so as to provide each individual with the best professional service available.

Although much standardization is possible through strict adherence to test routines, the lowest common denominator in diagnostic evaluations is the examiner. Test results are the product of the subject, examiner, test, and test circumstance, each of which has a certain influence. Examinations are clearly selected as a result of the experiences and biases of the examiner. Just as the answers we receive to questions are in part a function of the questions we ask and how we ask them, the diagnostic findings we obtain are in part a function of the tests we administer and the way they are administered. A defective communication pattern may be partially due to a defective testing pattern or a defective tester.

THE CLIENT AS A FACTOR:
CHILDREN, ADOLESCENTS, AND ADULTS

We see three major factors in any clinical transaction: the interpersonal dynamics, the sequence of goals, and the activities (see Figure 1.2). The most crucial factor in conducting a successful diagnostic session is the client-clinician relationship. When one person works with another, there is always human impact; even when clients are treated by computers, they come to accord human attributes to the machines. No matter how well prepared and rehearsed an examiner may be, if his/her approach to people is poor, failure will ensue. All tests, all examinations, all so-called objective diagnostic procedures are mediated by person-to-person contact.

We can be seduced into grave errors by test norms, percentile scores, and standard examination procedures: A human being is a total functioning unit, and the various tests are multiple and fragmented. Even if the instruments we use are relatively precise (which they are not), and we are deluded into thinking that the client is functioning with the same degree of precision in the testing situation, human elements may disturb the validity of the tests no matter how refined the scoring procedures or how calibrated the machines.

Impersonal, test-oriented clinical examination sessions can also make assessment more difficult because there is no absolute division between diagnosis and therapy. The first contact with a client initiates treatment. During a diagnostic session, the client is forming opinions and conceptions about the clinician and the total clinical situation. Barker and his colleagues have warned that

> while to the medical practitioner, diagnosis and therapy are often routine technical jobs, to the patient the situation never has such limited personal meaning. To him diagnosis and therapy are a route to highly important life conditions. (1953, p. 310)

Not all clients will require the full impact of this interpersonal dimension. Indeed, some individuals simply want to find out what is wrong and then rectify the situation. The point is, however, that the clinician should be able to discern what the client needs and then adjust his/her style appropriately.

Although all age levels present unique diagnostic problems, three groups in particular—young children, adolescents, and to a lesser extent, older or

Figure 1.2 Basic Constituents of the Clinical Transaction

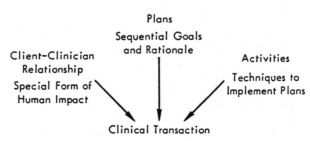

elderly clients—require special effort and expertise. Because the present chapter is generic in nature, we will mainly talk in general about relating to differing age groups seen in diagnostic evaluations. The more specific chapters that follow will provide additional suggestions for dealing with the different age groups in the context of evaluating particular disorders. A major reason for including this generic section is that many readers of the present text are students in training to become speech-language pathologists. It is often difficult for a young student to capture the ephemeral guidelines for relating to people of different ages. It is not as simple as just "being yourself" or talking one way to a child and another way to an adult. There are certain common errors students have made over the years that we can at least alert you to so that you may avoid them. These precepts, of course, are drawn from the experiences of the authors and there are obviously many more guidelines that could be added.

1. *Young Children:* Preschool and kindergarten children are often difficult to test and examine. Unlike most older children and adults, they just do not see the payoff for all the questioning and prodding. The main problem is dealing with the child's fear of the clinical situation. This apprehension may stem from one or more of the following related factors: (1) inadequate preparation for the examination by parents, (2) uncertainty as to what will be done to or with the child by the clinician, (3) vivid memories of trauma during visits to dentists and physicians, (4) the contagious anxieties and uncertainties experienced by the parents, and (5) stress and conflicts engendered by past listener reactions to the speech impairment. Children confront the clinical examination in a variety of ways, but the two most trying responses are shyness and withdrawal and, at the other extreme, aggressiveness and hyperactivity. The shy ones are the most difficult to deal with clinically because there is no output—no speech or language to evaluate. The lack of response per se is behavior too, however, and has meaning we must judge; the child is always telling us something even when no speech or language is produced. If the child cannot or will not respond to our attempts to discern his/her capabilities, we have to employ special procedures to produce involvement in tasks. Most clinicians advocate a low-key, easy-does-it approach with shy children, who must see that the diagnostician is not a threat and can be trusted. But that does *not* mean adopting a coy, childlike demeanor! We do not have to become a child to interact with one. Most authorities suggest the avoidance of questions and the interrogation mode (Hubbell, 1977; Van Riper, 1972). Van Riper makes several suggestions:

Questions are demands. They immediately place the child in a subservient role, with the questioner in the position of power. Even when the child responds appropriately, the resulting relationship is one which immediately puts the questioner into the same category with other authority figures who have been controllers, a relationship which often regenerates the conflicts the child has previously experienced in threatening communication. If you ask what something is called and the child cooperates, he must either think that you must be stupid not to know its name or that you suspect he doesn't know it (which implies stupidity), or that you must want him to do a little verbal dance for your pleasure. . . . Moreover, the eliciting of speech by questions often yields very impoverished samples. At best, you'll get just a vocabulary item, not a good speech sample. Or, if you ask him a yes-no question you'll get a yes or no answer, often the latter. If the question is more elaborate ("What did you have for breakfast this morning?" "What did you do in school today?") the child has probably forgotten or finds it difficult to formulate, or feels that it is none of your business, anyway. Especially with children for whom the acquisition of speech has been no easy accomplishment, any question tends to pose some threat. They have been bedeviled by too many questions from too many questioners and, when they have answered, their listeners have not always understood them or have rejected them. . . . How then should one begin? We suggest that you should simply greet the child, then do some simple self-talk, commenting on what you are doing, or perceiving, and with plenty of moments of comfortable silence interspersed until you have him playing with his box of toys. And then, in the role of the adult playmate, you can play with those in your own box—silently at first. No questions. No demands. Solo play! [See Figure 1.3.] Once the child is comfortable in this activity, you should begin to put some self-talk into your own solo play; first noises (those of trucks, animals, etc.), then single words, then short phrases and simple sentences. All of these refer to what you are experiencing at the moment. Usually the child will begin to follow suit. His noises and his self-talk begin to flow. Next you should shift to contact play very gradually. Let your toy truck occasionally touch his fire engine, or help him find a block, or put another one on his toppling pile, or straighten it up a bit so he can make it higher. When you feel the time is ripe in this tangential contact play, begin to accompany it with some noises or commentary, using parallel talk, telling him what he is doing, perceiving or feeling, again making sure you have more silence than speech. From tangential play, you can often proceed rapidly to intersecting play in which your activity becomes a part of his. (Let your truck go over the bridge he has built or feed your doll or toy dog a piece of the play fruit he has put on the play-house table.) Verbalize what you are doing. Next seek to achieve cooperative play, assisting him in what he is doing. (Have your truck bring him the blocks he needs to build his tower.) Usually by this time, the child is speaking very easily and often copiously, your own verbalizations primarily confined to reflecting what he has said. From this point onward, the communication can proceed fairly normally and naturally. There are, of course, many children for whom such a careful approach may not be vitally necessary, children who have learned that big people always seem to have to ask stupid questions, children who are willing to dance when the interrogative strings are pulled, children who relate easily. Yet even with these children this approach seems to work very well. The relationship established is less superficial, more satisfying. (1972, pp. 108–110)

Figure 1.3   Diagram of Interaction Between Clinician and Child (Van Riper, 1972; reprinted with permission.)

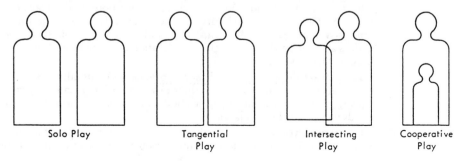

Solo Play   Tangential   Intersecting   Cooperative
                        Play   Play   Play

What do you do with the aggressive, active ones, the children who cannot or will not sit still, who demand to structure the situation in the way they desire? First, and most important, the clinician must retain control of the situation, especially if some structured tasks must be performed. This is basically done by defining the limits for the child using a firm, but accepting manner. The child must see clearly that the examiner cannot be tested, that the examiner is not threatened and has no intention of acquiescing. We do not mean a rigid intransigence, for it is often desirable to alter the testing situation to fit the child. To be sure, much of the behavior manifested by these children is for testing the limits of the situation; they want to know the rules of the game before they will cooperate. On some occasions, with a highly distractible child, we have had to reduce the stimuli in the room. With a few genuinely hyperkinetic children, we have resorted to mild physical restraint, generally holding the child so that he/she can deal with testing materials or toys for informal tasks.

In many cases with very young children, it is possible to have the parent participate in the interaction and this avoids any separation anxiety on the part of the child. The parents are typically willing to cooperate, the child is happy, and the parents can often get the child to do many things that the clinician would take several sessions of rapport building to accomplish. Parents can even be used to administer some formal tests that just involve turning picture plates and reading the cues on the backs of the pictures, while the clinician scores the child's responses. We have to choose our battles very carefully, and fighting an obstreperous child in a diagnostic session leads mainly to unsatisfying results for all concerned.

In dealing with children in the birth-to-two age range, *most* of the pertinent information will be gleaned from parents, both from interview data and by observing parent-child interaction. Not many one-year-olds do well with an unfamiliar clinician, and we need to focus on the parent-child dyad anyway since treatment will doubtless involve the entire family.

There are obviously many other considerations that could be discussed; additional suggestions will be offered in the chapters concerning various disorders. For the present, here are several basic precepts on the management of preschool children in a clinical examination:

a. Help the parents prepare the child for the diagnostic session. They can tell the child what will transpire, and maybe even bring along some stimulus items favored by the child (toys, picture albums, books, etc.).

b. Play, rather than small talk, is the natural medium of expression for children. This is especially important when dealing with potentially disordered youngsters. We have all known children in the three-to-five–year age range who are impressive conversationalists, but most children referred for communication disorders are not on this end of the conversational continuum. Try to arrange the diagnostic tasks with this in mind.

c. As a general rule, ask less and observe more. Children usually lack the insight and cooperation necessary to analyze their problem rationally and objectively. Naturalistic observations—assessing a child's behavior in natural environments— yields more useful information.

d. The prospective diagnostician should learn everything possible about normal children in order to provide a baseline for observations of youngsters presenting problems. This can be done by taking courses, studying relevant norms, but most of all by extensive scrutiny and interaction with children in daycare and preschool facilities. The prospective diagnostician should have a good idea of the typical or modal behavior for children at various age levels. One student claimed that a four-year-old client was in grave need of psychiatric appraisal and treatment. We remembered the child and were somewhat puzzled by this recommendation. We demanded a rationale. It seems that the child had an imaginary companion, a wrinkled green elephant that served as a scapegoat and alter ego. We chuckled and then sent the student scurrying to the Gesell profiles to see how common such fantasies are in four-year-olds.

e. Limit the choices you offer a child. Don't ask if he/she would like to go with you, do this or that, unless the alternatives do not conflict with the examiner's goals. The child will invariably say, "No!"

f. Be flexible in your use of tests and examinations. If you cannot employ the rigid standardized format for administration, use the test to obtain all the data you can. If the child refuses to name the test pictures or objects, you may be able to get a language sample from other items. Also, if there is no standard order for administration of tests and tasks, go with the items the child appears to be interested in at a particular time. For example, if a test has some objects associated with it and the child is attending to these items, start this examination even if you had initially planned it for later in the session.

g. Absolute honesty and candor are important in working with children. Do not make promises unless you can keep them.

h. The whole assessment does not have to be done in one session; marathon diagnostics tend to be counterproductive. Remember that all we can hope to obtain in one time frame is a sample of a child's behaviors. It is better to terminate (preferably on a pleasant, successful note) than to continue an unproductive session.

i. Watch your language complexity when talking to children. For obvious reasons, the examiner should avoid sarcasm, idiomatic expressions, ambiguous statements, and indirect requests (Blue, 1981).

2. *Adolescents:*   Experienced clinicians frequently report that adolescents, the classical teenagers, especially in grades 7 through 11, are often difficult to examine and resistant to treatment. The main problem seems to be getting through to them. There is no magic formula for this, but we would like to make some suggestions that we have found helpful in guiding our work with adolescent clients.

a. Acquire an understanding of the myriad pressures and changes the teenager is experiencing: rapid physical growth, sexual maturity, conflicts between dependence and independence, the development of self-confidence and interpersonal skills necessary to make decisions, a search for identity and life work, intense group loyalty and identification, and many more. It is a turbulent, trying period of behavioral extravagance and excess. Small wonder that teenagers are often overloaded with personal concerns and do not always welcome an overture of clinical assistance. Empathy that flows from understanding is a powerful force in establishing a working relationship.

b. Adolescents have an intense desire to be like others, not to stand out from the group in any way that would suggest frailty. Hence the adolescent may find it extremely difficult to reveal a speech impairment, even if help is desired. Often teenagers are simply sent for evaluation or treatment by parents. In some instances, the teenager with a chronic problem may have been in treatment for a long time and is weary at the thought of more therapy. Many will tend to cover up true feelings with a sullen bravado or a dense "it-doesn't-bother-me" shell.

Denial is a particular forte. "Coolness" and image are very important. You can neither beat this down nor simply dismiss it with a shrug. Nor is silence a particularly effective tool in dealing with adolescent resistance. We advocate a straightforward approach: Acknowledge the forces that are bearing on the individual; point up objectively the paths that others have taken; and provide information about the economic and social penalties that accrue to the communication-disordered person. The young client may need more time to become accustomed to the idea of therapy. Basically, try to demonstrate by your demeanor and what you say that you care about the client: A growing person needs lots of nourishment, and personal involvement and commitment are key factors.

c. Don't try to "swing" with teenage clients; empathy is not identification. Do not abandon your professional role for that of a teenager. Be yourself. As Will Rogers pointed out, if they don't like you the way you are, they are sure not going to like you the way you are trying to be.

d. Approach adolescents with tolerance and good humor. Do not be shocked or annoyed by their overstatements and superlatives; do not overreact to expressions of hostility or tempests of other emotions. In order to uphold their protective armor, they will sometimes resort to all sorts of strategies to confuse, defeat, or anger the clinician. The ability to laugh at yourself and to use humor in a gentle, needling manner is an asset. Remember, though, always treat the adolescent with honesty and dignity—don't make fun of intense or idealistic views.

e. Explain the diagnostic process as much as possible by explaining what we are about, the reasons for the various tests and examinations, and how we will use the information. We encourage the adolescent to challenge and question what we are doing. Finally, we usually give the client an idea of the route we would follow when therapy commences or even do some trial treatment activities.

f. If the client is highly critical of parents or school officials, we must keep the person's confidences and not act in a judgmental manner. We do not enter into the criticism or side with the client against others, nor do we try to defend the institution or retreat to moralisms.

g. Discuss the results of the evaluation with the client before talking with the parents or school personnel. Be sure to let the client know exactly what you intend to tell parents and teachers and determine any feelings the client has about these suggestions.

These recommendations have been distilled from our clinical experience and are not presented as magical touchstones for all diagnosticians or all clients; nor do they represent the full range of possibilities for successful interaction with teenage clients. We present them here to encourage other workers to develop clinical generalizations on the basis of their experience (O'Connor & Eldredge, 1981).

3. *The Elderly Client:* Older clients may present some rather special problems for the diagnostician or they may need no particular special handling. Although the concept of *elderly* is relative, we refer here to persons in their sixties or older. A word of caution: Although there are certain generalizations that are useful for planning and conducting evaluations, elderly people are not any more "all alike" than are children or adolescents.

The clinician should be alert to fatigue, disorientation, failing eyesight, and hearing loss. With advanced age, the person may find it more difficult to focus attention on a task and may have trouble remembering directions because of possible short-term memory decline. Many of these potential problems are exacerbated when the person has experienced a neurological insult, as have a good number of elderly clients. We need, therefore, to explain each step of our clinical procedures at greater length and repeat instructions when necessary to ensure understanding. Our pace should be geared to the client's abilities—or, if necessary, to a slower level (e.g., in cases of neurological damage). Organize the testing sequence carefully to reduce distractions, noise, or interference. Older people are often more cautious and have a greater need to be certain before they respond, so adapt the tasks with this in mind; following standard procedure may not be as important as providing an environment in which the person is able to perform at optimal level. Since many older clients tend to feel useless and discarded in our youth-oriented culture, and resentful that their bodies are betraying them, we may find it important to spend some time listening to their memories of past achievements. Older clients should always be treated with respect and not referred to by their first names. The clinician should also guard against using a louder vocal intensity and increased pitch range as if talking to a child. It is grossly offensive to infantalize an adult client. Many of our elderly clients will come to us with neurologically based disorders, serious vocal pathologies, and other medically related problems. There will be a tendency among many to talk about medical issues, since their problems have originated from this area. It is important for the diagnostician to be patient with these clients and listen to their concerns, without allowing conversation about medical issues to interfere with the testing. In most cases, clinicians will find older clients to be interesting, socially adept individuals to be treated with courtesy and respect. The number of people over 60 composes a significant proportion of the population, and we cannot afford to perpetuate the stereotype that old people are expendable or that they should be relegated to demeaning idleness. As with children and adolescents, the diagnostician should know as much as possible about aging. Many references pertinent to communication disorders in this population are readily available (Beasley & Davis, 1981; Cowley, 1980; Dancer & Thomas, 1983; Moore & Sherman, 1981; Mueller & Peters, 1981; National Council on Aging, 1982; Shadden, 1988).

PUTTING THE DIAGNOSIS TO WORK

Perhaps the most demanding of all diagnostic ventures is the ultimate synthesis of findings into a coherent statement of the nature of the problem. The skilled clinician draws the findings together using the data available, past experience, knowledge, and intuition to formulate a total picture of the condition. At this point, textbooks, research findings, and academic lectures fail to provide all of what is needed to succeed. Maturation of skills will only take place in an extensive practicum under the close supervision of a knowledgeable diagnostician. The essence of the synthesis process is a comparison of what is observed with what we expect to observe from our knowledge of the normal process. The incongruities between the observed and the normal provide the building blocks for completion of the picture. Figure 1.4 identifies a model of diagnosis as a synthesis of findings

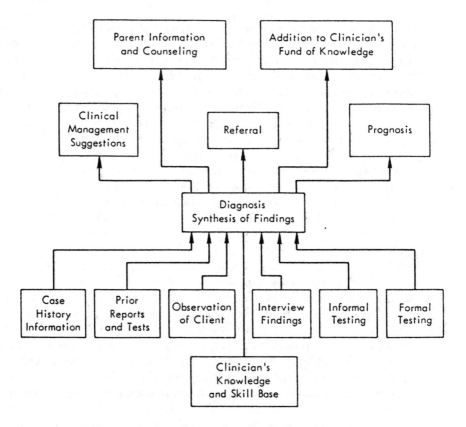

Figure 1.4   Paradigm of Diagnosis

and shows a number of outcomes to which the synthesis might lead. This figure points out several important concepts. First, the bedrock of the entire model is the clinician's knowledge and skill base. Without adequate training and experience, the administration of tests and tasks becomes meaningless.

A second important point in the model is the series of six boxes that are immediately above the clinician's knowledge and skill base. These boxes highlight the diversity of information that the diagnostician should ideally obtain in order to make a principled judgment about a client's disorder (case history, prior reports, observation, interview, informal testing, and formal testing). Interestingly, it is not unusual for prior reports and tests to be missing or unrequested, case history information to be returned by the client at the time of evaluation instead of prior to it, the case history forms to be incomplete or lost, and the interview cut to a ten-minute conversation because of time pressure. It is also not unusual for the clinician to spend the entire assessment time giving tests with little opportunity left for informal testing or observation of clients in relevant situations. Although it is difficult to obtain information from all six boxes in the model, we must try to get as close to the ideal as possible. In many settings, the evaluation will not take place unless the client has submitted all pertinent information and reports from other agencies have been received. It is certainly that way in many other professions (medicine, psychology, etc.). We must ask ourselves about the quality of the diagnostic evaluation that is done with incomplete information. What is the efficacy of performing an evaluation if we do not have access to critical information and are not willing to spend the time to carry on a decent interview and do informal testing and client observation?

A third area in the center of the model is the synthesis of findings. This is where we begin to see overlaps in the data from case history, interview, reports, observations, and testing results. We should look for common threads among all of these information sources and tie them together in the synthesis and diagnosis. Often, this is where certain informational components begin to disagree with one another, and this is also informative. For example, the parents indicate intense concern over their child's articulation in the case history and the interview. They also bring a host of prior reports that indicate the child has no clinically significant problem, and they look to you for guidance. If your own test results, informal task performance, and observations indicate that the child is performing within normal limits, the discrepancy between these components and the parent's perceptions is obvious. The prior reports also now gain significant importance in terms of counseling the parents and pointing out the disparity between their view and the perceptions of many professionals. Another example may point out the foibles associated with one or more of the sources of information. A child may not perform within normal limits on formal tests of language ability. Yet, that same child communicates well in informal tasks and observations of play interactions with caretakers and peers. The clinician must question the formal test results if the child's communication exceeds that which these measures suggest he/she is capable of achieving.

A fourth series of five boxes in the model points out some components that are important parts of a diagnostic evaluation that take place after the synthesis of information. As we mentioned earlier, a good diagnostician will make suggestions for treatment in terms of which goals may be logically selected for initial intervention. The parents need to be counseled regarding the results of the evaluation and any problems or feelings they express must be addressed. Often we are so zealous in performing the evaluation and scheduling time to do everything we feel is necessary that we give the client or parents short shrift in explaining our results. In many cases, the results we report to parents or clients represent a significant affective burden. For example, even though parents usually know in their hearts that their child has a communication disorder, they often hold out the hope that their child is really not disordered and will grow out of a language or articulation difference. By telling them that their child is indeed showing an impairment and is now officially in the ranks of the handicapped, we force them to come to terms with this problem. Diagnosticians frequently experience parents or clients who cry at the culmination of the evaluation session when they are told something that confirms the idea of a disorder and/or commits them to an undetermined length of time spent in rehabilitation. Other emotions such as anger and denial also emerge that must sometimes be dealt with at the end of the diagnostic session.

Emotions aside, it is enough of a challenge simply to communicate the complex evaluation results to people of different educational levels and abilities. A skilled diagnostician has the ability to summarize assessment results and recommendations on the correct level of abstraction for different parents and spouses.

Another aspect to deal with after synthesis is the possibility of referral. Many cases require a consultation by other professionals such as audiologists, laryngologists, neurologists, special educators, psychologists, and others. Often the assessment raises more questions than it answers, and this is perfectly acceptable. We need to know the parameters of the patient's problem, and many times this insight can only be gained from professionals who have expertise in areas with which we are not totally familiar.

Prognosis is another variable depicted in Figure 1.4. *Prognosis* may be defined as a prediction of the outcome of a proposed course of treatment for a given client: how effective treatment will be; how far we can expect the client to progress; and perhaps, how long it will take. Inasmuch as diagnosis is a continuing process, prognosis should, like treatment planning, have both long-range and immediate facets. Immediate prognosis covers what the person can do now, what steps in therapy are possible, and what is the best route to take. Prognosis for specific communication disorders will be discussed in subsequent chapters; in this section, we will present some generic purposes and a possible danger involved in predicting a client's response to treatment.

One basic purpose in making a prognosis is to economize our therapeutic efforts. There is only so much time and energy, and we must focus what there is on those clients who show the greatest promise of improvement. Patients and families also want to know what they may expect in terms of progress. Some general factors that the clinician must consider when making predictions include the following:

1. *Age:* The chronological age of the client is a gross predictor of treatment success. In general, the younger the client, the better the treatment outcome. This can be seen in childhood disorders where the earlier the intervention is begun, the more progress can be made prior to school entrance. The earlier we involve children in treatment, the more likely we are to prevent the formation of secondary problems such as social, psychological, and educational penalties (Shine, 1980; Starkweather et al., 1990; Wilcox, 1989). In adult cases, it is well known that patients who develop neurogenic disorders at younger ages (40–60) are generally given better prognoses than patients who develop these problems at later ages (70–90) (Rosenbeck, LaPointe, & Wertz, 1989). This, of course, is due to a variety of reasons that include psychological, motivational, and physical factors. Thus, age is a macrovariable that in and of itself is not a potent variable, but it subsumes many factors that do have an influence on prognosis.

2. *Length of Time Impairment Has Existed.* The length of time a client has had a communication disorder may relate to prognosis. Obviously, habitual activities (motor patterns, processing strategies, etc.) are more difficult to alter in clients who have performed them for a lengthy period. In addition to the habit patterns developed over time, the client has also learned complex ancillary

adjustment patterns to compensate for the communication impairment that may involve social, psychological, and motoric activities. These compensatory patterns eventually become part of the problem and must often be eliminated, as in the case of operant behaviors learned by stutterers (head jerks, timing devices, etc.).

3. *Existence of Other Problems:* It is axiomatic that the more problems a client has, the more difficult it will be to deal with the disorder. An aphasic client who is also hearing impaired will be more difficult to treat than one with the language disorder alone. A child with a cleft palate and articulation problems will be more difficult than one with the articulation problem alone. A child who is language impaired and mentally retarded is different from one who presents only a language disorder.

4. *Reactions of Significant Others:* A child with a communication disorder is going to make better progress in treatment if the parent takes an active role in the intervention. Many parents are interested in participating in treatment and will carry on home programs. On the other hand, if a child is brought to the clinic by a social worker and the parents do not appear interested in treatment, this child will probably take longer to succeed in remediation. If the spouse of an aphasic patient is disinterested in facilitating communication, the client may make slower progress. The same can be said about the cooperation of teachers, aides, daycare providers, siblings, peers, and anyone else who comes in significant contact with the client and is in a position to help with treatment. Generally, the more assistance available from significant others, the better the prognosis.

5. *Client Motivation:* Although we have no reliable way to measure motivation in a client, most diagnosticians can recognize it when they see it. If the client appears enthusiastic, interested, and eager to begin treatment, this is clearly a plus. If the client is an adult, was he/she self-referred? This may be a positive indication as opposed to a person referred by an employer or teacher or dragged to the evaluation by a domineering spouse. There may also be some positive prognostic value in cases where the client has something to gain from successful treatment (better social life, higher-paying job, etc.). Motivation is always difficult to quantify, but few would totally disregard the importance of this admittedly blurry construct.

Accurate prognoses can help establish our credibility with other professions. The ability to predict with reasonable precision is perhaps the highest form of scientific achievement. Needless to say, however, these predictions should be based on something more than clinical intuition. Impressionistic conclusions, especially when made by experienced workers, can often be startlingly accurate, but they should always be labeled as impressionistic: A prognosis should be supported by a substantial amount of information. We never say, "The prognosis is favorable," without some documentation, both impressionistic and scientifically based. It is much better to say, "The prognosis is good because the child is stimulable for all error sounds, trial therapy indicated good attention and a cooperative attitude, parents have committed to a home program, the client stated he wanted to change his speech, he has normal hearing, and language problems are not evident."

In what sense might a prognosis be dangerous? First, no one really knows the future. A client's prognostic variables might soon change with unforeseen circumstances (e.g., the uninterested parents become involved, the client develops motivation, the client makes a "breakthrough" in the ability to perform certain functions). This means that prognosis as a construct is dynamic, not static. A second danger in prognoses is that they may well influence a client's performance and/or perceptions. A clinician's certain expectations regarding the case's potential performance could inadvertently be communicated to the client or the family and negatively affect the course of therapy. They could also influence the level of effort exhibited by the clinician. The old notion of a self-fulfilling prophecy is still alive and well. We must always be willing to alter prognostic judgments in light of new data, and perhaps more importantly, we must be willing to restrain ourselves from making prognostic statements in the first place if we do not know what we are talking about. It is better to say, "I don't know how he will do in treatment. Let's see what happens," than to jaundice the whole enterprise with a negative prognosis that has no real basis or disappoint all concerned with a positive prognosis that was never realized. This is *not* an exact science!

PRECEPTS REGARDING THE CLINICAL EXAMINATION

In this chapter, we have presented some suggestions for general conduct of the diagnostic session. We dislike diagnostic formulas, and our purpose has not been to give out recipes, but rather to describe some way of approaching various problems without going too far astray. By way of summary, we now present a list of interrelated and overlapping precepts regarding the clinical examination.

1. We examine persons, not speech defects or speech defectives. Our primary concern is with communicators, not communication.
2. The clinical examination is conducted interpersonally; the catalyst of a diagnostic session is the person-to-person relationship between clinician and client.
3. There is an element of magic in every transaction between people. A diagnostic session can, in some instances, ameliorate a problem situation by engendering hope or be deeply disappointing to a client who hopes that a test or examination will resolve a difficulty.
4. A most important requisite for conducting a clinical examination is a thorough understanding of normalcy.
5. Diagnosis is the initial phase of treatment. The very first contact with a client— the manner in which he/she is treated during a clinical examination—is a crucial determining factor in response to therapy.
6. Diagnosis is not necessarily confined to a single session.
7. Treatment is often diagnostic; we can discover the nature of a client's problem in the initial stages of therapy.
8. The clinical examination is performed to provide a working image of the individual; it is accomplished by interviewing, examining, evaluating, and testing.

9. An important aspect in acquiring a working image of an individual is determining the person's self-perception and situation.

10. An individual makes certain adjustments to a problem (attempts to solve the difficulty) that may include a protective cover of defenses. These may be a part of the problem but must not be confused with the problem.

11. Behavior is a function of the individual and the situation. We should be aware that our test results reflect not just the client's abilities, but also his/her performance in the diagnostic setting rather than the natural environment.

12. Our diagnostic activities should include an assessment of a client's larger social context (home, family, peers, job, etc.).

13. Tests are only tools to provide a systematic guide for our observations. They enable the clinician to scrutinize a client in a structured manner.

14. Although for the examiner the testing situation may be very familiar and routine, for the client it is a novel experience.

15. Examination and testing can be iatrogenic. It can suggest problems to the client that he/she had not previously considered.

16. Even though a testing device is made up of a series of precisely defined tasks, administered and scored in a rigidly structured manner, a client's responses are not necessarily as precise.

17. It is as important to observe *how* the client responds during a testing procedure as it is to obtain a score. Informal evaluation tasks are as important or more important than formal, standardized procedures.

18. It is very easy to deify a particular testing instrument, to endow a scale or diagnostic concept with a special form of reality independent of its creator. Some clinicians embrace a diagnostic device with militant enthusiasm and attack all intellectual queries or criticism with apostolic zeal.

19. Impressions formed on the basis of the first careful evaluation of a client are generally accurate. There is a tendency to discount or deny our findings especially, for example, if they suggest a child is mentally retarded or that an adult aphasic is not capable of further improvement.

20. The needs of the client, not the work setting in which the clinician labors, should determine the scope of diagnostic activities. A good diagnostic is over when sufficient information about a client is gathered and should not be short-circuited because of administrative red tape, arbitrary guidelines of a facility, or government regulations. A good clinician will find ways to obtain critical information even if the evaluation extends into the realm of treatment.

BIBLIOGRAPHY

American Heritage Dictionary (1985). Boston, MA: Houghton Mifflin.

BARKER, R. (1953). *Adjustment to physical handicap and illness: A survey of the social psychology of physique and disability.* Bulletin 55, New York: Social Science Research Council.

BEASLEY, D., & DAVIS, G. (EDS.). (1981). *Aging and communication.* Baltimore: University Park Press.

BLACK, J., & HAGGEN, C. (1963). Multiple choice intelligibility tests, Forms A and B. *Journal of Speech and Hearing Disorders, 28,* 77–86.

BLUE, C. (1981). Types of utterances to avoid when speaking to language-delayed children. *Language, Speech and Hearing Services in Schools, 12,* 120–124.

BUSCAGLIA, L. (1982). *Living, loving and learning.* New York: Ballantine.

COWLEY, M. (1980). *The view from 80.* New York: Viking.

DANCER, J. & THOMAS, W. (1983). Beyond the boundaries. *Journal of the American Speech and Hearing Association, 25,* 25–30.

DEUTSCHER, M. (1983). *Subjecting and objecting.* Oxford, England: Basil Blackwell Publishers, Ltd.

EMERICK, L. (1984). *Speaking for ourselves: Self-portraits of the speech or hearing handicapped.* Danville, IL: Interstate.

EMERICK, L., & HOOD, S. (1975). *The client-clinician relationship.* Springfield, IL: Charles C Thomas.

FUCHS, D., FUCHS, L., DAILEY, A. & POWER, M. 1985. The effect of examiner's personal familiarity and professional expertise on handicapped children's test performance. *Journal of Educational Research, 78,* 3–14.

HAYNES, W., & ORATIO, A. (1978). A study of clients' perceptions of therapeutic effectiveness. *Journal of Speech and Hearing Disorders, 43,* 21–33.

HUBBELL, R. (1977). On facilitating spontaneous talking in young children. *Journal of Speech and Hearing Disorders, 42,* 216–231.

JOHNSON, D. (1972). *Reaching out.* Englewood Cliffs, NJ: Prentice Hall.

McCROSKEY, R., & MULLIGAN, M. (1963). The relative intelligibility of esophageal speech and artificial larynx speech. *Journal of Speech and Hearing Disorders, 28,* 37–41.

MOORE, J., & SHERMAN, D. (1981). Special considerations with the elderly patient. *Journal of Communication Disorders, 14,* 299–309.

MUELLER, R., & PETERS, T. (1981). Needs and services in geriatric speech-language pathology and audiology. *Journal of the American Speech and Hearing Association, 23,* 627–632.

National Council on Aging. (1982). *Service learning in aging: Implications for speech, language and hearing.* Washington, DC: National Council on Aging.

O'CONNOR, L., & ELDREDGE, P. (1981). *Communication disorders in adolescence.* Springfield, IL: Charles C Thomas.

OLSWANG, L., BAIN, B., ROSENDAHL, P., OBLAK, S., & SMITH, A. (1986). Language learning: Moving from a context-dependent to independent state. *Child Language Teaching and Therapy, 2,* 180–210.

ORATIO, A. (1977). *Supervision in speech pathology: A handbook for supervisors and clinicians.* Baltimore: University Park Press.

RINGEL, R., TRACHTMAN, L., & PRUTTING, C. (1984). The science in human communication sciences. *Journal of the American Speech Language and Hearing Association, 26,* 33–36.

ROGERS, C. (1942). *Counseling and psychotherapy.* Boston: Houghton Mifflin.

ROSENBEK, J., LaPOINTE, L., & WERTZ, R. (1989). *Aphasia: A clinical approach.* Boston: College-Hill.

SHADDEN, B. (1988). *Communication behavior and aging: A sourcebook for clinicians.* Baltimore: Williams and Wilkins.

SHINE, R. (1980). Direct management of the beginning stutterer. *Seminars in Speech, Language and Hearing, 1*(4), 339–350.

SILVERMAN, F. (1984). *Speech language pathology and audiology.* Columbus, OH: Merrill.

STARKWEATHER, C., GOTTWALD, S., & HALFOND, M. (1990). *Stuttering prevention: A clinical method.* Englewood Cliffs, NJ: Prentice Hall.

VAN RIPER, C., & EMERICK, L. (1984). *Speech correction: An introduction to speech pathology and audiology.* Englewood Cliffs, NJ: Prentice Hall.

VAN RIPER, C. (1972). *Speech correction: Principles and methods.* Englewood Cliffs, NJ: Prentice Hall.

WADE, K., & HAYNES, W. (1989). Dynamic assessment of spontaneous language and cue responses in adult-directed and child-directed play: A statistical and descriptive analysis. *Child Language Teaching and Therapy, 5,* 157–173.

YORKSON, K. & BEUKELMAN, D., (1981). *Assessment of intelligibility of dysarthric speech.* Tigard, OR: C.C. Publications.

chapter

2

INTERVIEWING

The clinician sets the process of recovery in motion at the very first contact with a client. This is accomplished through the vehicle of the spoken word—in short, the initial interview. Because the intake interview ushers the client into treatment, it is the key link in the evaluation process. In order to assess and treat persons with communication disorders, it is essential that we know how to talk with them in a manner that reflects our expertise and inspires confidence and trust.

THE IMPORTANCE OF INTERVIEWING

Although clinical evaluation obviously involves more than proficiency at conducting interviews, this skill is central to the role of the diagnostician. By means of verbal exchange, we gather data about the individual, transmit information, and establish and sustain a working relationship. The interview is also the means by which treatment is carried out and, as such, serves both as a tool and as a relationship (Figure 2.1). For the clinical speech-language pathologist, interviewing is an extremely important activity.

Although widely used, interviewing is one of the least understood aspects of the worker's role. Prospective clinicians are expected to acquire an impressive array of knowledge, but often it is merely presumed that they know how to communicate effectively with clients. The mastery of interviewing is either taken for granted or expected to accrue somehow as an artifact of required course work and practicum experiences.

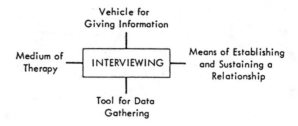

Figure 2.1 Interviewing Is Central in Speech Pathology

Some clinicians consider interviewing to be secondary; they use paper to replace personal interaction. An elaborate case history form containing a plethora of questions is mailed to the parents, and they are requested to fill it out and return it before the diagnostic appointment. The rationale for this procedure is that it saves the clinician time and alerts him/her to problem areas that can then be explored in the personal interview. Although the clinician certainly should get some idea of the problem before the diagnostic examination, there is no substitute for an indepth interview. There are several reasons for disenchantment with an approach that uses only paper-and-pencil techniques: (1) The questions on forms are often generic—they cover all possible respondents—and are thus ambiguous or not applicable to a particular client; a parent may not understand the relationship between the questions posed and the child's speech problem. Face-to-face interviews permit greater flexibility in formulating precise and germane inquiries. (2) The queries may be threatening or engender guilt, and the clinician is not present to observe these reactions or to support and assist the respondent as he searches for an answer. Does the mailed questionnaire allow time for the respondent to plan a defense? Is it more likely that we end up with a view of what the respondent wants us to see? More complete information can be obtained in an interview, where primary questions may be followed up with pertinent secondary inquiries. (3) If the respondent answers the question in one particular way, she may be prevented from developing any other possible answers. Spoken language does tend to create a reality for the individual, but writing lends an air of permanence. During an interview, however, the clinician can determine not only what a client says but also how she says it—for example, how does she assign priority to items, how does she associate items with one another, how does she reveal attitudes by vocal quality or body language?

THE NATURE OF INTERVIEWING

An interview is essentially a process, not an entity—a process of verbal and nonverbal intercourse between a trained professional worker and a client seeking services. More specifically, an interview, in a clinical diagnostic sense, is a *purposeful* exchange of meanings between two persons, a directed conversation that proceeds in an orderly fashion to obtain data, to convey certain information, and to provide release and support. The professional worker, by reason of his/her position and clinical expertise, is expected to (and usually does) provide the direction for the verbal exchange. Thus, an interview is not just an ordinary conversation in terms of a desultory exchange of opinions and ideas but rather a specialized pattern of verbal interaction directed toward a specific purpose and focused on specific content. The roles of interviewer and respondent are more highly specified in a professional interview than in a conversation. An interview differs from a social conversation in a number of other important respects: (1) The time and location of an interview is specified formally; (2) the inquiries are generally unilateral—the clinician may ask about the parents' relationship with their child, for example, but it is not expected that the client will reciprocate with questions about the worker's children; and (3) the clinician does not necessarily avoid unpleasant topics in the interest of social propriety.

In a good diagnostic interview, the clinician and client must become co-workers, multiplying their efforts by creating a mutual feeling of cooperation. It is futile to expect straightforward answers to simple questions, because clients are often unable to objectively evaluate their own life situations and effects of their behavior on the communication disorder. A good diagnostic interview always involves more than making queries and recording answers.

Interviewing is a unique kind of conversation. Perhaps for the first time the respondent can talk freely without fear of criticism or admonishment. The *clinician* knows that an interview is a unique and distinct mode of verbal exchange, but does the *client* need to know this? Probably not. Indeed, we typically advise students to refer to an interview as a "chat" or "a chance to share information" when they contact clients or parents to request an appointment time. An "interview" sounds rather ominous and frightening, perhaps even like a summons to account for one's failings.

In summary, a diagnostic interview is a directed conversation, carried out for specific purposes such as fact finding, informing, or altering attitudes and opinions. The clinician's efforts are directed toward the creation of mutual respect and team effort in the understanding and solution of the communication problem.

COMMON INTERVIEWING CONSIDERATIONS

Several factors can prevent the establishment of effective communicative bonds between a speech clinician and those he/she interviews. Although the list could obviously be expanded, we have picked several aspects that in our experience are the most common interviewing barriers.

Multicultural Considerations in Interviewing

More than ever before in our history, the United States has become a multicultural society. Soon after the turn of the next century, the country will no longer have a majority of white, European residents. The populations of Hispanic, Asian, and black individuals are the most rapidly growing segments of the society and within the next few decades, most of us will be from these groups. Although multicultural issues affect all aspects of any profession, there are some important factors to consider in interviewing that relate directly to our burgeoning multicultural society. First, as mentioned previously, the clinical interview represents the meeting of two or more individuals who each bring with them unique experiences, perceptions, views, values, and characteristics. When two people meet in a professional setting, the nature of the clinical relationship itself is sometimes problematic. That is, some people simply have trouble coming to a clinical situation, even if they are dealing with a clinician from the same culture as their own. When client and clinician represent differing cultural or racial backgrounds, there is an additional potential obstacle to overcome. Some clients may not feel as comfortable when they must reveal certain information to a stranger, and this discomfort may be intensified when the clinician represents a different race or culture. The solution for this is clearly not to make certain that clients and clinicians are culturally homogeneous. Given the diverse nature of our society, this would be impossible from a scheduling standpoint and unwise from a philosophical one. The best way to deal with cultural diversity in clinical situations is to make certain that clinicians have a sensitivity for cultural differences and a knowledge of multicultural issues in assessment and treatment. The American Speech-Language-Hearing Association has mandated that every accredited training program in communication disorders infuse multicultural information into each area of academic preparation and clinical practicum. Students need to have increased opportunity to deal with culturally different clients, parents, and children and to develop their interpersonal skills with and knowledge of these groups.

A second important implication of multicultural influence on interviewing concerns the specific information that is exchanged. We have indicated that much of the information exchanged in a clinical interview is of a highly personal nature and possibly charged with considerable affect. Many cultures (e.g., Native Americans, certain Asian groups) find it difficult to share personal information with unfamiliar people. The clinician must be sensitive to such cultural beliefs and not press the client to provide information too soon. In some cases, it will be necessary to conduct multiple interviews and establish a strong relationship with the clients before they will give information or take advantage of the clinician's suggestions for treatment. This issue alone is a strong indictment of some rigid policies in which an evaluation is expected to be completed within an hour or two, or Individualized Educational Program (IEP) goals are to be written within limited time frames. We must learn to consider that different cultures may require alterations in our methods if we are to serve them optimally.

An obvious multicultural influence on interviewing is the possibility of dealing with the many children and adults from bilingual backgrounds. In some cases, the clinician must be bilingual; and in others, the interviewer must make use of interpreters. The use of an interpreter, however, is a very specialized operation, and the clinician must be certain that the person has adequate knowledge and experience to perform this specialized task. In some areas of the country, there is an increased likelihood that the SLP will encounter a bilingual population and he/she should reflect on how these clients will be served appropriately in assessment and treatment. It is not possible to provide adequate services to these populations without a knowledge of and sensitivity to multicultural issues.

A final implication of multicultural issues on interviewing is the belief systems of the various cultural groups regarding disabilities. Some cultures believe that a handicapping condition is a situation that nothing can or should be done about, or that the help for this condition should come from a spiritual rather than a clinical source (Cheng, 1989). If the clinician charges into the interview making a host of recommendations without addressing cultural attitudes toward remediation, these suggestions may fall on unsympathetic ears. The clients may also be offended and not return for treatment. There is a growing literature in communication disorders and multicultural issues, and it is the ethical responsibility of every student and clinician to become familiar with this body of work (Cole & Deal, in press). We cannot serve our clients well unless we take this cultural information into account.

Fears of the Clinician

There are two points in a student clinician's career when anxiety rises to very high levels: the confrontation with his/her first therapy case and the first diagnostic interview. It is—and should be—an awesome responsibility to undertake the professional treatment of another human being. There is always an element of risk in offering help. As a matter of fact, if a student does not get somewhat tense in this situation, we suspect his/her suitability for the profession.

Perhaps the most common fear expressed by beginning interviewers is that clients will not accept them in a professional role because of their youth. They doubt they can bridge the age gap, especially when they deal with parents: "Who am I to be asking questions and giving suggestions to them when they are older and more experienced?" They sigh, "Won't parents consider me a pipsqueak? Won't they look down on me if I don't have children?" Most of this is pure projection on the student's part (Haynes & Oratio, 1978). If the interviewer indicates deep concern for the welfare of the child, then nearly every parent will respond in a positive manner, without scrutinizing the clinician for wrinkles, grey hairs, or diaper-pail hands. The clinician, of course, should not communicate the uncertainty felt in the interview situation, or he/she will never establish competence or inspire confidence.

Another common fear among incipient interviewers—and one that is also largely projected—is that the interviewee will become defensive or resentful during questioning. We have seen students omit a whole series of important questions when a client, especially a parent, responded curtly or showed mild annoyance. It is not uncommon for parents to feel ashamed because they think of their child's communication disorder as an outward and visible sign of their own failure, but few in our experience are resentful or defensive about the clinician's sincere efforts to determine the nature of the child's problem. The important point is, again, to make the interviewees feel that they have done the best they could do, and now, with some assistance from the clinician, they can do better. The clinician should *always maintain a nonthreatening posture in the clinical transaction.*

Many beginning interviewers are leery of questions directed at them. "What do you do when the client starts asking *you* questions?" the student interviewer frequently despairs. "Will I be able to explain to them adequately what they need to know? How will I know if I have gotten it across if they just sit there and nod?" We shall return to this important topic of clients' questions in a later section of this chapter.

Memory Failure

A common deterrent to communication in an interview is loss of memory. Clients simply will not remember things that the clinician needs to know in order to plan a program of therapy.

Emotional Barriers

Sometimes an interviewee cannot or will not give information because emotional blocks prevent free communication. Self-disclosure is often difficult, and the respondent may not be able to identify a payoff for revealing personal information.

The Language Gap

The clinician must remember that laypeople often have a markedly different way of talking about a speech, language, or hearing problem. If there is a language gap and the clinician does not take steps to close it, the interview will be unsuccessful.

The Lack of Specific Purpose

Many beginning interviewers have either purposes that are too broad and general or interviewing goals that are too nebulous. It is important to write out carefully and rather explicitly the purposes for the interview before meeting with the client. We must know *why* we want the answers to the questions we ask. Specifying the purposes of an interview is also an effective way to reduce the interviewer's uncertainty and anxiety. Kadushin summarizes the importance of planning in this way:

> To know is to be prepared; to be prepared is to experience reduced anxiety; to reduce anxiety is to increase the interviewer's freedom to be fully responsive to the interviewee. (1972, p. 2)

The clinician should keep in mind, however, that thorough planning does not mean the application of an inflexible routine.

AN APPROACH TO INTERVIEWING

We now present an interviewing approach, an eclectic product of our experience in social work, speech pathology, and clinical audiology, together with an intensive study of relevant bibliographic materials. No doubt the reader will want to modify this approach to suit individual settings. It is desirable to do so, for only through critical self-evaluation and modification can any clinician acquire an interviewing procedure that is uniquely personal.

There are three basic goals in diagnostic interviews: to obtain information, to give information, and to provide release and support. For the purpose of discussion, each goal will be considered separately, a procedure rarely possible to do in an actual interview.

Goal One: Obtain Information

Although it may seem obvious, it is worth restating that as clinicians we must listen before we speak. There are essentially three reasons for this: (1) It gives clients an opportunity to talk out problems, to ventilate fears and feelings, thus enabling them to profit better from the direction and advice that the speech clinician will offer; (2) it gives the clinician an idea of the nature and scope of the information the client will need; and (3) it allows the clinician to formulate hypotheses concerning the individual's communication disorder.

Setting the Tone.   The first important task of the clinician is to set the right tone for the interview, to get a structured conversation initiated and channeled in the proper direction. How does one go about that? Research by McQuire and Lorch (1968) has underscored the importance of proper structuring. Their findings indicate that the initial style of interaction may well determine the style of interaction for the entire interview (see also the work of Matarazzo & Wiens, 1972).

We find that defining the roles is an effective procedure for setting the tone:

> Mrs. Seelos, I'm Miss Sullivan, Terry's speech clinician. I really appreciate the opportunity to chat with you about Terry and the things we are doing in speech. First, though, you can be of great help to me since you know Terry so much better than I do. There are several things about his early development and how his speech seems to be at home that I need to understand before planning a long-range therapy program. Before you came in today, I made some notes for myself so that we could best use this half hour before my next session.

It is helpful to think of the interview as a kind of role-playing situation. The clinician defines the roles for the client and indicates the rules and responsibilities that accrue to these roles. She tells who she is, what she intends to do, and what she expects of the client. In other words, the interviewer structures the situation by explaining the purposes of the interview—why the information is wanted and what will be done with it. Initially, of course, the client accepts the respondent role because of the nature of the situation and the official sanction of the interviewer's position. Then it is up to the worker to demonstrate her empathy and clinical expertise in order to solicit further cooperation. Two problems sometimes arise here. First, some clients may be inhibited by such explicit role definitions; some respondents have had little experience in holding directed conversations. In this case, a clinician can prolong the small-talk phase, emphasize the nature of the interview as a chat, and gently ease into the more structured situation as the relationship develops. When two or more people meet together, even for serious purposes, a certain amount of social and idle talk seems to foster positive attitudes toward continued interaction. Czikszentmihalyi (1975) describes this feature of group interaction as "flow."

The second, more difficult problem concerns the site of the interview. Although it is generally best to conduct interviews in a clinical setting, sometimes this is not possible and one has to seek out the client or parents at home. This is rarely satisfactory, not only because of the distractions inherent in the situation (children, pets, and neighbors) but also because the interview frequently becomes a social visit.

It is vital that the interviewer convey sincere interest in the situation as the client sees it. The speech-language pathologist must demonstrate to the client that he/she is genuinely trying to comprehend what the problem is and what it means to the client personally. The clinician can show interest by carefully attending to the respondent: Assume a relaxed, natural posture; maintain eye contact; and offer minimal verbal encouragements that reveal you are listening ("Yes," "I see," etc.).

Rapport, of course, is not a separate substance that one pours into a session; it is mutual respect and trust, a feeling of confidence in the clinician, and a large measure of understanding. Empathy, warmth, and acceptance are crucial aspects; the worker must strive for the ability to understand sensitively and accurately the interviewee's situation. We should also try to be genuine, not contrived, with a professional character armor that signals "clinician on duty." As a matter of fact, it is helpful to avoid interposing a desk—a symbol of authority—between the respondent and the interviewer. The interview is more effective without such a barrier. In addition to the words spoken, a number of forces shape the tone of the interview. Some things are conveyed by the setting and by the dress, manners, and expressions of the participants. If our office is located in a boiler room or a storage area, we have already conveyed something of our attitude toward the client and his/her problem by the very physical space that we use. In professional interviewing, the goal is to provide an atmosphere that fosters communication between client and clinician (Staples & Sloane, 1976).

Asking the Questions.   Preferably, the clinician should use an interview guide rather than one of the more elaborate questionnaires—that is, instead of a formal set of questions written out to be read and answered, we should use a form that indicates areas to explore. The interview is much more spontaneous and meaningful if the speech clinician words questions in keeping with his/her understanding of the individual's situation rather than reading prepared questions. In most cases, formal questionnaires operate as another type of barrier or crutch for the insecure interviewer.

The specific content of the queries addressed to a respondent depend on, among other things, the age of the client, the nature of the problem, and the purposes of the interview. Most clinicians find that the younger the client being evaluated, the more important is the parent interview. Hodges et al. (1982) devised a *Child Assessment Schedule* that elicits a school-aged youngster's responses to items pertaining to school, friends, and family. Sigelman (1982) offers a multiple-choice technique (using pictures) that we have found useful in diagnostic interviews with mentally retarded persons. Because we intend to focus on style of interviewing in this chapter, we will not include lists of questions that pertain to particular disorders of communication. There are, however, seven general topics or areas of inquiry that are useful in any diagnostic session:

1. *What is the respondent's perception of the problem?* We seek here a global description of the communication disorder. In a parent interview, for example, we frequently open the session with an open-ended question, "Tell me why you brought Jamie to the speech clinic."

2. *When and under what conditions did the communication disorder arise?* The purpose of this question is to determine the history of the development and the onset of the problem. This line of inquiry is particularly important in evaluating a child with delayed language—we want to know as much as possible about the youngster's motor, social, and cognitive development.

3. *In what ways has the communication disorder changed since its onset?* When interviewing parents of a child exhibiting early signs of stuttering, for example, we are interested in how the speech disfluency has changed since first noticed.

4. *What are the consequences (the handicapping conditions) of the problem?* In what manner—socially, educationally, occupationally—does the communication disorder affect the person's life? In what ways has he/she adapted to the disorder?

5. *How has the client and family attempted to cope with the problem?* What lay remedies have been tried by the client and family? How has the client responded to them?

6. *What impact has the client's communication disorder had on the rest of the family?* When a child has a handicapping condition, it creates fertile ground for familial conflict (see Featherstone, 1980). In order to obtain a description of the child's ongoing behavior, and how he/she fits into the family regimen, ask the parents to describe a "typical" day, from the time the youngster gets up until he/she goes to bed.

7. *What are the client's (or parents') expectations regarding the diagnostic session?*

Students frequently ask what type of interviewers they should strive to be: directive, nondirective, behavioristic, psychoanalytic, neo-Freudian, and so forth. The best answer that we have been able to give—although it sounds facetious—is that they must use whatever techniques seem to be best for the job that they need to do. We often feel that a beginning clinician concentrates too hard on being behavioristic or Rogerian rather than focusing on what he must do to meet the needs of a particular client. Some writers feel that the direct interview is unpleasant, although there is no evidence to support this assumption. As a matter of fact, one research team (Richardson, Dohrenwend, & Klein, 1965) discovered that the lack of structure inherent in the pure nondirective interview produced anxiety in some respondents, especially the less-educated ones. Actually, the whole matter is an academic question, because a good diagnostic interview is characterized by a shifting of styles: objective questions that ask for specifics, subjective queries that deal with feelings and attitudes, and finally indeterminate questions such as "Tell me more" that keep the respondent going.

A far better question for the clinician to pose is, "Why am I asking these questions?" He/she should have the purpose clearly in mind. Classically, the interviewer should start with the least anxiety-provoking queries, mostly objective questions that have high specificity (Woolf, 1971), and then proceed to more subjective questions as the relationship develops.

Quite often, however, we find it useful to employ a "funnel" sequence of inquiry during the course of a diagnostic interview—starting with broad, open-ended questions and then progressing to more specific or closed questions (Stewart & Cash, 1974). Here is an example of a funnel sequence from a recent parent interview:

- How does Jimmy function in the family setting?
- How does he get along with his siblings?
- How does his older sister "help" him communicate?
- Can you describe an instance in which she talked for him?

The "inverted funnel" approach, proceeding from specific to general, is also useful. It is best to avoid the checklist or a long series of "tunnel" questions that call for information on one level of specificity and are all asked in a similar style (for example, "Did your child have earaches, fevers, head injury, etc.?").

The Presenting Story.   Most persons who anticipate visiting a clinic or discussing a speech problem with a public school speech clinician will have mentally rehearsed what they intend to say. In some cases, they may even have a pseudoconversation with the worker. We must allow this story to be unraveled, or the respondent will be left with a sense of frustration and lack of closure.[1] A question such as, "What seems to be the problem?" will permit the flow of conversation to begin. The clinician should remember that this is how the *client* perceives the problem—it is his/her unique way of looking at the situation. It may be grossly inaccurate, but the interviewer should hear it out; nothing turns a respondent off more quickly than for the interviewer to suggest by word or action that his/her views are silly or misguided. Sometimes the presenting story will become a motif that recurs again and again during the course of the interview.

This is generally a crucial point in an interview. The interviewee may cautiously extend a portion of herself verbally, carefully scan the interviewer's

---

[1] Often the interviewer will have to contend with events that occurred prior to the session—the family car failing to start, a burned breakfast, absence of a convenient parking place. A few words to reveal the worker's understanding of the distracting antecedents will generally assist the respondent in shifting to the topic of the interview.

response, and then decide whether or not to tell the whole story. Sometimes a respondent may even set up a straw man to see how the interviewer deals with it:

> Mrs. Dimitri, mother of Ivan, a fifth-grader who possessed a serious lateral lisp, appeared to see herself as a modern, informed parent. At our initial interview, she launched into a lengthy diatribe about the school reading program, explaining in great detail why Ivan couldn't read. We listened intently for a time and when she paused to recycle her complaints, we praised her for her concern and suggested that she bring this up at the next PTA meeting and with Ivan's teacher. Apparently Mrs. Dimitri expected a debate, and she was much mollified that we had heard her out. We then proceeded to an excellent review of her insights into the child's speech problem.

This is not the proper time for the clinician to debate an issue with the client. The story can be accepted initially on the level of feeling, and later in the interview—when rapport is stronger—the point can be discussed more fully. We feel very strongly that these initial stories, these primitive theories, should be respected as the best possible answer clients have been able to come up with. This does not mean agreeing with their conclusions; it just means we accept their judgment with understanding so that we can form a basis for further communication.

Actually, the presenting information can be a very rich source of clinical hypotheses to be explored during the course of the interview. How do the client and parent present themselves (Goffman, 1959)—as long-suffering, anxious, different? How do they associate ideas or items of information sequentially? What priorities do they assign to issues they raise? Do they seem to be realistic in their expectations regarding the diagnostic session and treatment?

Nonverbal Messages.   Respondents do not communicate by words alone, and the discerning clinician attends to body as well as oral language during an interview. As a matter of fact, some observers (Bosmajian, 1971; Harrison, 1974; Hinde, 1972; Mehrabian, 1972) suggest that a large portion of the total message—particularly that involving strong feelings—is carried by nonverbal cues. However, the diagnostician should resist the urge to interpret a client's every twitch; each instance of nonverbal behavior should be related to the *content* of the oral message and the *context* in which it occurs (Birdwhistle, 1970; Feldman, 1972; Knapp, 1972).

> If a parent leaves her coat on during an interview it may mean she feels vulnerable and the garment provides a bit of protective armor. It may also mean that she has a spot on her dress, or that all the hangers in the waiting room were taken again by forgetful students, or that the room is chilly. However, if she shifts her chair away from the clinician, sits with her arms and legs tightly crossed, avoids eye contact, and responds to questions with one-word answers, then it may be concluded that she is defensive and guarded in the clinical setting.

The issue here is to avoid making one item of nonverbal behavior the sole basis for interpretation; the interviewer should be on the lookout for patterns (Weitz, 1974).

Although research into the nonverbal facets of dyadic interviewing is still in its early stages, there are several useful questions that can assist the examiner's scrutiny of body language (Egolf & Chester, 1973):

1. What clues are evident during the initial contact with the client? Does he/she enter the room hesitantly and wait to be seated? What can be discerned from clothing or personal grooming? Does he/she avoid eye contact and shake hands limply?

2. Is the respondent's facial expression congruent with the content of his/her oral message? Does the face flush or show other emotions when discussing different aspects of the speech problem? Does he/she reveal tension by constant bunching of the jaw muscles?

3. How does the respondent use eye gaze during the course of the interview? As a general rule, persons maintain less eye contact when talking than listening, particularly when responding to questions that provoke reflection and recall. The amount of mutual gaze between two individuals is increased markedly when they like each other and are involved in a joint concern. Keep in mind, however, that unwavering eye contact by the clinician, particularly when asking questions, may be interpreted as a threat signal or an attempt to dominate (Argyle & Cook, 1976).

4. Attend to the client's body movements and postural shifts: What is the rate and extent of movement, and the degree of tension shown? Does the respondent's postural shifting congruently mirror that of the interviewer?

5. How does the client speak with his/her hands? Are the hands tightly clasped? Does he/she wring them or play continually with a ring? Are a number of "adaptors" used (Knapp, 1972), such as adjusting clothing, scratching, or inspecting the fingernails?

6. How does the respondent communicate by use of the available space? In which chair does a client choose to sit with respect to proximity with the interviewer?

7. What can be discerned by attending to nuances in the client's use of pitch, loudness, or vocal quality? Does the rate reflect apprehension, excitement, or depression? Is the respondent's recital of the presenting story punctuated by heavy sighs?

8. In what respect do the stigmata associated with various communication disorders (for example, stuttering, cerebral palsy) interfere with or confound nonverbal messages (Eisenberg & Smith, 1971; Goffman, 1963)? How does body language vary with respect to the factors of sex, age, and culture (Morsbach, 1973)?

The most important thing to look for may be lack of congruence between the respondent's verbal and nonverbal messages; in cases where the two conflict, body language is generally a more accurate indicator of how a person feels about an issue.

During a recent diagnostic session, we opened the parent interview by asking the parent to describe the nature of his child's speech problem (the child was multiply handicapped). Before the parent responded verbally, he made a short, chopping gesture with his right hand, stamped his right foot, and wrinkled his face in a fleeting expression of disgust. However, he then proceeded to tell us calmly what a wonderful relationship he had with his son. The nonverbal message occurred so swiftly that later we were uncertain if we had really seen it; when we played back the videotape, however, the graphic body language was evident even to the father. This vivid self-confrontation seemed to release some long-repressed feelings, and the father then talked at length about how disappointed he was in his son, how much attention his wife devoted to the child— often, he felt, at his expense, and what a financial drain the various treatment programs had been. The consequence of the interview was a referral to a family service agency where both parents received the type of counseling they needed.

Although persons vary in terms of their skill at "reading" nonverbal cues, it is possible to improve with training (Rosenthal et al., 1974). Since body language is continuous—there is no way to turn it off, not even for the clinician—the interviewer will want to investigate the topic of nonverbal communication more fully (Scheflen, 1972; Spiegel & Machotka, 1974; Leathers, 1976; Duncan & Fiske, 1977; Ekman, 1980).

Things to Avoid in the Interview.   Beginning interviewers commit several common errors that may make it more difficult for them to obtain needed information. The list that follows is not meant to be exhaustive, but it does cover the most glaring mistakes.

1. It is usually best to avoid questions that may be answered by a simple yes or no. Although open-ended questions do produce longer responses in general, it is interesting to note that respondents from lower socioeconomic groups, who have less education, become more anxious as the questions become less structured. Some clients are confirmed yes-people. No matter what the clinician asks, no matter what comments he/she makes, these respondents simply nod in passive agreement. Perhaps they are fearful of exposing their ignorance and feel that it is better to remain silent and be thought a fool than to say something and make it obvious.

We find that requesting clients to rate themselves on a simple scale is more effective than either-or questions. We frequently ask the client to tell us not whether something is difficult or easy but to what degree. A simple rating procedure, with low values (1 or 2) indicating relative ease and higher values (4 or 5) indicating relative difficulty, may be used.

2. Avoid phrasing questions in such a way that they inhibit freedom of response. Do not say, "You don't have any difficulty with ringing in your ears, do you?" or "You don't tell Billy to stop and start over again, do you?" Such leading questions are not effective interviewing. The beginning interviewer tends to be anxious about asking open-ended questions. He is afraid that silence will result and that this will damage his relationship with the client. So he will ask an open-ended question and then close it. For example, "How do you feel about David's stuttering; does it bother you?" Leave it open! Although open-ended questions consume more time and may produce some rambling and irrelevant responses, there are many advantages to recommend their use:

> They let the respondent do the talking while the interviewer plays his role as listener and observer. The freedom to determine the nature and amount of information the respondent will give may communicate to him that you are

interested in him, as well as his answers, and that you respect his ability to give accurate and relevant data. (Stewart & Cash, 1974, p. 28)

Try also to avoid abrupt shifts in your line of questioning. For example, if you are exploring the client's feelings or attitudes on a particular issue (subjective questions), don't suddenly ask an objective question. Inexperienced interviewers, fearful that they are too deep in an area, tend to jump around; often they persist with objective queries and, once a pattern of response is established, the client finds it difficult to shift to more elaborate answers.

3. Avoid talking too much. This is perhaps the most common mistake of the beginning interviewer. He/she feels that every pause must be filled up with verbiage. It is much better to rephrase what the respondent has said or make some comment like, "I see," "Tell me more," or "Anything else?" Sometimes a smile and an understanding nod are effective when it is felt that the client has more to say but needs some silent time to conjure it up. If there is a positive attitude—a good rapport—and the person feels comfortable in the situation, then these encouragements increase the length of the response; if the topic or situation is neutral, these comments tend to expand the message. However, if the topic is negative or the individual feels uncomfortable, the "hmm, hmm" may be taken as a criticism—that is, if the client *cannot* respond at length, he/she will feel pressured to do so.

Be careful not to fall into stereotyped verbal habits. One of our students used the words "very good" as reinforcement so frequently with a severely aphasic patient that one day, after making a particularly effective response to a problem, the patient—who had said very little since his stroke—finished the clinician's "very" with a resounding "good," surprising them both.

4. Avoid concentrating on the physical symptoms and the etiological factors to the exclusion of the client's feelings and attitudes. There is a little bit of physician in all of us; we yearn to play the role of omniscient healer. This is further compounded by instructors who dwell interminably on causation in a course dealing with speech disorders. But it is possible to track each suspicious symptom with such zeal that we fail to obtain a basis for understanding the emotional and environmental complications of a speech or hearing disability. The interviewer should remember to distinguish between items of information that are simply interesting and background information that is really important.

5. Avoid providing information too soon. There will be plenty of time to clear up misconceptions later in the interview. The surest way to cut off the flow of information is to stop a parent, for instance, after he says, "I just tell Michael to stop, take a deep breath, and start all over again," and counsel him on the proper responses to nonfluency.

6. Avoid qualifying and hemming and hawing when asking questions. Ask them in a straightforward fashion and maintain eye contact. Rather than asking, "Did you find that, well, you know, when you were, ah, shall we say . . . with child—did you experience any untoward conditions?," say "Did anything unusual happen during your pregnancy?" Instead of inquiring, "Did you discover, hmm, I mean, well, after your father, ah, passed away, did your

stuttering problem increase?," say, "What impact did your father's death have on your speech?"

7. Avoid negativistic or moralistic responses, verbal or nonverbal, to the client's statements (avoid even the response "good," as it implies a value judgment). The flow of information will stop rapidly and the relationship will be impaired severely if the individual senses that we find her or his behavior distasteful. We do not have to subscribe to a person's value or code of behavior to show compassion and understanding for her situation. Use inquiries that begin with "why" very sparingly—the word is often perceived as a challenge or a threat; it is too reminiscent of disciplinary sessions (Why were you late for class? Why can't you behave properly?). In a clinical setting, we must not let our values obscure our perception of the client's frame of reference (Benjamin, 1974). An interview is not the place to push the clinician's personal point of view. We have a student clinician who once wore a political button on her collar during a diagnostic interview. This can immediately alienate certain clients. Another student wore a button that said, "Jesus is the answer," which certainly would not have been the case for her non-Christian clients.

8. When the client causes the interview to wander, avoid abrupt transitions to bring it back to the point. Most of those whom you will interview have had little experience in directed, orderly conversation. They tend to follow chance associations and wander far afield. The experienced interviewer has the ability to make smooth transitions. How does one go about getting the interview back on track? The best way is by building a bridge to the respondent's previous statements; for example, "That's interesting, Mrs. Davis, maybe we can come back to that in a little while; now earlier you were mentioning that your child's loss of hearing occurred suddenly . . ." The goal here is to use respondent antecedents—things that the person has said earlier in the interview. If we use only the interviewer's antecedents—questions that the interviewer has asked before—the client will not feel understood and will sense that what he has said was of little consequence. The inexperienced interviewer asks lots of questions with no antecedents or with his/her own antecedents. This person is afraid of losing control of the interview and thus becomes preoccupied with formulating the next question.

9. Avoid allowing the interview to produce only superficial answers. We need ways to get deeper, more significant responses from our clients. There are several interviewing devices, termed _probes,_ that the clinician will find helpful. Several examples follow.

Crosshatch, or _interlocking,_ questions are useful when we need to elicit more detail about a topic that has been glossed over. There are often discrepancies that must be resolved. Essentially, the way to go about this is to ask the same thing in different ways and at different points during the interview. For instance, the father of a young stutterer responded in a superficial manner to our query about his relationship with the child. He assured us that he had a "loving relationship" with his son and then complained at length about the conditions in his work situation. Later in the interview, when we asked him to describe the sorts of things he did with the child, he was unable to mention a single one. We don't mean to imply that the clinician should attempt to catch the client lying and then demand an explanation. The clinician must check out discrepancies, however, in order to enhance understanding of the problem, since they could have a significant effect on the mode of treatment.

Pauses can be very helpful. When there is a lull in the interview, it may mean simply that the client has exhausted his/her store of information, that a memory barrier has prevented further recall, or that he/she senses lack of understanding by the clinician. It can also mean, however, that a sensitive area has been touched upon. Do not feel that pauses harm the interview. Much significant information can be forthcoming if we keep quiet and indicate with a smile or a nod that we expect more.

Another aid is to encourage *time regression and association*. Memories are weak. In order to pinpoint some significant data, we may have to take the person back in time to find a memory peg, such as a wedding, a natural calamity, or the like, that may call forth more information. One father, a long-time air force sergeant, catalogued everything in terms of the make and model of car he was driving. Another client, an inveterate bird-watcher, remembered incidents by the times he had seen the marbled godwit or the prothonotary warbler.

The *summary probe* is one of the best ways to keep the interview moving smoothly. The clinician periodically summarizes what the client has said, ending perhaps with a request for clarification or further information. Incidentally, the procedure also demonstrates to the person that the interviewer is indeed trying to understand his problem. We generally use "mini-summary probes"—echo questions—all the way through an interview:

RESPONDENT: After my husband's stroke, my whole world collapsed.
INTERVIEWER: You were overwhelmed by the sudden change in your life.
RESPONDENT: Yes, one day he was happily planning our trip to Sanibel Island . . . and then, in just a moment, he was paralyzed and couldn't talk. Now all our plans are up in the air . . . the new car, the checking account, he took care of all that.

The *stumbling probe* is a variation of the summary probe; we have found it helpful, especially with the reticent respondent. The interviewer rephrases a portion of the respondent's communication and then, attempting to interpret or comment upon it, she pretends to halt or stumble. For example, when interviewing the mother of a child allegedly beginning to stutter, the clinician might say; "Now, you were saying that Bruce first started to repeat and hesitate after he caught his finger in the car door. Under these conditions, it would be natural for you to . . . ah . . ." This really works. The respondent's need for closure will precipitate significant information and, perhaps more importantly, significant insights.

Finally, there is the *assuming probe*. (This stems from the old incriminating question, "Have you stopped beating your wife yet?") Such a technique should, of course, be used sparingly and only after some interviewing experience; at times, however, it is the only way to get information out in the open. If the client has avoided an important area, if he has left much unsaid regarding his speech or hearing problem and what it means to him, then it is up to the interviewer to bring this out. One adolescent boy who had been vehemently denying that his stuttering bothered him, unburdened himself when we said, "It bothers you so much that you don't want anybody to know, do you?"

10. Avoid letting the client reveal too much in one interview. You may have had an experience similar to this: A good friend encounters severe trouble and you come to his aid, helping him through the crisis. A curious thing often happens when your friend recovers his equilibrium. He feels obligated to you; he felt exposed to you as a raw human being during the crisis, and now he is embarrassed, somewhat resentful, and perhaps even hostile. It is as if you are now an outward and visible sign of his former debacle. Sometimes a beginning interviewer makes the mistake of trying to get everything in one sitting. The client, sensing perhaps his first really understanding listener, may want to pour out his whole sad tale of woe. Later, however, the individual will feel embarrassed and foolish, perhaps even exposed and guilty at revealing so much of himself to this comparative stranger.

Bringing an interview to a graceful close can sometimes be more difficult than getting it started. In our experience, an interview is more effectively terminated by summarizing what has been discussed and reviewing the specific actions to be taken. It is probably best not to consider new material at this time when neither the interviewer nor the client can devote sufficient attention to it. It is always important, however, to leave the door open for future contacts (see Kadushin, 1972, pp. 207–214; and Stewart & Cash, 1974, pp. 197–201 for more information on leave-taking).

11. Avoid trusting to memory. Record the information as the interview progresses. Tell the client that you will take some notes during the interview so that you can plan her treatment program more effectively and make recommendations for other services. Such note taking or even recording devices are rarely questioned. Indeed, we have found that clients expect you to write down some of the information they are giving you; they doubt that you would be able to remember all of their answers. You obviously would lose your relationship, however, if you scribbled furiously while the client was revealing some sensitive information. It is axiomatic that the respondent's confidence will be respected. The clinician's manner should suggest that all information received is to be held strictly confidential or will be shared only with client permission.

Prepare a report of the interview as soon as possible. Commit your observations to paper while the encounter with the respondent is still fresh in your mind (see Chapter 13 for information on writing reports).

Goal Two: Give Information

The most common complaint of patients in hospitals and clinics is that they have not been kept informed of their condition and progress. Interviewing 214 patients, Pratt, Seligman, and Reader (1958; p. 229) report: "Patients who were given more thorough explanations were found to participate somewhat more effectively with the physician and were more likely to accept completely the doctor's formulation than were the patients who received very little information." We have formulated a fundamental principle in this regard: *There is never too little information, there is instead misinformation.* Not one of us can stand uncertainty. All too frequently the information, if not supplied by the professional worker, will come distorted from other sources. When not correctly informed, parents become misinformed and this leads to confusion, misunderstanding, and further compounding of the problem. It is our responsibility, therefore, to provide accurate, unemotional, objective information on the status of the individual's speech and hearing problem. This is generally accomplished during the postdiagnostic conference (Martin, 1977).

Summarize the findings of the clinical examination in simple, nontechnical language; use common terms compatible with the person's background. We prefer to begin, if possible, with results that show a client's area of normal functioning, to review findings that indicate what is good before describing deficiencies. Relate comments to normative values whenever possible. Clarify and help the respondent to ask questions by using examples and simple analogies. If the interviewer is in doubt concerning the client's understanding of the diagnostic material (clients will rarely ask if they don't understand), he/she should talk more slowly, employ longer descriptions, and use more redundant language (Longhurst & Siegel, 1973). Recapitulation of a conference by audio or videotape playback fosters even greater understanding (Marshall & Goldstein, 1969).

The Questions Clients Ask.   An interview is much more than a clinician posing questions and recording the client's answers. It is an important forum for *exchange,* a reflexive, dynamic experience of sharing between the diagnostician and the informant. Indeed, we find that a client—especially a parent of a young child being evaluated—is frequently eager to probe the worker's expertise. But often the questions she asks may have a hidden meaning or purpose. The clinician must evaluate the informant's inquiries and decide what the person is *really* asking. Is there an unstated concern behind the questions? Luterman (1979) distinguishes the questions clients ask into three categories: *content, opinion,* and *affect.* We will describe and illustrate these three types of inquiries with excerpts from an initial interview with the mother of a three-year-old child brought to the speech clinic as a beginning stutterer.

1. *Questions dealing with information or content.*   In this instance, the client seeks an informative or factual response from the clinician. The question usually takes the form, "I want to know about something and I hope you have the right information."

MRS. BELL: The type of choppy speech [disfluency] Jesse has—is it common among children his age?

CLINICIAN: It sure is. Most children between the ages of two-and-a-half and five do a lot of repeating and hesitating.

2. *Questions with predetermined opinions.*   Here the client has an opinion regarding a particular subject and wants to determine if the clinician agrees with it. The clinician must be careful not to merely demolish the client's opinion until she understands *why* and *how strongly* the client holds it.

MRS. BELL: Um, on TV a couple of times, I've seen a demonstration of the airflow technique for stuttering. What do you think of it?

CLINICIAN: Those demonstrations are very dramatic, aren't they? What's your impression of the technique as it applies to Jesse?

3. *Questions that are "faint knocking on the door."*   In this case, the client is not asking for information or for the clinician's opinion, but rather for emotional support and reassurance. The question conceals a feeling the individual is either unaware of or reluctant to reveal.

MRS. BELL: Do you think my divorce and remarriage had anything to do with Jesse's speech problem?

CLINICIAN: It's pretty easy for parents to feel guilty about something they might have done to cause their child to begin stuttering.

No doubt the reader has already detected a flaw in the triad: On the surface, each question posed by Mrs. Bell could be classified in any of the three categories. How does a clinician know *what* the client means? The clinician doesn't know in every case, but we try to determine the purpose of a question by scrutinizing *how* a client asks it—by vocal inflection and body language—and by the context in which the inquiry appears. Interestingly, as long as the clinician is *trying to understand,* a client will not be alienated by an inaccurate interpretation (Chinn, Winn, & Walters, 1978).

In our experience, speech clinicians do a good job of responding to content questions, probably because the bulk of their training focuses on information. However, many beginning clinicians find it difficult to respond appropriately to a client's expression of emotion. Although Luterman is discussing clinical audiologists, his remarks pertain to many speech clinicians as well:

> Professional training programs rarely provide any information or experience for the student in how to deal with parents. They concentrate instead on providing considerable information and practicum experience with the handicapped child. As a result of that imbalance in emphasis, the young therapist feels very insecure in dealing with parents, who may be older and more experienced in the care of children. So the therapist begins to adopt defensive strategies to "distance" the parents, the most common one being to impart information. The content-based relationship is completely controlled by the teacher and subtly puts the parents down by increasing their feelings of inadequacy. That one-sided way of dealing with parents becomes habitual with time, and older teachers rely on content strategy almost exclusively. In some circles that approach is considered very professional. It is only when professionals feel secure as people that they can allow more intimacy and more freedom in their relationship with parents. (1979, p. 48)

Avoid superficial statements of reassurance. Most people can see through this sort of sham. The individual's anxiety and uncertainty will be better relieved once he begins to understand his particular speech problem; the best antidote to fear and uncertainty is knowledge. Be sure, however, to avoid iatrogenic errors. Do not use terms or suggest consequences that will precipitate more stress for the client. One parent was told his child's hearing problem was caused by atrophy of the hearing nerve. It is difficult enough to have a hard-of-hearing child without worrying about mysterious nerves atrophying, something about which the parent can do very little. Do not communicate your negative expectations regarding the outcome of therapy to the client. We are convinced that what the clinician thinks a client can do, that he shall do. In other words, the client's behavior expands to fit the clinician's concept of his potential. Do we precondition our own therapeutic behavior when we make a prognosis? Is this communicated to the client and his relatives in some manner and on some level? We think it often is.

Below are six basic principles for imparting information to clients that we have found useful:

1. Emotional confusion may, and often does, inhibit the person's ability to understand cognitively what you are trying to say. Just because you have once reviewed the steps of therapy is no reason to expect that their importance will be grasped.
2. Refrain from being didactic; do not lecture your clients. Focus on sharing options rather than giving advice.
3. Use simple language with many examples and illustrations. If you must err, err in the direction of being too simple rather than complex. And repeat, repeat, repeat the important points—rephrasing each time.
4. Try to provide something that the client—especially a parent—can do. Action reduces the feelings of futility and anxiety. The activity should be direct and simple and should require some kind of reporting to the clinician.
5. Say what needs to be said pleasantly—but frankly. Do not avoid saying something that must be said on the assumption that the client cannot take it or that you will be rejected. People often display an amazing reserve of courage in difficult situations (Buscaglia, 1975).
6. Remember, however, that the one who finally communicates what the client may have been dreading to hear is often hated and maligned. If you are the first to say the feared words, you may become the focus for all the hostile, negative feelings thus aroused. As a professional worker, you will have to be strong enough to be the lightning rod for these emotions.

Clients and their parents expect to receive help from the clinician but will often resist change. No matter how maladaptive a client's behavior may seem from an objective point of view, it represents her best solution; in fact, she will often resist attempts to alter her equilibrium, precarious as it may appear to others. Change is stressful. Diagnosis and treatment imply change; therefore, assessment and therapy are stressful.

According to Carkhuff and Berenson (1976) and others (Ginott, 1965; Gordon, 1970), the key feature of *creative listening* is the ability to scan a client's comments and respond in a way that fosters understanding and releases the potential for growth. Creative listening represents empathy in action: Before anyone can or will listen, he must first be listened to.

The particular kind of understanding we are referring to involves two facets, a *cognitive* aspect (the content) and an *affective* aspect (the feelings). In order for genuine understanding to take place, both must be included in the interviewer's response to the client's statement. If the clinician is successful in crystallizing both aspects of his/her response, this provides an *interchangeable base* that allows the interview to move forward to levels of helping that involve direct action. Here are some examples taken from diagnostic interviews:

CLIENT: (in response to a query regarding his marital status): No, I'm single . . . who would want to marry a clod who stutters like me?

CLINICIAN: You feel rejected because of your speech problem, is that right?

PARENT: We tried to be good parents, we really did . . . but somehow we messed up in helping Peter learn to talk.

CLINICIAN: You feel a sense of failure, perhaps even guilt, that your child has a speech problem.

CLIENT: I stutter so badly that life is worthless . . . I can't get a job . . . the business of living just doesn't seem to meet expenses.

CLINICIAN: You feel thwarted and frustrated by your speech problem; sometimes you wonder if you can go on . . .

Note the clinician's responses carefully. She does not simply repeat the client's comment; she attempts to restate it in clarified form. Observe that the interviewer used the second-person singular "you" in referring to the client's affect to show empathy. Feelings are commonly stated first, since they are more important than content. We sometimes add a tag question ("Is that right?") to check on the client's intake of our responses.

Goal Three: Provide Release and Support

The clinician does not, of course, wait until the end of the interview to provide release for the frustrations and fears of the client. Most of the parts of the interview already discussed will serve this purpose. By helping the individual talk out his problems, the worker is providing an excellent escape mechanism for pent-up feelings. We maintain that our purpose is not just to remove discomfort but also to promote a state of comfort and well-being.

More than advice is needed during interviews for the purpose of helping clients take some specific action or move in a particular direction. They need help in sorting out the confusing choices before them. To support a respondent's real strengths, we need to make it clear that we understand what the situation means to him and that we uncritically sympathize with his feelings and attitudes. We can restore the client's self-esteem and ability to function more appropriately if we convey our interest in him as a person and our solid acceptance of his importance. If the client feels appreciated and understood, he can sometimes drop his self-protective behavior and see how the experience will eventually be of benefit.

There is an unfortunate tradition of "sweetness and light" in client counseling. A person has a problem. The person is sad and depressed, and we try to cheer her up. Sometimes this degenerates into a debate, with the interviewer attempting to persuade the person that she should not feel miserable. When people feel depressed, anxious, and fearful, they do not want to count their blessings. They want you to feel miserable, too. They want you to share and identify with them on their own level. Thus, the interviewer is given a basis for communicating with the person. We start where she is, accept it as the proper place to start, and agree that it is a sad state of affairs that would make anyone sad and depressed. Then, using this bond of identification, which becomes a basis for communication, we can assist in solving the problem. The main ingredient is *empathy*, the capacity to identify oneself with another's feelings and actions. The best way to demonstrate our attempt to understand a client's point of view is by listening creatively. In our judgment, of all the skills inherent in effective interviewing, the most important is the ability to listen carefully and empathically. This skill can be learned, although beginning clinicians find it difficult to employ remarks that facilitate a client's expression of feelings (Volz et al., 1978).

How does one handle emotional scenes? They are bound to arise at some point in your interviewing experience. Some clinicians excuse themselves from the room and allow the respondent to recover his/her dignity alone. Others try to change the subject to something less emotional. Both of these approaches may, with certain clients, give the impression that the clinician is rejecting their feelings. It is more effective to indicate one's understanding of the feelings that are being expressed and accept them as natural human reactions. For example, "That's okay to let it come out, Mrs. Moody; you have been holding it back too long. Sometimes it helps to get it out in the open."

Not all clients seen by the speech clinician will need or even want extensive supportive interviewing. In some cases, the procedures discussed here would be grossly inappropriate. Visualize an interview as ranging along a continuum from affective concerns such as feelings and attitudes to objective matters such as goals and advice. Some respondents simply need objective information so that they can take over and modify their behavior. The clinician's role in some interviews may consist of simply listening to and supporting a client. We quite agree that love alone is not enough in a helping transaction; a good relationship is a *necessary* but not a *sufficient* condition for good interviewing. However, it may sound trite, but it is true that the secret of care *of* a client is caring *for* the client. The sense of being understood by a helping professional is a powerful stimulant to the client's growth (Llewelyn & Hume, 1979; Sherman & Fields, 1982).

IMPROVING INTERVIEWING SKILLS

We hope the material in this chapter will be useful to students majoring in clinical speech pathology and to our colleagues working in various settings. However, no one ever became proficient in interviewing solely by reading about it. Nor, it seems, are interviewing skills enhanced by increasing knowledge about communication disorders (Janz, 1982; Wolraich et al., 1982). It took us many years of constant searching and experimenting to evolve the interviewing approach presented here. And, with the indulgence of our clients and many long-suffering parents, we continue to explore for better ways.

We have included below a series of activities and projects for your own practice. Let them serve as the beginning steps in a continual learning effort toward improved interviewing. You will find that the time devoted to such training exercises is well spent. Now, consider these steps for improving your interviewing skills:

1. Read widely from a variety of sources. We have included a list of selected references to get you started. Find out what people are like by reading in sociology, psychology, anthropology, and philosophy. This is, of course, a lifetime project, which we feel is delightful since there is always a new frontier, an open horizon on which we can set our sails. Our profession has arisen so abruptly, grown so rapidly, and been so concerned with the urgent scientific and clinical issues that it has ignored the most important issue—the development of a philosophical basis for our work. A speech and hearing clinician without a rationale is like a ship without a rudder. The fundamental and mandatory basis for sound, purposeful therapy is an overall point of view, a workable theory that does not necessarily include the specific activities that will be used to carry it out. Nothing is so pathetic as the clinician who, in a willy-nilly manner, empties a bag of therapeutic homilies on the client's lap, hoping somehow that one of them will work. Only a sequential system of logically interrelated theorems will enable us to evaluate our clinical effectiveness.

2. Listen to all sorts of people, to their dreams, their rationalizations, their insights—or lack of them—and their gripes. Get acquainted with the way common people think and talk by following the examples of Caldwell (1976) and others (Coleman, 1974; Least-Heat-Moon, 1982; Morris, 1972; Steinbeck, 1961; Terkel, 1980; Walters, 1970).

3. Form small heterogeneous groups of students majoring in speech pathology and audiology. Conduct some sensitivity and values clarification training, particularly as it relates to your self-concept, your assets and liabilities, your responses to people, and your relationships with your own parents and other older adults (Kaplan & Dreyer, 1974). In order to provide assistance to others, we must know our own foibles and potential blind spots and have them under reasonable control. Remember, too, that the way our academic preparation teaches us to explain a situation will tend to determine the way we perceive it.

4. Role playing is still one of the best methods to prepare for interviewing (Finn & Rose, 1982; White, 1982). Set up several typical interview situations in front of a class and play, for example, the roles of the reluctant parent, the spouse of an aphasic patient, or the hostile father. Discuss the interaction, and replay the situations with others assuming the roles. Write out interview purposes prior to the role playing and determine, or have the class determine, how effectively the interviewer accomplished avowed purposes. Whenever the viewers feel that the interview went wrong or the responses were ineffective,

Figure 2.2 Checklist of Interviewing Competencies

Interviewer: _____   Date: _____

Client/Respondent: _____

I.   *Orienting the Respondent*
     A. Attends to comfort (coats, seating, and so on)
     B. Engages in appropriate "flow" talk
     C. Explains purposes, procedures
     D. Structures roles

II. *Engendering Communication*
     A. Attending behaviors (demonstrates receptiveness)
        1. Relaxed, natural posture
        2. Appropriate eye contact
        3. Responses that follow the client's comments (restating, overlapping the client's message)
     B. Open invitation to share (open-ended questions)
     C. Nondistracting encouragement to continue talking
        1. Verbal ("yes," "I see," and the like)
        2. Nonverbal (nodding, shifting posture toward client)
     D. Obtains an overview of the presenting problem

III. *Use of Questions and Recording*
     A. Orderly, sequential questions
     B. Nondistracting note taking

IV. *Active Listening*
     A. Reflects feelings (empathic statements)
        1. Matches affect
        2. Matches content
     B. Periodic summarizing of affect and content messages

V.   *Monitoring Nonverbal Clues*
     A. The diagnostician's
     B. The respondent's

VI. *Skills in Presenting Information*
     A. Transmission of information
        1. Content
        2. Style and language
     B. Responds to questions appropriately
     C. Appropriate use of humor, "flow" talk

VII. *Closing the Interview*
     A. Summary, review of findings
     B. Recommendations
     C. Supportive comments

VIII. *Analysis of Information*
     A. Major themes in the client's presentation, association of ideas, inconsistencies, and omissions
     B. Descriptive report

Note: This checklist is designed to help monitor the performance of beginning interviewers. It can be used as a self-rating device or a format for supervisory feedback. (See also Enelow & Swisher, 1972; Maier, 1976.)

see how many different ways it could have been handled. This builds up the beginning interviewer's repertoire of adaptive responses. You can do a surprising amount of interpersonal role playing in your spare time. While we are waiting for a class to begin, for a light to change, or for our father-in-law to cease talking, we frequently imagine ourselves in various interviewing situations and then explore alternate statements, probes, and so forth.

5. Make recordings of your first few interviews, then analyze them carefully with your clinical supervisor or a colleague (Adler & Enelow, 1966; Cannell, Lawson, & Hausser, 1975; Irwin, 1975). We believe that multiple interviewers simply do not work (although seeing multiple interviewees—such as a mother and father at the same time—can be useful and productive); hence, we would suggest that your supervisor not observe your performance in the same room, especially for your first ventures. In a dyadic interview, there are only two possible directions for communication ($1 \times 2 = 2$). When a third party is added, potential interactions are increased to six ($1 \times 2 \times 3 = 6$). Add yet another person and the possibilities for communicative exchange reach unwieldy proportions ($1 \times 2 \times 3 \times 4 = 24$). We have found that when the supervisor stays in the room, the student has a tendency to seduce him/her into taking over as interviewer; and if the supervisor refuses to assume the mantle, he/she can only sit there looking at the clients as if they were bugs in an insect collection. We have no role sanction in our social structure for the silent scrutinizer, and this presence can seriously impair the effectiveness of the interview.

Play back your interview again and again, revising statements, underscoring errors, and scanning for the good parts. Have typed protocols prepared from some of these tapes—the errors really leap out at you from the printed page—and discuss them with your instructors, fellow students, or colleagues.

Use the set of questions devised by Stewart and Cash (1974, pp. 201–202) as a guideline for evaluating your performance. Explore also the methods prepared by Iwata et al. (1982) and Molyneaux and Lane (1982) for the assessment and training of clinical interviewing skills. Finally, we suggest you evaluate your diagnostic interviews using the Checklist of Interviewing Competencies (Figure 2.2). Obviously, no beginning clinician will remember, let alone exhibit, all the skills delineated in the checklist; practice only a few at a time, and provide constructive feedback for each other.

We would like to end this chapter with a challenge to the reader. We challenge you to utilize the interviewing approach delineated above, find the errors, the things that just don't work for you, and then develop your own methods. We have given you the foundation blocks. Can you use them to make stepping-stones?

BIBLIOGRAPHY

ADLER, L., & ENELOW, A. (1966). An instrument to measure skill in diagnostic interviewing: A teaching and evaluation tool. *Journal of Medical Education, 41,* 281–288.

ARGYLE, M., & COOK, M. (1976). *Gaze and mutual gaze.* London: Cambridge University Press.

BENJAMIN, A. (1974). *The helping interview* (2nd ed.). Boston: Houghton Mifflin.

BIRDWHISTLE, R. (1970). *Kinesics and context.* Philadelphia: University of Pennsylvania Press.

BOSMAJIAN, H. (Ed.). (1971). *The rhetoric of nonverbal communication.* Glenview, IL: Scott, Foresman.

BUSCAGLIA, L. (1975). *The disabled and their parents: A counseling challenge.* Thorofare, NJ: Charles B. Slack.

CALDWELL, E. (1976). *Afternoons in mid-America.* New York: Dodd, Mead.

CANNELL, C., LAWSON, S., & HAUSSER, D. (1975). *A technique for evaluating interviewer performance.* Ann Arbor, MI: Institute for Social Research.

CARKHUFF, R., & BERENSON, B. (1976). *Beyond counseling and therapy.* New York: Holt, Rinehart & Winston.

CHENG, L. (1989). Service delivery to Asian/ Pacific LEP children: A cross-cultural framework. *Topics in Language Disorders, 9,* 1–14.

CHINN, P., WINN, J., & WALTERS, R. (1978). *Two-way talking with parents of special children.* St. Louis: C. V. Mosby.

COLE, L., & DEAL, V. (in press). *Communication disorders in multicultural populations.* Rockville, MD: American Speech-Language-Hearing Association.

COLEMAN, R. (1974). *Blue-collar journal: A college president's sabbatical.* Philadelphia: Lippincott.

CZIKSZENTMIHALYI, M. (1975). *Beyond boredom and anxiety.* San Francisco: Jossey-Bass.

DUNCAN, S., & FISKE, D. (1977). *Face-to-face interaction: Research, methods and theory.* Hillsdale, NJ: Lawrence Erlbaum Associates.

EGOLF, D., & CHESTER, S. (1973). Nonverbal communication and the disorders of speech and language. *Journal of American Speech and Hearing Association, 15,* 511–518.

EISENBERG, A., & SMITH, R. (1971). *Nonverbal communication.* New York: Bobbs-Merrill.

EKMAN, P. (1980). *The faces of man.* New York: Garland Press.

ENELOW, A., & SWISHER, S. (1972). *Interviewing and patient care.* New York: Oxford University Press.

FEATHERSTONE, H. (1980). *A difference in the family: Life with a disabled child.* New York: Basic Books.

FELDMAN, S. (1973). *Mannerisms of speech and gesture in everyday life.* New York: International Universities Press.

FINN, J., & ROSE, S. (1982). Development and validation of the interview skills role playing test. *Social Work Research Abstracts, 18,* 21–27.

GARRETT, A. (1972). *Interviewing: Its principles and methods,* 2nd ed. New York: Family Service Association.

GINOTT, H. (1965). *Between parent and child.* New York: Macmillan.

GOFFMAN, E. (1959). *The presentation of self in everyday life.* Garden City, NY: Doubleday.

GOFFMAN, E. (1963). *Stigma: Notes on the management of spoiled identity.* Englewood Cliffs, NJ: Prentice Hall.

GORDON, T. (1970). *Parent effectiveness in training.* New York: Peter H. Wyden.

HARRISON, R. (1974). *Beyond words: An introduction to nonverbal communication.* Englewood Cliffs, NJ: Prentice Hall.

HAYNES, W., & ORATIO, A. (1978). A study of client's perceptions of therapeutic effectiveness. *Journal of Speech and Hearing Disorders, 43,* 21–33.

HINDE, R. (1972). *Nonverbal communication.* New York: Cambridge University Press.

HODGES, K. et al. (1982). The development of a child assessment interview for research and clinical use. *Journal of Abnormal Child Psychology, 10,* 173–189.

IRWIN, R. B. (1975). Micro-counseling interviewing skill of supervisors of speech clinicians. *Human Communication, 4,* 5–9.

IWATA, B. et al. (1982). Assessment and training of clinical interviewing skills: Analogue analysis and field replication. *Journal of Applied Behavior Analysis, 15,* 191–203.

JANZ, T. (1982). Initial comparisons of patterned-behavior description interviews vs unstructured interviews. *Journal of Applied Psychology, 67,* 577–588.

KADUSHIN, A. (1972). *The social work interview.* New York: Columbia University Press.

KAPLAN, N., & DREYER, D. (1974). The effect of self-awareness training on student speech pathologist–client relationships. *Journal of Communication Disorders, 7,* 329–342.

KNAPP, M. (1972). *Nonverbal communications in human interaction.* New York: Holt, Rinehart & Winston.

LEAST-HEAT-MOON, W. (1982). *Blue highways: A journey into america.* Boston: Atlantic–Little, Brown.

LEATHERS, D. (1976). *Nonverbal communication systems.* Boston: Allyn & Bacon.

LLEWELYN, S., & HUME, W. (1979) The patient's view of therapy. *British Journal of Medical Psychology, 52,* 29–35.

LONGHURST, T., & SIEGEL, G. (1973). Effects of communication failure on speaker and listener behavior. *Journal of Speech and Hearing Research, 16,* 128–140.

LUTERMAN, D. (1979). *Counseling parents of hearing-impaired children.* Boston: Atlantic–Little, Brown.

McQUIRE, M., & LORCH, S. (1968). A model for the study of dyadic communication. *Journal of Nervous and Mental Diseases, 146,* 221–229.

MAIER, N. (1976). *Appraising performance: An interview skills course.* La Jolla, CA: University Associates.

MARSHALL, N., & GOLDSTEIN, S. (1969). Imparting diagnostic information to mothers: A comparison of methodologies. *Journal of Speech and Hearing Research, 12,* 65–72.

MARTIN, A. (1977). Post-diagnostic parent counseling by a speech pathologist and a social worker. *Journal of American Speech and Hearing Association, 19,* 67–68.

MATARAZZO, J., & WIENS, A. (1972). *The interview: Research on its anatomy and structure.* Chicago: Aldine-Atherton.

MEHRABIAN, A. (1972). *Nonverbal communication.* Chicago: Aldine-Atherton.

MOLYNEAUX, D., & LANE, V. (1982). *Effective interviewing: Techniques and analysis.* Boston: Allyn & Bacon.

MORGAN, H., & COGGER, J. (1973). *The interviewers manual.* New York: Psychological Corp.

MORRIS, T. (1972). *The walk of the conscious ants.* New York: Knopf.

MORSBACH, H. (1973). Aspect of nonverbal communication in Japan. *Journal of Nervous and Mental Disorders, 157,* 262–277.

NIDEFFER, R. (1976). *The inner athlete.* New York: Crowell.

PRATT, L., SELIGMAN, A., & READER, G. (1958). Physicians' views on the medical information among patients. In E. Jaco (Ed.), *Patients, physicians, and illness.* New York: Free Press.

RICHARDSON, S., DOHRENWEND, B., & KLEIN, D. (1965). *Interviewing: Its forms and functions.* New York: Basic Books.

ROSENTHAL, R. et al. (1974). Body talk and the tone of voice: The language without words. *Psychology Today, 8,* 64–68.

SCHEFLEN, A. (1972). *Body language and social order.* Englewood Cliffs, NJ: Prentice Hall.

SHERMAN, J., & FIELDS, S. (1982). *Guide to patient evaluation.* 4th ed. Garden City, NY: Medical Examination Publishing Co.

SIGELMAN, C. K. (1982). Evaluating alternative techniques of questioning mentally retarded persons. *American Journal of Mental Deficiency, 86,* 511–518.

SPIEGEL, J., & MACHOTKA, P. (1974). *Messages of the body.* New York: Free Press.

STAPLES, F., & SLOANE, R. (1976). Truax factors, speech characteristics and therapy outcome. *Journal of Nervous and Mental Disorders, 163,* 135–140.

STEINBECK, J. (1961). *Travels with Charley.* New York: Viking.

STEWART, C., & CASH, W. (1974). *Interviewing: Principles and practices.* Dubuque, IA: W. C. Brown.

TERKEL, S. (1980). *American dreams: Lost and found.* New York: Pantheon.

VOLZ, H., et al. (1978). Interpersonal communication skills of speech-language pathology undergraduates: The effects of training. *Journal of Speech and Hearing Disorders, 43,* 524–542.

WALTERS, B. (1970). *How to talk with practically anybody about practically anything.* Garden City, NY: Doubleday.

WEITZ, S., (Ed). (1974). *Nonverbal communication: Readings with commentary.* New York: Oxford University Press.

WHITE, R. (1982). Observer's presence and self-focused attention in role-rehearsal activities. *Perceptual and Motor Skills, 54,* 839–842.

WOLRAICH, M., et al. (1982). Factors affecting physician communication and parent-physician dialogues. *Journal of Medical Education, 57,* 621–625.

WOOLF, G. (1971). Information specificity: A correlate of verbal output in diagnostic interview. *Journal of Speech and Hearing Disorders, 36,* 518–526.

chapter

3

PSYCHOMETRIC CONSIDERATIONS IN DIAGNOSIS AND EVALUATION

Let us interest you in purchasing a standardized test to use in assessing communication disorders. It has the following characteristics:

1. Test administrators have trouble agreeing on whether a response on the test is correct or not.
2. Clients seem to perform differently on the test each time they take it.
3. The test does not really focus on the aspects of communication that are relevant to treatment or diagnostic decision-making.
4. The test manual is vague about how to administer the instrument and how to interpret the results.
5. The test does not really examine the true process that you are attempting to assess.
6. The test was normed on 200 normal, white children from Idaho.

No serious student or professional would buy such an instrument because it would provide little valid and reliable information to use in assessment. Do tests in communication disorders ever have this many shortcomings? Unfortunately, *many* formal tests in our field suffer from the problems listed above and *more* (McCauley & Swisher, 1984a, 1984b; Muma, 1983, 1984, 1986; Muma, Lubinski, & Pierce, 1982)! Our point here is that if test developers clearly spelled out the psychometric inadequacies of some of the instruments they designed, consumers would never purchase them. This, however, is not likely to happen. The authors of these tests no doubt begin with the notion of designing a useful instrument; however, when conceptual and psychometric limitations manifest themselves, the test designers are typically reluctant to scrap the whole enterprise. The test is submitted, warts and all, to a publisher because even though it suffers from inadequacies, it represents a significant amount of work in its development. The publisher will not often point out inadequacies because it relies on authors to submit quality work. It is therefore up to the consumer to carefully evaluate any instrument in terms of psychometric adequacy before purchasing it. The main reasons for consumer awareness then are that (1) the test designers and publishers will not alert you to inadequacies, and (2) there are plenty of tests available that are simply worthless. We must become educated in evaluating any instruments that we buy, not only because purchasing an inadequate test is a waste of our money, but it is more importantly a waste of our time. It also affects our clients because they must spend money paying for the administration of these tests and also invest their time to take the tests. A client can be misdiagnosed, mislabeled, and mistreated on the basis of testing with psychometrically poor instruments. One can readily see that psychometric adequacy of standardized tests is a significant issue and one we must deal with in a textbook on diagnosis and evaluation.

It is important to note that it is not only standardized instruments that require some measure of psychometric adequacy. Although most authorities apply psychometric principles only to standardized, norm-referenced tests, it is the feeling of the present authors that most of the informal or descriptive measures that we use in communication disorders are also susceptible to considerable error. Just because we are not using a standardized test does not relieve us of the responsibility of checking the validity and reliability of the instruments we are using. The same psychometric rigor applied to standardized examinations could easily be applied to our informal evaluation procedures (Hegde, 1987). Informal measures can clearly vary in the degree to which they are valid and reliable. *Validity* is the degree to which a procedure actually measures what it purports to measure. Reliability typically refers to agreements of judges or the degree to which a person's behavior remains consistent over time. Validity can be compromised in both formal or informal procedures. For instance, we can ask a person with velopharyngeal incompetency to blow a pinwheel and time how long it spins to get an indication of velopharyngeal closure. This measure may have some reliability in that two clinicians could time the pinwheel with a stopwatch and agree on how long it spins. Perhaps the client could even be reliable in terms of blowing the wheel in a similar fashion over several trials and making the wheel spin a fairly consistent length of time each trial. The problem, however, is validity. We know that blowing a pinwheel may not at all relate to the ability to maintain velopharyngeal closure during speech production. Reliability is useless if the measure being taken is not valid.

There are many potential problems with reliability as well in the use of informal measures. For instance, many of the behaviors that we observe, count, or time are often not clearly defined and this contributes to a lack of reliability. In order to have good agreement, two examiners would have to be looking for the same behavior and coding it in a similar manner. The difficult aspect of informal assessment is that many behaviors are transient (phonemes, disfluencies, facial grimaces, laryngeal tension, slight head jerks, etc.), while others may be ill-defined and subjective (pitch changes, topic changes, cohesive adequacy, voice quality changes, stress alterations, intelligibility, severity, etc.). In research reports, it is incumbent on the investigator to provide evidence that behaviors studied are both valid and reliable. Clinicians must pay the same attention to these issues if they use informal measures so that these measures can be replicated over time as indications of treatment progress. Without validity and reliability, informal measures are nothing more than the "artsy," subjective judgments of one person that may tell us little about client performance.

COMMON TYPES OF TESTS

Most textbooks on psychometric issues focus on norm-referenced tests. *Norm-referenced tests* are also called standardized tests or formal tests, depending on the author's preference. Just because a test is standardized, however, does not mean that it is norm-referenced. *Standardization* can only imply that the procedures for test administration are standard while no norms may be provided with the instrument. In developing *norm-referenced tests,* the authors have designed some tasks they feel are relevant (valid) and have administered the instrument to large groups of subjects who they believe represent the population on whom the test is to be used. From these large-scale administrations, the designers are able to calculate normative data that reflect the performance of the large sample. When an individual is given the test, his/her score is compared to the performance of the normative sample, and it is determined how similarly this person performed relative to the large group. The purpose of norm-referenced tests is to determine if an individual obtains a score similar to the group average or, if not, how far away from the average the score is. If the individual scored within two standard deviations above or below the mean, he/she is said to reflect performance within "normal limits." If the score was more than two standard deviations above or below the mean, the performance is said to be exceptional, since only about 5 percent of the normative population scored in a similar manner. Thus, norm-referenced tests have the major purpose of determining if there is a problem, or if there is a significant enough difference from standard performance to warrant concern with regard to normalcy. We will have more to say in a later section regarding some qualifications that must be taken into account when considering this purpose of standardized tests.

The other type of test typically mentioned in psychometric texts is the *criterion-referenced instrument.* Salvia and Ysseldyke (1981, p. 30) describe such tests as follows:

> Rather than indicating a person's relative standing in skill development, criterion-referenced tests measure a person's development of particular skills in terms of absolute levels of mastery. . . . Items on criterion-referenced tests are often linked directly to specific instructional objectives and therefore facilitate the writing of objectives. Test items sample sequential skills, enabling a teacher not only to know the specific point at which to begin instruction but

also to plan those instructional aspects that follow directly in the curricular sequence.

The criterion-referenced test, then, serves a different purpose from a norm-referenced instrument. It attempts to define specific skills in assessment and treatment and emphasizes individual performance, while the norm-referenced tests focus on group similarity (Muma, 1973). There are precious few criterion-referenced measure in communication disorders. Most of our formal instruments are norm-referenced, so the focus of the rest of the chapter will be on these types of tests.

VALIDITY: THE FOUNDATION OF THE TEST OR MEASURE

As we mentioned before, a test can be reliable, but lack validity. Validity basically refers to the extent that a test measures what it sets out to measure. If we say we are going to measure a child's language comprehension, we try to select a test that can accomplish this goal. If the test is measuring something other than the child's language comprehension, then the test is invalid for our purpose. So many of the behaviors we assess in communication disorders are extremely complex and involve multiple systems. Language, for example, has many divisions (semantics, syntax, morphology, phonology, pragmatics), and it is influenced by other systems (cognitive, social, psychological, neurolinguistic, etc.). If we develop a test of "language ability" that can be administered and scored in 20 minutes and has the child imitate, name pictures, and point to photographs, we have not really looked at language ability completely. We have taken a few tasks and we are willing to make judgments about a very complex linguistic system based on the child's ability to perform these operations, which are non-communicative and only peripherally related to normal language use. This is tantamount to a cardiologist making clinical judgments about a significant heart condition only by feeling the patient's pulse. It just is not valid, especially when we have the technology available to do a thorough evaluation of heart function using EKG and other measures. The major point here is that without validity, we are fooling ourselves as we look at complex behaviors. Even if we can demonstrate that the items on the test are reliable, it does not matter. We have only developed a reliable way of looking at "garbage." This point is made painfully clear by several authors who raise ethical concerns regarding the administration of tests that lack validity (Messick, 1980; Muma, 1984). If we use such tests, we not only waste time and money but can arrive at erroneous judgments about our clients resulting in incorrect goal selection, or worse, placement in inappropriate programs.

Classically, three types of validity are discussed: construct, content, and criterion-related validity. *Construct validity* is "the degree to which a test measures the theoretical construct it is intended to measure" (Anastasi, 1976, p. 151). To obtain this type of validity, "the test author must rely on indirect evidence and inference" (Salvia & Ysseldyke, 1981, p. 108). Thus, a test in any area of communication disorders must ideally reflect the underlying construct it is attempting to assess.

The second type of validity, _content validity_, is derived by

> . . . a careful examination of the content of a test. Such an examination is judgmental in nature and requires a clear definition of what the content should be. Content validity is established by examining three factors: the appropriateness of the types of items included, the completeness of the item sample, and the way in which the items assess the content. (Salvia & Ysseldyke, 1981, p. 102)

Typically, expert judges are involved in examining the content of the test in order to make the determination of content validity.

A final type of validity is _criterion-related._ There are two types of criterion-related validity. First, _concurrent validity_ is a measure of how an individual's current score on one instrument can be used to make an estimate of his/her current score on some other criterion measure, typically another test in a related area. _Predictive validity_ is a measure of how an individual's current score on one instrument can estimate scoring on a criterion measure taken at a later time. A critical variable, however, is the validity and reliability of the criterion measure selected for use in criterion-related validity. The instrument you design must be valid and so must the criterion measure.

The three types of validity mentioned above would ideally be used in concert to determine the overall validity of a test instrument. There is, however, a tendency among some test designers to believe that only one or two types of validity are required to validate an instrument and perhaps the three types of validity are equally powerful and thus interchangeable. This is _not_ the case. The most potent type of validity is construct validity. Construct validity is viewed by most authorities as the _keystone_ of test development (Messick, 1975, 1980; Muma, 1985). We have separated this section on validity from the rest of the psychometric background in this chapter and discussed it first because it is probably the most important issue in psychometric adequacy. It does not matter how popular a test is, how easy it is to administer, or how much statistical hocus-pocus is found in the examiner's manual. If it lacks validity, it is nothing more than a wasteful, empty exercise.

RELIABILITY

The notion of reliability is critical to formal as well as informal measures. If one were to develop a valid norm-referenced test or informal measure, it would be useless if the test developer could not demonstrate that different examiners could use it with similar facility and that clients performed consistently from one occasion to another. Several types of reliability are classically discussed.

1. _Interjudge Reliability:_ This refers to the agreement of two independent judges on the occurrence and type of responses performed by a

client. Almost every clinician has had the experience of asking another speech-language pathologist to take a look at a difficult case. We question our abilities to judge aberrant vocal qualities and pitches. We often want another opinion on a child's intelligibility or pragmatic abilities. Stutterers often present many complex avoidances and timing devices that we ask our peers to scrutinize, just to make sure we are on the right track. Sometimes, even in standardized tests, we ask the opinions of others to check some arbitrary scoring convention we have used because the manual did not tell us what to do in enough detail. All of this has to do with interjudge reliability.

The types of responses we ask children and adults to make in diagnosis and evaluation tasks are many and varied. Some responses are relatively straightforward and easily agreed upon by two independent judges. For example, if we ask a client to point to one of four pictures in response to an auditory model (e.g., "Point to 'running'"), most judges would agree on the correctness of the client's response. Other types of responding may not be quite as clear to judges. For instance, judges may not be able to agree on the occurrence of a distorted /s/ or /r/ phoneme.

Judges may have difficulty determining if a response was correct if the client initially makes the wrong response and then self-corrects it. Does the test provide guidelines for examiners in terms of accepting a self-corrected response as "correct"? In informal tasks, it is often difficult for judges to agree on certain behaviors such as the amount of time spent in symbolic play. An adequate operational definition of symbolic play would be necessary and criteria for when such play begins and ends would be required if two judges are to agree on time sampling of behavior. Thus, we can see that the behaviors judges must agree upon vary in terms of their observability, definition, and subjectivity. If judges cannot agree on what they are observing, then the test or procedure is unreliable. There are some obvious contributing factors that decrease interjudge reliability:

a. *Incomplete or Ambiguous Definitions:*   If a behavior is to be counted, timed, observed, or interpreted, there must be an adequate definition of the behavior so that independent judges can agree on behavioral occurrences. For example, if one goal of treatment is to reduce behavior problems in a language-impaired, mentally retarded client, the measurement of this construct must be guided by a specified definition. Do behavior problems include only tantrums, or do actions such as pushing the materials away, whining, repetitive vocalizations, and refusal to participate in tasks also constitute behavior problems? One can readily see that two examiners could experience major disagreement on this measure unless the definition is quite precise. The two judges need to know what to count or time and what behaviors to exclude from the concept of behavior problems. Sometimes the operational definition selected by an examiner may not be universally agreed upon, and this may affect the *validity* of the measure. Even if the definition is somewhat incomplete, however, reliability can be increased by limiting the behaviors under scrutiny so everyone can agree when they occur. One of the present authors was once completing a study on misarticulation of the /s/ phoneme. The experimenters had difficulty agreeing on whether an /s/ distortion occurred in the school-age subjects. It turned out that one experimenter was counting /s/ distortions strictly by acoustic criteria (when it *sounded* distorted). The other experimenter was counting /s/ distortions when the sound was acoustically correct, but the child evidenced some slight tongue protrusion (*visual* distortion). When the experimenters agreed to count only the auditorily distorted productions, the agreement was much better. No matter if the measure is a formal, standardized test or an informal evaluation measure, interjudge reliability is critical to psychometric adequacy of the test. Formal tests should include data on interjudge reliability. Test manuals should include detailed definitions of the behaviors to be scored and as many guidelines as possible about potential response modes that may be difficult for the examiner to interpret as a correct or incorrect response. Some tests (Porch, 1967) have multidimensional scoring systems in which the client's response is not merely judged for correctness, but also for how the response occurred and levels of acceptability. If the scoring is complex enough, the test developer may even recommend taking a training course in test administration. This is routinely done in relation to tests of intelligence where there are many judgment calls to be made about client responses and some consistency in these decisions is required.

b. *Training:* For any procedure to be reliable, the judges need to receive similar training on how the observation, coding, and interpretation of the data are to be accomplished. Most researchers put reliability judges through training periods, sometimes lasting several hours, prior to actual computation of the reliability scores. It makes good sense that prior to using any procedure, a clinician will have adequate exposure to the methods and some practice using them.

c. *Practice:* Reliability is a function of practice. Both formal tests and informal evaluation measures require practice before they can be efficiently administered and scored. If one judge has much experience with a particular test or measurement and another judge has had none, lack of reliability can be expected. The more we perform procedures, the more systematic and consistent our decision-making becomes.

d. *Response Complexity:* Generally, the more complex the response, the greater the lack of reliability. If the system you are using to examine teacher-child interactions has a host of teacher and child variables, it will be more difficult to use than one with fewer aspects to examine. Another common example is the poor reliability associated with narrow phonetic transcription. The more molecular we become in what we do, the more difficult it is to obtain adequate reliability. In this age of writing generative phonologies from children's spontaneous samples, you can imagine how many specific disagreements could occur between two clinicians. First, there is error in just transcribing the sample. Second, there is error in detecting the specific errors within the transcript. Third, there is further error in trying to arrive at a list of phonological processes or idiosyncratic rules that account for the child's sample. Finally, there is error in determining the frequency or percent of occurrence of each rule derived from the sample. The result could be a catalogue of chaos. The more guidelines these clinicians have in making decisions, the better the reliability; also, the less complex the decisions, the better the reliability. This is why some authors have developed specific guidelines and definitions to use in phonological analyses (Ingram, 1981; Shriberg & Kwiatkowski, 1980).

e. *Live Scoring versus Tape Analysis:* Scoring behaviors "online" is always more difficult than being able to replay audio or videotapes for second and third opportunities to examine a behavior. Probably, videotape scoring would tend to be more reliable simply because it is difficult to accurately observe behaviors in rapid sequence and take the time to note their occurrence on an observation form (which further takes away from one's ability to observe).

MEASURING RELIABILITY

1. *Interjudge Reliability:* There are several ways to compute reliability. One method involves statistical procedures known as *reliability coefficients* or *correlation coefficients* (Hegde, 1987; Salvia & Ysseldyke, 1981). Typically, formal tests compute such correlations on judges' scores to determine whether the scores vary consistently (move up and down together). It is preferable for standardized tests to have interjudge reliability coefficients of 0.90 or above to show good agreement among examiners. For example, if Judge *A* scored a series of tests 89, 62, 53, 36 and Judge *B* scored the same tests 90, 60, 50, 35, there would be general agreement and a correlation of 0.99. The closer a coefficient of reliability is to 1.0, the more reliable the scoring. Some reliability coefficients take into account variance in the examiner's judgments (e.g., intraclass correlation; Winer's Coefficient of Reliability). Other test developers have used a simple correlation coefficient (e.g., Pearson Product Moment) that is far less effective in evaluating reliability (Bartko, 1976). In the previous example, the judges did not agree exactly on any of the test scores, but there was a general trend for the two judges' scores to go up and down together. There was also a tendency for the scores to be rather close (within three points of each other). This type of reliability may be acceptable for general responses, but if we want to gain insight into more specific behaviors, the correlation coefficient is too general a measure. For instance, if we wanted to count specific articulatory errors, it would be important to agree on the type of error produced. It also would be important for the judges to be counting the *same* errors. The following scenario is possible. A child is asked to produce 10 words for two judges who are going to count misarticulations. Both judges come up with five misarticulations. If the two judges made these kinds of responses over many subjects, they would appear to represent perfect agreement (1.0 in a correlation). Further analysis, however, reveals that Judge *A* found errors in the first five words and Judge *B* found errors in the last five words. In essence, they did not agree on *any* of the misarticulations, but they came up with the same total number. This example points out the importance of a

different type of reliability measure called *point by point* or *percent exact agreement.* In this type of reliability, a formula such as the following is used:

$$\frac{\text{Agreements}}{\text{Agreements} + \text{Disagreements}} \times 100.$$

Thus, one takes the total number of specific agreements and divides this number by the total number of agreements plus the disagreements and arrives at a percentage of exact agreement. In this way, we get a good idea of the behaviors judges rate in exactly the same way. Any clinician can compute such a simple formula and determine interjudge reliability for almost any clinically relevant behavior in a diagnostic or treatment context. It is good to check our perceptions every once in awhile to see if we are fooling ourselves with regard to the occurrence of client behaviors. This type of reliability is especially important in behaviors that lend themselves to error because of subjectivity. Unfortunately, this includes many of the relevant measures in communication disorders.

2. *Test-Retest Reliability:*   Some behaviors are highly stable over time. We would hope that most of the responses we assess to gain insight into various processes underlying communication are of this variety. If we are attempting to examine language comprehension, we assume that client performance on one day will be similar to that on another day. Vocal differences found one week would be observed the next week. If it were not for these behavioral consistencies, we would have difficulty justifying treatment. A person's voice is either disordered, or it is not. Clearly, there are behavioral fluctuations in some disorders (e.g., stuttering, voice problems that vary with fatigue, etc.), but in others one can expect a fairly consistent occurrence (e.g., articulation errors, language errors). Tests are supposed to be designed to probe a particular error in such a way as to show consistent problems with a client's communication. If an aphasic showed drastically different performances from week to week, it would be impossible to formulate a treatment program since the targets would always be changing. If a person's IQ were not relatively stable from week to week, it would be impossible to diagnose mental deficits. If a laboratory test for cancer varied from day to day in its diagnosis of your tissue samples, it would be unuseable. It is easy to see that test-retest reliability has much to do with the behavior being evaluated, and also with the test items chosen to reveal the skill you are testing. Reliability coefficients are also used to examine test-retest reliability and those close to 1.0 indicate stability in performance on a particular task. One could also use the point-by-point procedure to determine if the errors made on one day are similar to those made at a later time. It depends on how molecular the clinician wants to be in examining client performance.

3. *Split-Half Reliability:*   Many formal test developers want to evaluate the internal consistency of the items on their instrument. In essence, they want to determine if both halves of the test tend to be reliable or agree in terms of scores obtained.

SOME QUANTITATIVE BACKGROUND FOR TEST INTERPRETATION

There are some basic concepts in measurement that are necessary in order to appreciate most standardized tests. Many traditional quantitative aspects will not be covered, since they are rarely found on tests we use (e.g., mode, median, semiquartile range, types of curves, kurtosis, skewedness, etc.). Although we are omitting these measures, we are certainly not suggesting they are of diminished value. We simply want to discuss aspects that are useful for interpreting most tests in communication disorders. For more detailed accounts of these concepts, the reader is referred to other sources (Anastasi, 1976; Messick, 1980; Salvia & Ysseldyke, 1981).

CENTRAL TENDENCY, VARIANCE, AND THE NORMAL CURVE

Whenever someone takes a test, he/she earns one or more scores. Part of test interpretation involves placing the score(s) of an individual in the context of others who have also taken the test.

The most common measure of *central tendency* in formal tests is the mean or arithmetic average of the normative sample. This is computed simply by adding up all the scores of the standardization sample and dividing by the total number of scores. As a clinician, you will probably not have to compute many mean scores on clients you test. They will be given to you in the manuals for the formal tests that you use to examine differing age groups on a particular skill, and you will use this information as a reference point to compare the score of a specific child or adult you have tested. For example, if we have tested a four-year-old on a vocabulary test, we are interested in how his/her score compares to the normative sample of four-year-olds who took the same test as part of the standardization procedure. Some tests report data on other measures of central tendency (e.g., mode, median), but the most frequently reported scores are means, and they are perhaps the most meaningful to a clinician.

The other important score we must deal with in order to make sense of normative data is some measure of variability (variance) in the standardization sample. The *variance* is "a numerical index describing the dispersion of a set of scores around the mean of the distribution" (Salvia & Ysseldyke, 1981, p. 50). In computing the variance, the statistician first derives the amount by which each person's score deviates from the sample mean (e.g., if the score is 70 and the test mean is 60, the deviation is 10). After this is done for each subject in the sample, the deviation scores are all squared (multiplied by themselves). Then, these squared scores are added up and divided by the total number of subjects minus one. This results in the variance. One can easily see that we are essentially obtaining a very gross measure of the average amount of variation from the mean (squared) by computing the variance. The variance is not particularly meaningful in test interpretation, but its square root, the *standard deviation,* is used since it is a more interpretable measure of variation. Thus, if the variance is 25, the square root of this is 5, which is the standard deviation. This is more interpretable because it is in the same unit as the mean, instead of squared values as in the variance. If the mean on a test is 50 points and the standard deviation is 5 points, one can actually use these numbers together to gain a picture of variability. If we used a mean of 50 points and the variance of 25, we are no longer talking about the same types of numbers (points) since the variance is the average number of points of deviation squared.

In most cases, whenever researchers gather data on a particular skill from a large sample of people, the scores tend to form what statisticians call a *normal curve*. This means that there will be a tendency for most of the scores to fall around an average value, while some scores will be scattered toward very high and very low values. If researchers weighed a random sample of 2,000 adults between the ages of 20 and 40, they would probably find an average weight with most people clustered around this value and a much smaller number of people who were very fat or very thin and deviated markedly from this value. This is where means and standard deviations are helpful in describing the performance of a given population of subjects. Figure 3.1 shows a normal bell-shaped curve that could theoretically depict the performance of a sample of people on any variable. For our purposes, let us say that the curve represents scores on a vocabulary test. There are several important things to note. First, the line in the center of the normal curve at the score of 45 represents the mean performance or the average score in the distribution. Notice that it is the tallest line in the curve because it represents the largest number of people (9) who earned this score. The lines on either side of the mean are shorter and represent smaller numbers of subjects (8) who earned these scores (e.g., 40 and 50). The shorter lines indicate that fewer subjects earned the scores that are progressively higher or lower than the mean of 45. The two subjects scoring 10 and the two subjects scoring 80 are in the tails of the normal curve and are called "outliers."

If we said that the standard deviation for scores in Figure 3.1 was 10, we would mean that +1 standard deviation would be located at 55 and −1 standard deviation would be located at 35. Taking the example further, +2 standard deviations would be at the score of 65 and −2 standard deviations

Figure 3.1 Example of Normally Distributed Data

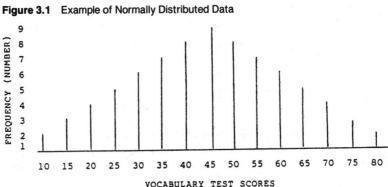

VOCABULARY TEST SCORES

would be at 25. Now look at the top panel of Figure 3.2 which depicts the percentage of cases under portions of the normal curve and the standard deviations at the bottom. We can see that about 68 percent of cases in the sample would probably score within −1 and +1 standard deviations from the mean. This means that on the vocabulary test, about 68 percent of the subjects would earn scores somewhat between 35 and 55. If we considered the cases scoring between −2 and +2 standard deviations, about 96 percent of the subjects would earn scores in the area between 25 and 65. Finally, if we looked at cases scoring between −3 and +3 standard deviations, around 99 percent of the cases would earn scores between 15 and 75. Thus, the use of means and standard deviations helps researchers and test developers to determine scoring patterns that are characteristic of the majority of a particular population.

It has often been stated in the assessment literature that scores falling at or below −1.5 to −2.0 standard deviations from the mean are thought to be abnormal enough to be clinically significant (Ludlow, 1983; McCauley & Swisher, 1984b). This, of course, indicates that the score in question was lower

Figure 3.2   Relationship of Various Types of Derived Scores to the Normal Curve

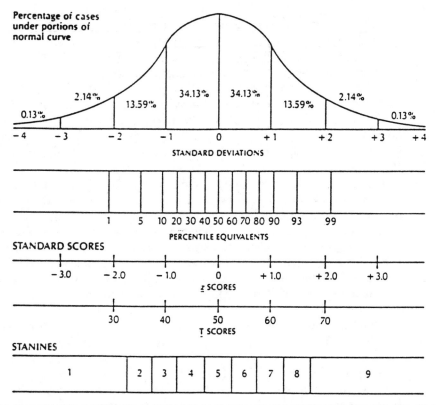

From: Carrow-Woolfolk, E. (1985) *Test for Auditory Comprehension-Revised*, DLM Teaching Resources, Allen, TX. used with permission.

than some 96 percent of the population included in the standardization sample. Thus, it should be clear that we use the means and standard deviations of the normative sample as a context for comparing an individual client's score on a standardized test. If the client's score falls below a particular standard deviation level (e.g., −2.0), we may decide to make a judgment about lack of normality in performance. This is why it is important to understand some basic facts about means and standard deviations. All distributions, however, are not normal. Some are skewed positively (many low scores) or negatively (many high scores), others have much variation (platykurtic) or very little variation (leptokurtic). It is significant to realize that most standardization samples tend to be normally distributed and this is important for the statistical analyses that are applied to them. There are many special problems in dealing with abnormally distributed data that are beyond the scope of the present text. It is enough if we are clear about normally distributed data and ways to describe these distributions.

Types of Scores Found on Formal Tests

There are several kinds of scores the diagnostician will encounter when dealing with standardized, norm-referenced tests. The first type of score is the *raw score*. The raw score is the actual number you arrive at when grading the client's test. Many times the raw score amounts to the number of correct responses that the client gave to the test items. So, if the test has 75 items on it and the client got 50 of them correct, the raw score might be 50. On some tests, the raw score is not simply the number correct, but some other number (e.g., maybe each test item is worth two points). At any rate, you score the test and arrive at some number that the test manual typically refers to as the raw score.

Most standardized, norm-referenced examinations include a manual to be used by the diagnostician in scoring and interpreting the test results. These test manuals typically contain a series of tables that are designed to convert raw scores into more interpretable numbers. Raw scores by themselves are not readily meaningful. For instance, the raw score of 50 out of 75 does not tell us anything about how our client's score compares to the performance of the normative sample. Perhaps this is normal performance for the client's age group and perhaps it is not. Thus, we must convert the client's raw score into a more meaningful type of number to allow comparison to the normative sample. Another reason to convert the raw scores to some other type of derived score is that one cannot compare the results of two different tests using raw scores. For instance, if a child obtains a raw score of 50 out of 75 on a vocabulary test and then earns a raw score of 125 out of 200 on a metalinguistics test, it would be difficult to compare these results. If, however, the raw scores were converted to some derived score, we can generally compare the performances on the two measures.

One type of converted score is called the *percentile rank*. Percentile ranks reflect the percentage of subjects or scores that fall at or below a particular raw score. For example, if a child scored in the 20th percentile, this means he/she scored as well or better than 20 percent of the children of the same age in the normative sample. Likewise, if a child were in the 90th percentile, the score was as good as or better than 90 percent of the children taking the test.

Another way to look at it is that only 10 percent of the normative population scored higher than a child who performed in the 90th percentile. If you look at Figure 3.2, you will see that percentile ranks are arranged under the normal curve. It can be seen that the 50th percentile rank basically represents the middle performance of the normative sample. A percentile rank of 10 is slightly more than −1 standard deviation below the mean. Remember from the prior discussion that some authorities view performance below −1.5 or −2.0 standard deviations to constitute clinical significance or abnormality. Some authorities suggest that consistent performance below the 10th percentile is cause for clinical concern (Lee, 1974) because this is between −1 and −2 standard deviations. One can see that conversion of the raw score into a percentile rank allows the clinician to put an individual client's performance into the context of the normative sample. It is meaningless to say the client got a raw score of 90, but it is much more valuable to be able to say a client scored in the 90th percentile.

Another way to derive more interpretable data from a client's raw score is to convert it into a _standard score._ There are a number of types of standard scores the diagnostician will encounter on formal tests; however, we will discuss only the two most common types, _z-scores_ and _T-scores._ Standard scores transform the raw scores into sets of scores that have the same mean and standard deviation. A z-score has a mean of 0 and a standard deviation of 1. One can see from Figure 3.2 that the z-scores are exactly equivalent to the standard deviations in the normal curve. Thus, a z-score of −1.0 is in the same place on the curve as a standard deviation of −1.0. A raw score can be converted to a z-score by subtracting the raw score from the mean of the normative sample and dividing the resulting number by the standard deviation of the normative sample. Test manuals typically include tables for the conversion of raw scores into z-scores so the clinician will not have to perform the mathematical operation him/herself. It is easy to see that when a client's raw score is converted to a z-score, it is much more interpretable. For instance, it is meaningless to say a client had a raw score of 59 on a test because that score cannot be related to the normative sample. If, however, the client has a z-score of −2.0, we can look at Figure 3.2 and see that this is equivalent to performing at −2.0 standard deviations, which is a clinically significant abnormality according to the criteria mentioned earlier.

Another standard score is the _T_-score. It operates in basically the same way as the z-score; however, the mean is 50 and the standard deviation is 10. Thus, a client with a _T_-score of 30 would be performing equivalent to −2.0 standard deviations.

A final type of standard score depicted in Figure 3.2 is the _stanine._ Tables for conversion of raw scores to stanines are not found as often in standardized tests. Salvia and Ysseldyke report that

> Stanines are standard score bands that divide a distribution into nine parts. The first stanine includes all scores that are 1.75 standard deviations or more below the mean, and the ninth stanine includes all scores 1.75 or more standard deviations above the mean. The second through eighth stanines are each .5 standard deviation in width and the fifth stanine ranging from .25 standard deviation below the mean to .25 standard deviation above the mean. (1981, p. 73)

It can be seen from this discussion that standardized, norm-referenced tests provide the diagnostician with a variety of possible scores to use in the interpretation of a particular client's performance. We must remember, however, that even though standard scores are useful to the diagnostician, they are valid only if the score distribution in the normative sample is normal. Percentiles do not require a distribution to be normal and can be computed on any distribution shape, thus they have fewer requirements than standard scores for accurate use and interpretation.

The Age and Grade Score Trap

Many formal tests include tables for converting raw scores into age-equivalent and/or grade-equivalent scores. Thus, a nine-year-old child who earns a raw score of 50 might be said to have an age-equivalent score of 7-5 (seven years, five months). A fourth-grader might earn a grade-equivalent score of 2-2 (second grade, second month). It is easy to be seduced into using these types of scores because they appear to relate to development. On the surface, these age and grade equivalents seem to place the child in a developmental context with peers who took the same test. It is tempting to say that the nine-year-old mentioned above is really at the seven-and-a-half-year-old level, or the fourth grader is performing at the second-grade level. All of these assumptions would be wrong. Most authorities who focus on psychometric interpretation indicate that age-equivalent and grade-equivalent scores are the *least* useful and *most dangerous* scores to be obtained from standardized tests because they lead to gross misinterpretations of client's performance (McCauley & Swisher, 1984b; Salvia & Ysseldyke, 1981). Basically, age-equivalent scores indicate that the client's raw score approximated the average performance for a particular age group. In the example above, the nine-year-old earned a raw score that was the average of the children in the seven-year-old group of the normative sample. A similar relationship holds for grade-equivalent scores.

There are several commonly discussed problems with age- and grade-equivalent scores. McCauley and Swisher discuss these problems:

> For most tests, as age increases, similar differences in age-equivalent scores are the result of smaller and smaller differences in raw scores. Therefore, an age-equivalent score that is 6 months behind an individual's chronological age may indicate a larger difference in actual test performance for younger test takers than for older ones. . . . The 1-year delay . . . reported for Paul, who is 4 years old, may have resulted from 12 missed items; whereas a 1-year delay for a 10-year-old child taking the test might be due to only one or two missed items. This causes the reliability of age-equivalent scores to be poorer for developmentally more advanced test takers. A second psychometric problem with age-equivalent scores is that they are not necessarily based directly on evidence collected for children of that chronological age. . . . Instead, a given age-equivalent score is often calculated indirectly either by interpolating between two ages for which data are available or by extrapolating from ages for which data are available to older or younger ages, for which data were not gathered. For example, Paul's raw score . . . probably fell between the average scores of the 3-year-olds and 4-year-olds in the normative sample, and he was assigned

the age-equivalent of 3-2 by interpolation although no children of age 3-2 were sampled in the normative studies. (1984b, p. 340)

Such psychometric problems lead to a number of misinterpretations of age-equivalent scores. First, as Salvia and Ysseldyke (1981) indicate, they lead to "typological thinking": "The average 12-0 child does not exist. The child is a composite of all 12-0 children. Average 12-0 children represent a range of performances" (p. 68).

A second misinterpretation is that laypeople and some professionals may believe that a nine-year-old child who earns an age-equivalent score of 7-0 is *performing like* a seven-year-old. This is probably not true. Although the nine-year-old may have earned the score obtained by the average seven-year-old, the test items that the client answered correctly and incorrectly may be totally different from the normative sample of seven-year-olds. As McCauley and Swisher (1984b, p. 341) state: "Similarly, a 60-year-old suffering from aphasia might receive an age-equivalent score of 10 years on the vocabulary test. It is unlikely, however, that such a client would make the same kind of errors as the 10-year-old or that he would exhibit similar communication skills."

A final danger in using age-equivalent scores is their use in attempting to define impairment in a client. The assumption is often made that a child exhibits a disorder if his/her age-equivalent score is lower than his/her chronological age (e.g., a four-year-old earning an age-equivalent score of 3-0). It is important to understand that these age-equivalent scores do not take into account the variation in performance expected in a particular age group. If a child performs below the average score for his/her age group, it may be within the range of normal variation for that group and not an indicator of impairment at all. McCauley and Swisher provide a graphic example shown in Figure 3.3.

> Paul—and all of those 4-year-olds whose scores fall in the shaded area of the curve—would be said to have received an age-equivalent score of 3 years or less. However, when the variability shown by the 4-year-olds as a group is taken into account using z scores, the same score may not be found to be sufficiently different from the average obtained by this group to suggest impairment. Certainly, if a z score better than −2.0 were considered within the normal range, almost all of the scores falling in the shaded area on the figure would be considered normal, despite their correspondence to age-equivalent delays of up to a year or more. Thus, age-equivalent delays do not necessarily indicate delay or impairment. (1984b, p. 341)

It is almost universally agreed, then, that the least useful and most perilous types of scores are the age-equivalent or grade-equivalent scores. They tend to distort a client's performance and lead to misinterpretations by laypeople and professionals alike. Most authorities advocate the use of percentile ranks and standard scores for test interpretation since they do not suffer from the problems mentioned in relation to developmental scores. Perhaps the percentile rank is the easier of the scores to use in communicating with parents and spouses because most people can readily understand this concept. Clinicians who are consumers of formal, standardized, norm-referenced tests would be

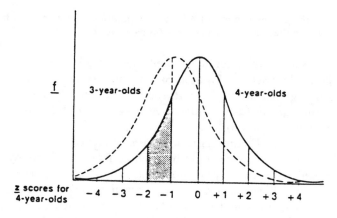

From McCauley, R. and Swisher, L. (1984). Use and Misuse of Norm-Referenced Tests in Clinical Assessment: A Hypothetical Case. *Journal of Speech and Hearing Disorders*, 49, 338–348. Used with permission.

Figure 3.3 Hypothetical Distributions of Scores Received by Two Groups of Children. The Shaded Area of the Distribution for 4-Year-Olds Includes Scores That Would Yield Age-Equivalent Scores of 3 Years or Less but z Scores of − 2 or Better.

wise to refuse to purchase examinations that offer only age-equivalent scores and omit standard scores and percentile ranks.

Standard Error of Measurement and Confidence Intervals

Two final concepts that we will deal with regarding standardized tests are the notions of *standard error of measurement* and *confidence intervals*. When used with the concepts previously discussed (mean, standard deviation, standard scores), these measurements give the diagnostician some very powerful quantitative tools to use in evaluating test performance.

Even though a standardized test may be developed very carefully, a client's responses to test items may not really reflect the underlying ability the examination is attempting to tap. Statisticians realize that *any* measure is susceptible to error. Error is ubiquitous—it is in everything we measure, and especially in evaluating human performance. Thus, we know that no test is perfectly reliable (1.0) and that some distortion is present in any measurement device. Some statisticians use the terms *observed score* and *true score* to refer to the actual raw score the test taker earns and the "ideal" score the person would have earned if there were no error in the measuring instrument. The true score, then, does not really exist; it is only hypothesized. We would ideally like the observed score to be highly similar to the true score, and this is the case in using tests that have high reliability. As the reliability of a test decreases, the disparity between true and observed scores increases. A statistic called the standard error of measurement (SEM) has been developed to increase our precision in determining whether the observed score of a client is reasonably close to his/her possible true score.

Although the SEM and associated confidence intervals can be calculated from one of several statistical formulas, many tests provide tables from which to arrive at this information. Basically, the calculation of SEM involves three things (McCauley & Swisher, 1984b, p. 339): "(a) an estimate of the test's reliability, (b) the mean and standard deviation of scores obtained by the normative sample to which the test taker's score is to be compared, and (c) the test taker's observed score." We should be able to look up the SEM in a test manual and find a table that indicates the confidence intervals around the client's true score for at least a 95 percent level of confidence. Thus, if a subject had an observed score of 50 on a test and we calculated the true score and it was 53, there would be a pretty good correspondence between the observed and true scores. If we look up the 95 percent confidence interval in a table included in the test manual, we might find that the confidence interval is 5. Next, we subtract 5 from the subject's true score and arrive at 48 and add 5 to the true score and get 58. Thus, we have a range from 48 to 58 with the subject's true score in the middle. We can have confidence that the subject's true score would fall in this range 95 times out of 100 test administrations. McCauley and Swisher (1984b, p. 340) point out the importance of using confidence intervals, especially when attempting to determine cutoff points for abnormality. Figure 3.4 shows a normal curve with an observed and true score for a particular subject expressed in z-scores. If one were to use the traditional cutoff of −2.0 standard deviations as an indication of abnormality, the observed score would clearly fall below this point and the client would be considered impaired. The 95 percent confidence interval, however, straddles the −2.0

Figure 3.4   A Normal Probability Curve Showing the 95% Confidence Interval and Estimated True Score (•) for an Observed Score (○)

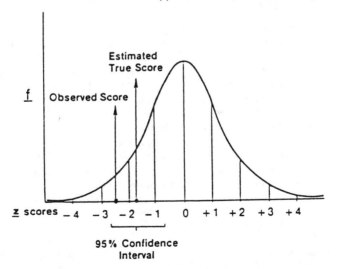

From McCauley, R. and Swisher, L. (1984). Use and Misuse of Norm-Referenced Tests in Clinical Assessment: A Hypothetical Case. *Journal of Speech and Hearing Disorders*, 49, 338–348. Used with permission.

standard deviation cutoff. We see that the client's observed score is below the cutoff and the calculated true score is above the cutoff. If this were the case in making a clinical decision, it would be difficult to say that the client is exhibiting impairment just because of the observed score. There is enough error in the test to suggest that the client's true score might be above the cutoff and this suggests normal performance. Only in a case where the true score and its associated confidence interval do not overlap an arbitrary cutoff would this type of decision be clear. This problem becomes especially important in cases where psychometrists are attempting to determine if a child is mentally retarded. If an IQ below 70 is indicative of mental retardation, it would be important for the client's true score *and* confidence interval to be well below 70 to make a judgment. If the confidence interval overlaps the cutoff, it is possible that the true score could lie in the area above the cutoff even though the observed score is below it. Important decisions should not be dealt with lightly and clients should be given the benefit of the doubt, especially where program placements are concerned.

CRITERIA FOR EVALUATING STANDARDIZED TESTS

We would be remiss if we did not report the most common considerations in evaluating formal tests. These criteria have been reported by many authors but basically flow from the *Standards for Educational and Psychological Tests* compiled by the American Psychological Association in 1974. We will paraphrase these considerations here, but the reader should know that the actual standards go into much more detail. The criteria should be used by a consumer of formal tests in communication disorders to make principled decisions about selection and purchasing of instruments.

1. The test should be accompanied by a comprehensive manual that provides detailed information on (a) the rationale behind the test, (b) the development of the test, (c) the specific purposes for which the test is to be used and not used, (d) the qualifications of the test administrator, and (e) specific instructions for administering, scoring, and interpreting the test.
2. The test manual should also provide information on construct, content, and criterion-related validity. The emphasis should be on construct validity, and reporting of the other types without this one is unacceptable.
3. The test manual should include a section that reports interjudge, test-retest, and internal consistency (split-half) types of reliability.
4. Descriptive statistics including means and standard deviations for all groups studied in the normative sample should be included along with tables to use in converting raw scores into standard scores and percentile ranks. Information on the standard error of measurement and computation of confidence intervals should also be included.
5. The sizes of the normative sample should be reported. Most authorities suggest that if the test has subgroups, the number of subjects in each group should not be less than 100.
6. The normative sample should be fully described in terms of race, socioeconomic level, geographic residence, and normality on relevant variables (e.g.,

IQ, hearing, medical). If any subjects are included in the sample to represent disordered groups, these individuals should be described in detail in terms of relevant variables.

We could go into much detail on any of the above points or subpoints, but it should be clear that selection of a standardized, norm-referenced test should not be just an arbitrary decision on the part of a diagnostician. Every month we are inundated with flyers and catalogues attempting to sell tests. The choice of whether to purchase one of these instruments is significant in terms of cost and more importantly in terms of serving our clients well. Try to examine these tests at conferences and conventions, read reviews in professional journals, and/or examine the *Buros Mental Measurements Yearbook* (Conoley & Kramer, 1989) for critical reviews. The test brochures and catalogues never tell us enough to make an accurate judgment. If possible, order a test "on approval" and pay for it only if you are satisfied with its psychometric adequacy and what it will actually tell you about a client. Most reputable publishers allow a customer to return an instrument that he/she would not use.

COMMON ERRORS IN THE USE OF NORM-REFERENCED TESTS

With very few exceptions, norm-referenced tests are designed to help the clinician determine if a client is performing within normal limits on a particular behavior. We compare an individual's score to the normative data and decide if our client is impaired or not. Muma (1973) has said that the purpose of formal tests is to solve the "problem–no problem" issue. Often, the clinician could do this just by observation alone, but many institutions (e.g., school systems) may require some formal test score to include in a client's record instead of relying solely on clinical judgment. Public Law 94-142 requires that more than one standardized test be used in assessment. At any rate, solving the problem–no problem issue is a rather narrow payoff for taking the time to administer and score a standardized test. As a result, some clinicians try to make more of the test results than they should. Formal tests are designed to go only so far, and if we make other judgments about our clients based on these data, we are violating the assumptions of the tests. Following are some of the common ways that clinicians misuse standardized tests:

1. *Measuring Treatment Progress with Norm-Referenced Tests:* We mentioned earlier that the purpose of norm-referenced tests is to determine if a client is performing similarly to a large standardization sample. The tests were not designed for the purpose of measuring progress in treatment. If the clinician administers a formal test at the beginning of treatment and readministers the test (or even an alternate form of the test) after a period of treatment, the resulting scores can lead to gross misinterpretations. First of all, the formal test samples a broad range of behaviors and may sample the behavior trained in therapy in only a few trials. Thus, much of the time spent in test administration

would be devoted to assessing behavior that is unrelated to therapy. It would be much more logical to examine the trained behavior in detail using an informal format that focused more fully on the particular behavior of interest. Second, a subject who scores abnormally low on an initial administration of an instrument will tend to score higher on a subsequent administration of the same test. This is a well-known phenomenon called *statistical regression,* which states that subjects earning extreme scores (either high or low) will tend to regress toward the mean of the sample population on subsequent administrations. Thus, a client may receive a higher score, not because of treatment effects but due to statistical regression. Third, clinicians may unconsciously "teach to the test" and prepare the client to do well on a second administration by practicing items in a format similar to the formal test. Fourth, all tests include elements of unreliability. It could very well be that an increase in an overall score on a formal test is simply the result of chance. We urge clinicians not to use standardized, norm-referenced tests as measures of progress. Criterion-referenced tests and informal probe tasks are the best way to gauge treatment progress.

2. *Analyzing Individual Test Items for Treatment Target Selection:* After administering a norm-referenced test, it is always tempting to examine the client's responses to particular test items and try to determine some kind of pattern of impairment. For example, on a receptive vocabulary test one might find that particular prepositions are in error. A natural tendency would be to include the understanding of prepositions in a treatment program based on the analysis of the formal test performance. There are several problems with this. First, clients cannot be expected to take tests that are of an inordinate length. As a result, a formal test must be relatively brief in order to be practical. On the other hand, most formal tests are broadly based in that they cover a number of areas (e.g., syntax, morphology, vocabulary) or one area that has several facets to it (e.g., assessment of all relevant bound morphemes). This creates a dilemma for the person developing a test instrument. In order to cover all of the areas of interest, or even all aspects of one area, the test developer must be very selective in deciding how many items to include and how many times a particular behavior will be sampled. In assessing bound morphemes, for instance, the test developer must determine how many times each morpheme of interest will be sampled and in what contexts. Often, a particular form will be sampled only two or three times in order to make the length of the test manageable. Herein lies the trade-off: Making a test of reasonable length necessitates the use of small samples of each behavior of interest. Thus, it would be difficult to make a judgment about a particular grammatical morpheme (e.g., plurals) based on only two or three occurrences. This is especially true when client responses on formal tests can be due to a variety of reasons. As much as test developers would like to believe that an incorrect response indicates lack of ability on a particular item or that a correct response suggests mastery of an item, it is well known that test takers are human. Clients make lucky guesses, are distracted during test administration, do not fully understand instructions, and experience a variety

of internal states (fatigue, boredom, pains, urges to go to the bathroom, etc.) that could affect test performance. Be wary of selecting treatment objectives from any norm-referenced test.

3. *Forgetting That Formal Tests Almost Always Distort What They Are Designed to Examine:*   Almost every construct one might desire to measure in communication disorders is highly complex. Whenever we deal with human behavior and try to translate a complex activity into a single score, there is a considerable amount of information lost in the process. Is it valid to say the child's vocabulary is a 74 because he/she earned this score on a test? Does this tell us how many words are in the lexicon, or are understood? Does it tell us how words are retrieved? Does it tell us if the child's internal definition of the word is equivalent to an adult's? Do we know how the word is used for communication? Do we know how the word will be used in sentences or written language? We could continue to ask questions about how deeply we have examined the child's vocabulary by obtaining a formal test score, but you probably have the idea by now that such a score is quite superficial. Standardized tests have a number of ways they tend to distort constructs we wish to examine. First, almost all tests that are standardized imply a circumscribed method of administration. The testing must be done in a particular setting, specific instructions must be given, and items must be administered in a particular order. Also, the client's responses must be graded as pass or fail, based on the criteria set forth by the test developer (some tests do not classify client responses as pass/fail, but these are few in number). The vast majority of formal test scenarios involve a highly artificial, regimented way of assessing performance.

A second source of distortion is that most of the tests designed to assess communication rarely examine *real* communicative efforts. The interactions are typically artificial. The client has no real communicative intent, communications are often about trivial topics (e.g., telling the examiner what is going on in a picture while both client and clinician look at it), and the topic of each task is constantly changing as the clinician flips the test plates. Thus, we must *always* remember that we have not examined real communication until we have analyzed the client's communication in a natural situation.

A third source of distortion is the fragmentation of integrated systems often seen in formal testing. As Muma (1973) points out, many systems interact with one another in communication and to single out a particular area to analyze is in many cases ludicrous. For instance, how can one separate semantics from cognition, syntax from semantics, syntax from morphology, phonology from syntax, motor speech skills from language, intonation from meaning, or structural language from pragmatics? Even though this can be done on the formal test level, it certainly cannot be done on a construct validity level. We cannot evaluate a system or subsystem independent of the context in which it typically operates. If we do, we have not really evaluated the system of interest. Always be aware that when we use an artificial task from a formal test, we are a dimension or more away from looking at the reality of communication.

CONCLUSION

Some students and clinicians feel frustrated when confronted with the type of information presented in this chapter. This is especially true if the person has emphasized formal tests in his/her approach to diagnosis and evaluation. People also may feel a bit guilty if they have misused norm-referenced tests or have used instruments and techniques uncritically without ensuring their validity and reliability. These practices, unfortunately, are probably the rule rather than the exception. Other people might feel lost if all of their traditional tools are suddenly taken away from them and they ask, "What are we supposed to do without our tests?" There is no simple answer. One obvious response would be that we can still use tests for the purposes they are intended to serve, but we need to tighten up our criteria for test selection, use, and interpretation. The other response would be that we need to develop and use more informal methods for diagnosis and evaluation that will give us insight into the nature of a client's problem and the means for treating it. In many areas of communication disorders, we are beyond the basic question of the problem–no problem issue. We need ways to describe client performance and gain insight into individual differences, dynamism, ecological relevance, processes, and patterns of behavior (Bates, Bretherton, & Snyder, 1988; Bronfenbrenner, 1979; Chafe, 1970; Donaldson, 1978; Muma, 1978, 1981, 1983, 1984). The field of communication disorders is moving more toward descriptive and criterion-referenced measures rather than norm-referenced tests. This, however, does not absolve each of us from the ultimate responsibility of incorporating sound scientific principles into our measurements. An informal probe or task used to describe client behavior is just as susceptible to psychometric and examiner error as a norm-referenced test. Students, professors, and working clinicians need to adhere to high standards of measurement and refuse to use inadequate test instruments or descriptive procedures that cannot be effectively replicated.

BIBLIOGRAPHY

American Psychological Association, American Educational Research Association, & National Council on Measurement in Education, *Standards for Educational and Psychological Tests,* Washington, D.C.: American Psychological Assn.

ANASTASI, A. (1976). *Psychological testing.* New York: Macmillan.

BARTKO, J. (1976). On various intraclass correlation reliability coefficients. *Psychological Bulletin, 83* (5), 762–765.

BATES, E., BRETHERTON, I. & SNYDER, L. (1988). *From first words to grammar.* Cambridge, MA: Cambridge University Press.

BRONFENBRENNER, U. (1979). *The ecology of human development.* Cambridge, MA: Harvard University Press.

CHAFE, W. (1970). *Meaning and the structure of language.* Chicago: University of Chicago Press.

CONOLEY, J., & KRAMER, J. (1989). *The tenth mental measurements yearbook.* Lincoln, NE: University of Nebraska Press.

DONALDSON, M. (1978). *Children's minds.* London: Fontana.

HEGDE, M. (1987). *Clinical research in communication disorders.* Boston, MA: Little Brown.

INGRAM, D. (1981). *Procedures for the phonological analysis of children's language.* Baltimore: University Park Press.

LEE, L. (1974). *Developmental sentence analysis.* Evanston, IL: Northwestern University Press.

LUDLOW, C. (1983). Identification and assessment of aphasic patients for language intervention. In

J. Miller, D. Yoder, & R. Schiefelbusch (Eds.), *Contemporary issues in language intervention*. Rockville, MD: American Speech-Language-Hearing Association.

McCAULEY, R., & SWISHER, L. (1984a). Psychometric review of language and articulation tests for preschool children. *Journal of Speech and Hearing Disorders, 49,* 39–42.

McCAULEY, R., & SWISHER, L. (1984b). Use and misuse of norm-referenced tests in clinical assessment: A hypothetical case. *Journal of Speech and Hearing Disorders, 49,* 338–348.

MESSICK, S. (1975). The standard problem: Meaning and values in measurement and evaluation. *American Psychologist, 30,* 955–966.

MESSICK, S. (1980). Test validity and the ethics of assessment. *American Psychologist, 35,* 1012–1027.

MUMA, J. (1973). Language assessment: Some underlying assumptions. *Journal of the American Speech and Hearing Association, 15,* 331–338.

MUMA, J. (1978). *Language handbook: Concepts, assessment, intervention.* Englewood Cliffs, NJ: Prentice Hall.

MUMA, J. (1981). *Language primer.* Lubbock, TX: Natural Child Publisher.

MUMA, J. (1983). *Language assessment: How valid is the process?* Double miniseminar presented at the annual convention of the American Speech-Language-Hearing Association, Cincinnati, OH.

MUMA, J. (1984). Semel and Wiig's CELF: Construct validity? *Journal of Speech and Hearing Disorders, 49,* 101–104.

MUMA, J. (1985). No news is bad news: A response to McCauley and Swisher. *Journal of Speech and Hearing Disorders, 50,* 290–293.

MUMA, J. (1986). *Language acquisition: A functionalistic perspective.* Austin, TX: Pro-Ed.

MUMA, J., LUBINSKI, R., & PIERCE, S. (1982). A new era in language assessment: Data or evidence. In N. Lass (Ed.), *Speech and language* (Vol. 7). New York: Academic Press.

PORCH, B. (1967). *Porch Index of Communicative Ability.* Palo Alto, CA: Consulting Psychologists Press.

SALVIA, J., & YSSELDYKE, J. (1981). *Assessment in special and remedial education.* Boston, MA: Houghton Mifflin.

SHRIBERG, L., & KWIATKOWSKI, J. (1980). *Natural process analysis.* New York: John Wiley.

chapter

4

ASSESSMENT OF CHILDREN WITH LIMITED LANGUAGE

In this textbook, we will divide the language-disordered population into two groups, based on presenting linguistic development level. One group is children with limited language (nonverbal, single word, early multiword). The other group is comprised of syntax-level clients whose problems are largely grammatical and/or pragmatic. This is similar to an approach to assessment that was suggested by McLean and Snyder-McLean (1978), in which they recommended certain evaluation areas based on the child's utterance length. Carrow-Woolfolk and Lynch (1982) also recommended determining a child's mean length of utterance (MLU) and then suggested specific analysis procedures. Table 4.1 describes three types of children with limited language and the assessment areas associated with each type. Note that we have not divided our assessment approaches specifically by age groups—a client with limited language can be from any age group; there are even nonverbal teenagers and adults. Thus, we focus on the communicative level and not the chronological age of our client. Since most of these clients are children, however, we will refer to them as such in this chapter.

First, there are children who are largely nonverbal. They use vocalizations and perhaps gestures, but their caretakers report no real use of language to control their environment. Obviously, in dealing with a nonverbal child, a "test of language ability" would be too advanced. Faced with the virtual elimination of an entire shelf of standardized tests, the clinician must focus on more informal assessment procedures. There will be no lengthy transcripts here, just assessments of more primal things like cognitive skills, caretaker-child interaction, adaptive behavior, social development, phonetically consistent forms, phonetic inventory, and other things not found in most formal test batteries.

Table 4.1   Summary of Assessment Areas for Early Communicators

Evaluation of Nonverbal Communicators

1. General developmental test/Adaptive behavior scale
2. Specific language test to focus on communication
3. Biological prerequisites (audiometry, neurological, medical)
4. Case history—preevaluation questionnaire, interview
5. Caretaker-child interaction evaluation—sample
6. Communicative intent inventory (types, frequency, level)
7. Phonetically consistent form analysis (phonetic inventory/syllable shape)
8. Cognitive analysis—play analysis, screening tasks, formal scales
9. Lexical comprehension—parent report and/or tasks to get lexicon size

Evaluation of Single-Word Communicators

1. Biological prerequisites
2. Case history
3. Caretaker-child interaction analysis
4. General developmental test/Adaptive behavior scale
5. Specific language test to focus on communication
6. MLU from spontaneous sample
7. Communicative intent inventory (types, frequency, level)
8. Form/Function analysis of single words
9. Analysis of presyntactic devices
10. Lexical production—parent report and sample to determine lexicon size
11. Lexical comprehension—parent report and tasks
12. Phonetic inventory and phonological process analysis from sample

Evaluation of Early Multiword Communicators

1. Biological prerequisites
2. Case history
3. Caretaker-child interaction analysis
4. General developmental test/Adaptive behavior scale
5. Specific language test to focus on communication
6. MLU from spontaneous sample
7. Form/Function analysis of semantic relations
8. Phonetic inventory and phonological process analysis from sample
9. Comprehension analysis of simple commands

A second group of children is made up of those who speak largely at the single-word level. The single-word stage has been reported in the developmental literature (Nelson, 1973), and according to some authorities, the child may accrue a lexicon of about 50 words before starting the use of word combinations for generative language. Clearly, the assessment of a single-word child is different from that of a nonverbal one. We can look at the structure of the lexicon and we can search for some evidence of a transition into multiwords by watching for presyntactic devices (PSD) as reported by Dore et al. (1976). The clinician should also determine the functions behind these early single-word utterances by interpreting the verbalizations in light of contextual and gestural cues (Dore, 1975; Halliday, 1975). Other areas listed in Table 4.1 may also be evaluation targets.

A third type of child is one who is using early multiword combinations. For this type of child, it is clear that some basic cognitive capacity for using a symbol system exists. It becomes more important with an early multiword child to focus on the types of word combinations used and the functions for which the child uses the utterances. The phonetic inventory and phonological process analysis also become important for this type of case, because a child's language can only be functional if it is intelligible to listeners. Thus, for the child using early multiword utterances, we must examine the language, but not necessarily in the same way as we would a sample of a child who has a longer length of utterance.

There are then at least three categories into which we can place children with limited language. Within the categories are different assessment targets, many of which cannot be evaluated using formal test instruments. The clinician's first step is to determine the most common language behaviors and decide in which category to place the client. The next step involves considering the high-probability diagnostic areas associated with the category. Finally, the clinician can use some of the specific procedures referred to later in this chapter that will allow evaluation of the appropriate areas.

Although we have characterized language-disordered children by their general linguistic development level, some students may be tempted to describe language-impaired children by etiology (e.g., mental retardation, hearing-impairment). We agree with those who suggest that classification of language disorder by etiology does not relate productively to assessment (Aram & Nation, 1975; Bloom & Lahey, 1978; Newhoff & Leonard, 1983). The various etiological groups are highly heterogeneous, and referring to a child as "mentally retarded" means little in terms of predicting what the child might be like. Also, the language disorders manifested by these various groups may not be significantly different. Therefore, the language samples gathered from children who are hearing-impaired, mentally retarded, learning-disabled, autistic, or language-delayed with normal intelligence may be highly similar. In essence, there does not appear to be a "language of the mentally retarded" that is critically different from the language produced by members of many other causation groups. Diagnostic grouping, then, does not necessarily provide the clinician with valid guidelines for assessment of language skills.

WHAT MAKES LANGUAGE ASSESSMENT DIFFICULT?

Language assessment in children is one of the most difficult and challenging tasks faced by the speech-language pathologist, and many clinicians are insecure about their diagnostic ability in this area. One complicating factor for the diagnostician is the previously mentioned heterogeniety of the language-disordered population (Aram & Nation, 1975; Wolfus, Moscovitch, & Kinsbourne, 1980).

A second variable that makes diagnosis difficult is the difference in the degree of severity found in the language-impaired population. The children range from those who are nonverbal and lack social and cognitive bases for language to youngsters who inconsistently omit or misuse grammatical morphemes. Thus, for each evaluation, the clinician must be prepared to assess the broad representation of linguistic and prelinguistic behaviors.

A third variable is the complex nature of language itself. Most introductory courses discuss language as being comprised of various domains. In fact, many textbooks are organized in terms of language areas such as semantics, syntax, morphology, phonology, and more recently, pragmatics. Complicating the problem further is the fact that authorities in the area of linguistics are not in total agreement regarding certain aspects of these domains of language.

In addition, there is the proliferation of assessment devices and procedures available on the market. We are inundated with flyers and catalogues, many reputing to offer "the best language assessment device." How does one select a test? Is one test really enough? The fact that people have designed tests of language for children, oftentimes with very inclusive titles, suggests that it is possible to find out all one needs to know from a single test. Unfortunately, the disclaimers that some authors place in their test manuals regarding the shortcomings of the instruments are forgotten and the perhaps overly ambitious title remains in the mind of clinicians and parents. Also, tests are based on different theoretical points of view or models. The differing theoretical underpinnings result in dramatically different types of tasks and areas of emphasis on tests. The plethora of tests, then, is a source of confusion to many clinicians.

It is also difficult to know what to do in language assessment because language development and disorders encompass so much more than just linguistic ability. In the literature on language acquisition, for instance, one routinely reads about cognitive development, neurolinguistics, linguistic theory, adaptive behavior, play development, social development, self-help skills, phonology, motor ability, caretaker-child interaction, and other areas that may not appear to be directly related to linguistic symbols but are critical to language development. Because language itself has many domains (semantics, syntax, phonology, morphology, pragmatics, etc.) and the related areas are numerous, language assessment may take on quite different guises, depending on the focus of the evaluation. This is clearly a source of confusion for clinicians and requires a very broad base of skill and knowledge.

These difficulties probably contribute to many clinicians' uncertainties in the area of language assessment. Models, as we indicate in the following section, are sometimes helpful in reducing the difficulties in understanding an area and assisting diagnosticians in developing workable clinical procedures.

COMPONENTS TO CONSIDER IN LANGUAGE ASSESSMENT

If we were to travel around the country and eavesdrop as speech-language pathologists evaluate children, we would find a confusing conglomeration of activities being performed under the aegis of linguistic assessment:

A clinician has a child repeat sentences.
A child plays silently while the clinician takes notes.
A child is trying to obtain a toy and the clinician resists.
A clinician is having a child point to one of three pictures.

A clinician is giving instructions telling a child to act out a scene with dolls.

A child is trying to get a piece of candy with a string tied around it by pulling the string. The clinician is scribbling on a clipboard.

A clinician is watching a child and the parents play.

A clinician is pushing a car back and forth with a child and suddenly pushes a horse on wheels back to the child instead of the car.

A child is trying to complete open-ended sentences presented by the clinician.

A child is describing pictures for a clinician behind a cardboard barrier.

What does it all mean? Are all these clinicians really performing language assessments? How does a clinician know which thing to do with a particular child? If one thing is clear today, it is that language assessment requires more varied skills and diversity of educational background on the part of the clinician than ever before.

When one contemplates language assessment or acquisition in the 1990s, it is not enough to consider structural components (semantics, syntax, etc.) alone. Conceptions of language have changed considerably since the 1950s when in some quarters the syntactic component was the primary emphasis (Chomsky, 1957). Behavioristic thought in the 1950s and 1960s viewed language as just another behavior. Also, in the 1960s Osgood's model of language was applied in a "specific abilities" orientation (Bloom & Lahey, 1978). Tests and language training programs were developed that emphasized specific psycholinguistic abilities such as auditory memory span and auditory sequencing. Thus, language has traditionally been fractionalized in one way or another since investigators first began to theorize about it. One can see this isolation of components reflected in society as a whole with the specialization of workers after the Industrial Revolution, the rise of medical specialties, and the institution of particular designations in the behavioral sciences (Toffler, 1981). The decade of the 1970s, however, brought with it a larger view. In society as a whole, the emphasis on ecology was in full flower and people began to talk about the reciprocal influence of different components formerly thought to be isolated. We began to consider the far-reaching effects of a single act toward one element in the ecology on the entire ecosystem. A movement toward holistic medicine was observed and an inter/multidisciplinary staffs treating exceptional children attempted to view "the whole child." After years of fractionalizing the world (and language along with it) into "little boxes," we began to put it together again.

It is not realistic to assess or train only isolated components of the total communicative process. An analogy to fragmenting the communicative process is conceptualizing an automobile as individual parts and systems. One can assess the fuel system of a car, but from that evaluation the functioning of the car will not be known until it is driven in real conditions. So, when someone begins to think of language as just linguistic elements, some very important aspects of the process are being ignored. Language does not exist in a vacuum. It occurs when humans who possess a reasonable amount of symbolic ability (intelligence) use a communication system in a social environment. In the late 1970s, the language area called *pragmatics* received renewed emphasis. The focus on pragmatics has had far-reaching implications for assessment and treatment of both child and adult language disorders. It has also influenced the study of child language acquisition. Although pragmatics is "an area" of language, it really permeates all of the other areas of linguistics; and the present authors view it as somewhat of a unifying force. Pragmatics deals with the use of language in context and all of the changes in the structure of an utterance in response to differing communicative situations.

Most current conceptualizations of language are more integrative than linguistic models of the past three decades. By *integrative,* we mean that language depends on biological, cognitive, and social variables that are both prerequisite to communication and significant determinants of how linguistic structures are used in day-to-day situations (Bloom & Lahey, 1978; Carrow-Woolfolk & Lynch, 1982; Hubbell, 1981; McLean & Snyder-McLean, 1978; Muma, 1978). The present chapter will also take this integrative point of view because it helps to make language acquisition and assessment more understandable.

The clinician engaged in a language evaluation must have some framework upon which to gather and organize the data. For years, authorities have been *model building.* Many people, however, tend to think that the theoretical models that are built in paneled dens across the country are exclusively the stuff of intellectualization and idle theorizing. There is a point, however, where some models begin to have clinical relevance. When a clinician has some sort of guiding principle to use in assessment and treatment, the model appears as a relevant clinical concept. As Nation and Aram (1982) indicate, you cannot operate effectively unless you have some organization of your data base. Models, then, are *organizing principles.* The way that the clinician conceptualizes language and communication will largely dictate how language disorders are assessed and treated. For instance, a strict behavioral model of language and communication would not necessarily consider cognitive or social prerequisites. It does not deal with intent or other unobservable phenomena. If a clinician subscribed exclusively to this model, there may be no evaluation of the cognitive or social areas. Models that emphasize modalities of input and output such as Kirk and Kirk's (1971) model do not particularly focus on linguistic aspects such as syntax, morphology, and pragmatics. Prerequisite areas (cognitive, social, biological) are also ignored. These are just two examples of how the model of language that is adopted by a clinician can constrain thinking and clinical behavior. Thus, all models are not equally useful to a clinician and certain important aspects of the language process can be missed. There are some cautions. First, general semanticists have said for decades that the "map is not the territory." So it is with models. They are not the knowledge or behavior they represent. Clinicians should never forget that it is what they know that is important, far beyond any model. Models are perspectives and guides for organizing clinical information, nothing more. If the clinician is confronted with a real child who is performing at odds with a model's prediction, the validity of the child's behavior is not questionable, but the applicability of the model in this case is certainly a bit dubious. Do not, as they say, let the tail wag the dog. A second caution is that at the present time no one knows for certain all the details of exactly how language is developed, processed, or most efficiently assessed. Any model is likely to be inaccurate or at least incomplete. Clinicians, like theorists, must be open to change in their conceptualizations of language and its evaluation.

Before discussing assessment of language in children, it is important to review some aspects of language in a developmental perspective. Figure 4.1 lists some of the components of language development included in the integrative models of a number of authors (Bloom & Lahey, 1978; McLean & Snyder-McLean, 1978). We will briefly expand on each domain in Figure 4.1.

Language has some obvious biological prerequisites. A child must have an intact nervous system and be physiologically capable of using the auditory-vocal channel for speech output or gestures for nonspeech output of language. This prerequisite area should not be overlooked, since cognitive, social, and linguistic development depend on it. The diagnostician will gain most of this information from parental interviews and from professional reports by physicians, neurologists, or other specialists. Some neurological and biological information may be gained by the SLP through observations, interviews, and the oral peripheral examination. If the clinician has any doubts about the child's neurological, medical, or physical status, a referral should be made to the appropriate professional. A highly important biological prerequisite to oral language learning is an intact auditory system. It cannot be emphasized enough that any language assessment should include an audiometric evaluation to ensure that the child has the auditory/biological prerequisites for language. There is nothing more disheartening than to have performed language treatment for a long period of time and then to discover that the child has had a hearing loss. The auditory problem might have received early attention and resulted in greater treatment progress.

Figure 4.1 Selected Components Involved in Language Acquisition and Use

Biological	Cognitive
Intact vocal tract	Representation (symbolic ability)
Intact sensory system	Concepts underlying language
Intact motor system	
	Social
	Interaction with others
	Stimulation with model by caretakers
	Reasons to communicate with others
	Joint referencing with caretakers
	Linguistic
	Structural aspects
	—Semantics (word meaning)
	—Syntax (word ordering)
	—Morphology (word endings)
	—Phonology (sound ordering)
	Functional aspects
	—Listener perspective
	—Discourse rules
	—Contingency

A second prerequisite area that is referred to in most integrative models is cognitive development. Cognitive prerequisites are important on at least two levels. First, language is an abstract symbol system, and the user must be capable of symbolic representation which is a higher cortical function (Morehead & Morehead, 1974). Thus, just to appreciate language, a certain degree of cognitive ability is necessary. On a second level, language has been said to "map" or "code" aspects of reality that the child understands (Bowerman, 1973; Brown, 1973; Nelson, 1974). The implications for assessment and treatment are that (1) a child who is not capable of symbolic/abstract representation is not likely to be as successful in learning a language, and (2) the language a child is trained to use in treatment should reflect the youngster's cognitive holdings (e.g., what he/she knows about the world). We talk about objects and relationships in the world that we know about.

The third prerequisite area is the social basis of linguistic acquisition. The social area is important for two major reasons. First, language is learned in a social context. We learn it from our caretakers by (1) hearing a model of what the language sounds like, (2) seeing how the language is used by others in our environment, and (3) using the language ourselves as we learn it in real interactions with caretakers. Another social aspect that is important to consider in a language model concerns the functions that language serves for the child. In essence, we want to know why the child speaks. What are the intents behind his/her communications? Is language used to regulate, inform, question, and so on? Also, joint referencing takes place when a child can identify which referent or event the caretaker is referring to in an utterance (McLean & Snyder-McLean, 1978). This joint referencing activity takes place socially when an adult directs a child's attention to utterances and events or when the caretaker becomes involved in an activity that the child is already interested in. In an assessment, these social prerequisites can be evaluated by interviewing the caretakers, observing caretaker-child interactions, and simply taking a sample of the child's communication to determine why he/she talks. We will deal more specifically with these variables later in this chapter.

These three prerequisite areas are important both individually and interactively. One can readily see that if biological prerequisites are not attained, a child's cognitive and social development may be affected. Likewise, a child with no obvious biological abnormalities may not possess the cognitive prerequisites for language and the social behavior may be affected. Certainly, in cases where any of the three prerequisites, individually or interactively, is affected, language development has the strong possibility of being delayed. It is interesting that so far we have not even discussed language and its traditional areas of semantics, syntax, phonology, and pragmatics. Yet, in a nonverbal child, there is really no language to assess. It is not unusual to receive lengthy diagnostic reports on nonverbal children that focus primarily on the cognitive, social, and biological prerequisites to language.

The portions of most integrative models that clinicians are most familiar and comfortable with are the linguistic-structural aspects. There are many introductory language acquisition textbooks that provide a good review of these areas, and the present authors will not go into them here (Bloom & Lahey, 1978; Brown, 1973; Carrow-Woolfolk & Lynch, 1982; Dale, 1976; Devilliers & Devilliers, 1978; Haynes & Shulman, 1992; Owens, 1988; Trantham & Pederson, 1976; Wood, 1981).

THEORETICAL CONSIDERATIONS IN LANGUAGE ASSESSMENT

Following the lead of Muma (1973, 1978, 1983), we would like to echo some basic diagnostic precepts that we feel should underpin language assessment. First, the best language assessment device, as Siegel (1975) stated, is a well-trained clinician who keeps up with current developments. There is no "best" language test, just as there is no ideal language treatment program.

Second, language is a multidimensional process that has many facets of structure and use. There are also the prerequisite areas discussed earlier to consider in evaluation. The existence of the multidimensional process makes it unrealistic to separate structure and function or syntax from semantics or pragmatics. The most ecologically valid methods of analyzing the process are preferable. Whenever we fractionalize the communicative process, we are no longer really looking at it.

Third, Muma (1978) has reminded us that whatever we do in assessment must apply to treatment of the language disorder. If we administer tests and then do not consider these results in planning our treatment, the time spent in assessment is wasted. Our assessment and treatment procedures should also be based on similar assumptions about the communication process.

A fourth important concept was also articulated by Muma. He stated that the diagnostic paradigm seems to have two levels or issues associated with it. The most basic issue is the problem–no problem issue. Standardized tests help to solve the problem–no problem issue by comparing a child's test performance to that of other children. This type of testing emphasizes group similarity and minimizes individual variability. The "nature of the problem" issue, however, must be addressed through description of the individual child's communicative performance. This is best accomplished through nonstandardized, descriptive techniques that are more ecologically valid. Fortunately, the problem–no problem issue is solved by many parents when they have referred their child for evaluation. They typically know something is wrong when they compare the communication of their youngster with his/her peers. A standardized test can confirm this, but it rarely can be prescriptive in terms of specifying treatment targets (Millen & Prutting, 1979).

A fifth important notion has to do with sampling. All we ever do in a diagnostic evaluation is obtain a sample of communicative behavior. There are several important implications that stem from the sampling issue. First, the samples we obtain should be "representative" of the child's communicative performance. The notion of representativeness has been with us for a long while, and we must not forget that a sample we obtain may or may not represent a child's typical or "best" performance. Second, speech pathologists have subscribed for years to the idea that an evaluation can and must take place within a one- or two-hour block of time. This kind of thinking can result in frustrated clinicians when they do not obtain the data they need in the allotted time, or if the child is uncooperative. Evaluation is ongoing, and there should be no pressure to find out all there is to know in a limited time frame. The medical profession does not feel compelled to diagnose in a limited time with short, abbreviated procedures. Physicians order examinations that they feel are appropriate, and the diagnostic process takes place over as much time as is necessary. This is not to say that we should emulate the lengthy testing procedures of the medical profession, but on the other hand, we should not become like purveyors of fast food. Third, whenever possible, the clinician should attempt to obtain multiple samples. Many children behave differently in the clinical setting than they do at home or in the preschool. There have not been many comparisons of language in preschool settings with clinical environments, but we suspect that there are important differences as in the following example:

> Tyrone had said nothing during the two-hour evaluation session. He is a foster child who was brought to the clinic by a caseworker from the state Pensions and Securities Office. The caseworker said that Tyrone did talk and could not explain why he was so taciturn upon meeting us. He seemed shy and reluctant to participate even in play with the clinicians. We decided to make an observation the next week at Tyrone's daycare center. We sat unobtrusively in a corner and watched Tyrone carom off the walls like a buzz saw going awry, pulling pigtails and spewing broken crayons. He yelled at his classmates and when the teacher asked who wanted to play ball, Tyrone was one of the first to initiate his loud request. Lucas (1980) has observed that some preschoolers take on the role in the classroom of "stater of the rules." They tell other children, "You can't do that," "The paper has to be over here," and so on. (We often wonder what types of people these children develop into when they become adults. Know any?) Tyrone frequently made rule statements to the other children. We half felt that we had seen a "medicated" Tyrone at our clinic. Our goals for treatment would have been far different had we not observed Tyrone in more than one setting. It may have been appropriate, based on our first impression, to begin work on increasing child-initiated language.

What we have just described is not an isolated case. We have often made the recommendation to clinicians in the field to observe children in other settings before deciding on treatment goals. In many cases the feedback from these professionals has been, "I thought he was a different child when I saw him in the classroom."

A sixth basic premise of language assessment is that for every technique or test that the clinician uses, she must realize that certain assumptions are implied about child language. To use an instrument, you should "buy the assumptions" that underlie it. Whenever we receive the myriad flyers and announcements of new language-assessment instruments, we should remember that each is based on assumptions. We should ask ourselves, "What do I have to believe about language to use this instrument?"

Finally, we feel compelled to say that the quality of the information obtained is proportional to the amount of time the well-trained clinician spends in evaluation. In short, there is no free lunch. A 20-minute screening test that is easily administered and scored will simply not yield as much information as various analyses of a 20-minute spontaneous interaction. These suggestions should not be taken to mean that we are opposed to the use of standardized tests. We do, in fact, recommend the use of such instruments for the purpose they are most able to accomplish: to determine if a child is performing similarly to other children of his age group. Standardized tests, however, cannot make a principled clinical judgment; clinicians make decisions. Assessment has aspects of both art and science (Allen, Bliss, & Timmons, 1981). We advocate the use of a combination of standard measures coupled with nonstandardized tasks and more naturalistic sampling of communicative behavior (Lund & Duchan, 1988). We believe that exclusive reliance on either type of procedure will not provide as complete a picture of a child's performance as the use of both types. Additionally, school systems and other institutions often require some form of standardized testing.

SPECIFIC ASSESSMENT AREAS: PROCEDURES, CONSIDERATIONS, AND DIRECTIONS FOR FURTHER STUDY

In the sections that follow, we will discuss specific techniques for assessing important aspects of communication in the child with limited language. We try to provide guidelines and references for the clinician to use in learning about these various aspects of language assessment. In cases where we cannot adequately summarize a procedure, we refer the reader to a primary source with the hope that he/she will critically evaluate and perhaps learn techniques that will be clinically useful.

At the beginning of most sections, we will provide a brief sketch of some important developmental trends reported in the existing research. It is imperative that the clinician appreciate that each assessment technique mentioned is basically grounded in the research on communication development. Even though it is beyond the scope of this chapter to present a complete view of any aspect of language acquisition, we would be remiss if we did not touch upon some "highlights" of the process that are related to language assessment. The areas discussed are only suggestive of some linguistic and prelinguistic attainments of children between birth and age four. These particular achievements are discussed to provide a context for the assessment suggestions that follow later in the chapter. Many fine textbooks are available that summarize research in language acquisition and the reader should become familiar with this information prior to engaging in any language assessment (Bloom & Lahey, 1978; Brown, 1973; Carrow-Woolfolk & Lynch, 1982; Dale, 1976; Devilliers & Devilliers, 1978; Haynes & Shulman, 1992; Hubbell, 1981; Muma, 1978; Owens, 1988).

Preassessment and Pertinent Historical Information

Preassessment. In most major clinical settings, prospective clients are required to complete some sort of case history information prior to being seen by the speech-language pathologist and/or other professionals. It is especially unnerving to meet a client for the first time before receiving the completed case history information, because the clinician has little idea about how to prepare for the evaluation. The client could be totally nonverbal or have only subtle language problems. It is critical for speech-language pathologists in any work setting to avoid performing an evaluation without access to important historical information that will allow the clinician to plan the evaluation in such a way as to maximize the use of time and resources during the initial contact with the child and parents.

Gallagher (1983) suggested a preassessment procedure for use with language cases and outlined the advantages of such a process for the clinician in planning and conducting evaluations. Preassessment is more than the typical process of having the parents fill out a case history form. The notion of preassessment includes finding out some clinically useful data that could affect the way the initial evaluation is conducted. We use a preassessment form in our university setting that contains components from a variety of research projects (George & Yivisaker, 1984; Gallagher, 1983). Clients are asked to complete the form and return it prior to scheduling the evaluation appointment. In cases where the parents cannot read or have difficulty completing the form, an interview session is scheduled prior to seeing the child in which the parents are questioned about each item on the preassessment. The important thing is that the clinician has a fairly good picture of the child's cognitive, social, play, and communicative behavior before the evaluation session. We also include a short adaptive behavior scale focusing on motor skills, self-help skills, and personal-social abilities to provide additional information on noncommunicative behaviors that relate to cognitive, social, and language development. Gallagher (1983, p. 14) gives a concrete example of the value of preassessment information:

> One child who was particularly sensitive to the communicative partner had an MLU value of 1.6 in the clinician-child sample and an MLU of 3.96 when she talked with her brother. One boy produced his most structurally complex utterances while he was playing with water toys in a plastic pan filled with water, an activity his mother had indicated "he would talk most about." One boy's most structurally complex language performance was obtained when he played with a younger friend who was his neighbor. For one child, it was talking about pictures in a family album.

None of these language facilitating situations would have been known to the clinician if the appropriate questions had not been asked on a preassessment instrument. The clinician can plan ahead and have family members bring specific stimulus items, toys, or interactants that would provide the best sample of the client's communication abilities.

The Parent Interview.   The clinician will find many questions raised by the parent responses on the preassessment packet. The interview is a good place to clarify any missing information or inconsistencies in the parent's responses. The information obtained from caretakers of limited-language children is highly important. First of all, many of these children may not have the linguistic means or cognitive development to express themselves well and the parent or guardian must be relied upon to provide pertinent background details and estimations of present skill levels.

As mentioned in Chapter 2, we do not recommend that the diagnostician write down specific questions prior to the evaluation. Appendix A contains an interview protocol for the assessment of the limited-language child. The protocol is divided into broad areas covering the prerequisites to language, as well as the beginnings of linguistic development. Much of the specific information can be filled in from responses to the preassessment packet, and the interview can simply follow up on areas of interest to the clinician. The interviewer should ask questions in the broad areas, obtaining information in each subarea. The exact wording of questions is not provided because of the variability of interview situations. Parents represent differing levels of education, intelligence, socioeconomic status, and experience, and we have found it more feasible to tailor interview questions to each individual case. The protocol was designed only to "jog the mind" of the clinician to ask questions in specific topic areas. When remarkable information is reported in any area, the interviewer should formulate appropriate follow-up questions to clearly illuminate the area of interest. The major interview areas represent biological, social, and cognitive prerequisites to language, as well as linguistic level, and they were gleaned from a variety of child language-acquisition and language-impairment sources. The interviewer should especially focus the interview on the most applicable portions of the protocol and not ask unnecessary questions. For instance, if a child is using a wide variety of multiword utterances and is communicating effectively in the environment, it would be inappropriate for the interviewer to spend inordinate time on cognitive and social prerequisites.

One of the most revealing questions about the child's home environment is the item that asks the parent to describe a typical day in the life of the child. It is often surprising how much clinically useful information can be uncovered in the answer to this question. For instance, parents may report many hours spent watching television, or in solitary play outside, or in self-stimulatory activities that have been allowed to continue despite their lack of productivity. Often, a pattern emerges that shows that the child spends precious little time in meaningful social interactions. Another pattern that reveals much about a child's problem is a lack of a schedule or rules in the household. One mother reported that her nonverbal three-year-old child typically went to bed at 11:30 P.M. after a late night talk show and liked to sleep until 9:30 A.M. The child also ate all his meals while walking around inside the house, refused to wear pajamas, threw frequent tantrums, and was prone to writing on the walls. This scenario suggests that the parents and child may be in some need of counseling regarding behavior management. Much of this information would not have been gleaned from the preassessment packet or a formal test, but it would be quite important when it comes to making recommendations for treatment. If, for example, we wanted these parents to begin to withhold desired items from this child to create communicative opportunity, they would have extreme difficulty with this procedure because there appear to be few existing rules in the home. Tantrums would inevitably increase, and the treatment plan would have a high probability of being aborted by the family.

The protocol in Appendix A is designed for the well-informed child language clinician. The question areas will mean nothing to the interviewer who does not know the relevance, rationale, and research that underlies each major area and subheading. Finally, no single item on the protocol is significant in its own right. We are looking for patterns among the major areas. It should be remembered that the areas are divided in the protocol only for convenience and that in reality, the domains are interrelated. In obtaining the information, the interviewer should

1. Tape-record the interview and take notes after obtaining permission from the client to do so.
2. Frame questions on the correct level of abstraction for the parent.
3. Use many examples when asking questions, and do not use frequent yes/no questions. For instance, ask questions such as, "How does Randy let you know he wants something?" "Tell me what he likes to do when he plays." "What kinds of sentences have you heard him say?" "Under what circumstances does he try to communicate with you?" If the parent is not providing enough specific information, the clinician can ask some specific questions such as, "Does he seem to use objects for the purpose they were intended—for instance, does he use a comb to comb his hair?"
4. Ask the parent to give you *examples* of behaviors and language you are interested in.
5. Use the space provided on the protocol to make a brief note of remarkable findings in any area.

Assessment of Social Prerequisites and Caretaker-Child Interaction

Language development takes place in a social context. From the moment of birth, a child interacts with his/her caretakers and is bombarded with visual, auditory, and tactile stimuli that occur in this relationship. It is especially important in cases of nonverbal, single-word, and early multiword children to observe them interacting with their caretaker. There are two reasons for this. First, we want to observe the child with someone that he/she is familiar with and comfortable being around. It is often the case that the best sample of the child's communication is obtained in this portion of the evaluation. When unfamiliar clinicians attempt to establish rapport with a child in strange surroundings, it may be quite difficult to observe natural communication, especially in a limited time period. Occasionally, we have seen children who refused to interact with us in an evaluation. In these cases, the caretaker-child interaction provides the only data base available. In the early years of our field, we were frequently told that the initial step in an evaluation was to separate the child from his mother. Often, this resulted in a catastrophic reaction on the part of the child and little information was gained from the evaluation (other than the fact that the child did not "separate well from his mother"). We must not lose sight of our goal—to observe the child's communicative and prelinguistic skills through talking and play. If the caretaker can provide a more effective demonstration of certain skills than the clinician, then we must take advantage of this opportunity and not feel that we have failed as clinicians. Rather, we have succeeded in getting the data we were after as the result of making a sound clinical judgment. Establishing a relationship with a child can always be accomplished in the initial treatment sessions, when we are not under as severe time constraints. Thus, the caretaker-child interaction can provide a rich sampling of the child's communication. As we will soon indicate, it can also give the clinician a meager, constrained, and repetitive sample.

A second goal of observing the caretaker-child interaction is to note the quality of the language model provided by the caretaker. Research has shown that caretakers alter many aspects of their communicative behavior when interacting with their child. Suprasegmentally, they may raise their fundamental frequency, increase their pitch range, speak more slowly, and use double primary stress patterns (Garnica, 1974). The caretaker is less disfluent when talking to an infant and pauses at major linguistic constituent boundaries. Linguistically, the mean length of utterance is reduced, and the vocabulary and syntactic complexity are simplified (Snow, 1972). In addition to being exposed to a simpler language model, developing children are given an introduction to the reciprocity of communicative interchange. Snow (1977) has shown that even with infants as young as three months of age, mothers engage in turn-taking reciprocal behavior. Early on, the child's "turn" is a nonverbal action that is biologically programmed, such as a smile, sneeze, or burp. The mother simply responds to this with some sort of language response and often takes the child's turn for him/her linguistically. As the child develops, the caretaker demands that the youngster's turn more closely resemble the adult correct model.

As important as the model itself are the circumstances under which it is developed. The youngster benefits cognitively from interacting with the caretaker. Mothers and fathers typically show the child "how the world works" in terms of demonstrating the functional use of objects, body parts, attributes of objects, and many other conceptual aspects of the environment. Children have been shown to follow their caretaker's line of visual regard (look at objects their parent is focused on) very early in development (McLean & Snyder-McLean, 1978). Adults also show the child how to play with a variety of objects and even stimulate symbolic play. We see then that caretakers demonstrate language structure, language use, concepts, and the reciprocity of communication. Children are highly sensitive to their social environment and they learn that language is a tool to be used for a variety of social and nonsocial purposes (Dore, 1975; Halliday, 1975). With young children, it is clear that their early exposure to language and their early use of it is highly social.

The clinician needs to answer many questions about the caretaker-child interaction. Does the caretaker talk about the "here and now" (Holland, 1975) or about things removed in time and space? What kind of joint referencing takes place in the interaction? Does the caretaker talk about and participate in things that are of interest to the child? Does the caretaker direct the child's play to things that he/she feels are significant, disregarding the child's preferences?

Is there a balance between when the parent joint references with the child and other times when the child joint references with the parent? Does the parent force the child into limited or respondent modes of communicative function? It is not unusual to observe parents of early language-disordered children who ask incessant questions (e.g., "What's this?" "What color is this?") or require the child to constantly imitate (e.g., "Say 'ball'"). We are not intimating that the parent's interactive style is in any way causally related to the child's language disorder. In fact, a parent's way of talking to a child could be the result of the disorder rather than a cause. Whatever the relationship, the caretaker's model, as it presently exists, may not be conducive to language development and should be changed. The only way to determine this is through the observation of caretaker-child interaction. There are various important dimensions to consider in the assessment of social development.

Specific aspects of the child's behavior are also important to examine in the caretaker-child interaction. Socially, the child's eye contact and willingness to participate in reciprocal nonverbal activities should be observed. A child who does not tolerate or seek out the participation of another person may not have any need for a communication system. Perhaps this child might need to work on some prelinguistic social skills prior to developing language. Language is, after all, a social tool and a child who is not "social" has little need of a code to use with people she does not even communicate with nonverbally.

> Natalie entered the examination playroom and her attention settled on the juice. She ran to the table and tried to remove the top of the glass container. When she could not, she proceeded from item to item, pausing only a few seconds on each. When the clinician called her name loudly, she did not respond. Small noises in the hallway occurred several times and she paused, transfixed on the door with her head cocked to one side like a dog listening to a distant sound. The clinician physically caught her and tried to engage in reciprocal play with a car. Natalie would not look the clinician in the eye and the car was thrown across the room behind her. Throughout the two-hour session, the child never maintained eye contact longer than two seconds and never participated cooperatively with the clinician. More importantly, even when it was clear she wanted something out of reach, she never sought out help from the other human being in the room. The mother reported that Natalie plays alone most of the time or with animals outside in the rural farmyard. It is doubtful that this child has much need for social interaction, let alone a communication system.

Appendix B provides an example of a checklist the clinician could use in examining caretaker behaviors during interaction in the evaluation session. Note that the "score" is not important; however, the clinician's impressions of the caretaker modifications could lead to treatment recommendations involving work with interaction patterns.

Adaptive Behavior Scales. Adaptive behavior scales typically rate a child's development of motor skills, social behavior, self-help skills, and language ability. Either children are given tasks to perform or the parents are asked to respond to items on the protocol. The advantage of such scales is that they help to broaden the perspective of the SLP beyond exclusively examining language ability. Although we will assess social cognitive development as it relates to language, much of a child's adaptive behavior depends on cognitive and social attainments. We can obtain a better overall picture of the child's level of functioning, and this information, when coupled with our other assessment data, can be valuable. Also, many conditions (e.g., mental retardation) may show a child to be of generally low functioning in most areas, and language is only part of the problem. Knowledge of adaptive behavior will also be important to the clinician in making referrals. Language treatment activities can also be designed to incorporate motor, social, and self-help areas so the child is learning a variety of needed skills plus the language associated with them. Several adaptive behavior scales are available (Balthazar, 1973; Lambert et al., 1981; Project RHISE, 1979).

Assessment of Cognitive Attainments
Associated with Communication

Conceptual holdings are thought to be important to linguistic acquisition for several reasons. First, language is a representational act. It represents reality or stands for objects and relationships in the world. Second, language is an abstract symbol system. In order to appreciate abstract symbols, we must be able to represent them mentally. Third, language is a tool that we use in social interactions. Tool use implies certain conceptual underpinnings, such as the apprehension of relationships like means–end. Fourth, language use involves talking about objects, events, and relationships in the world. It is necessary that one knows the properties of these objects and relationships in order to talk about them coherently. As Nelson (1974) said, we use words as "tags" for the concepts that we have.

Perhaps the most well-known researcher in the area of children's cognitive development has been Jean Piaget. A most significant period in language development occurs between birth and two years. By the age of two, a child is typically beginning to use multiword utterances and has clearly demonstrated the symbolic capacity for dealing with language. Piaget calls the period between birth and age two the *sensorimotor stage* of cognitive development because most learning takes place through active sensorimotor exploration of a child's environment. There are many sources available that describe this period of cognitive growth in detail (Beard, 1969; Ginsburg & Opper, 1969; Morehead & Morehead, 1974). We hope to present a flavor for some of the developmental landmarks that a child is thought to pass on the way to becoming representational. The implication for the diagnostician is that these landmarks may be assessment targets for severely language-disordered children. It should be emphasized that not all of these cognitive attainments have been shown to directly or strongly correlate with language acquisition. However, many authorities have advocated the administration of Piagetian assessment batteries that examine cognitive attainments in the sensorimotor period (Newhoff & Leonard, 1983; McLean & Snyder-McLean, 1978; Ruder & Smith, 1974). Some skills examined on these scales seem to be "logically related" to language development, and others have been shown to have a statistical relationship to linguistic acquisition. There is, however, a difference between correlation and causation. Actually, some authorities feel that the relationship between specific cognitive developments and specific language acquisitions has not been clearly shown (Leonard, 1978). Others support the notion of more specific cognitive skills being related to linguistic acquisition (Gopnik & Meltzoff, 1987; Lifter & Bloom, 1989). In reviewing the cognitive development literature, however, there seem to be certain skills that are included on cognitive assessment scales and often referred to by authorities as being potentially language related.

One cognitive skill that is logically related to language development is that of object permanence. Up to a certain point in development (before object permanence is obtained), an infant will not appear to be able to represent an object mentally when it is not in physical view. They seem to "forget" about the object, even if it is one that they desire. If you cover an object with a cloth, a child of a certain age and cognitive level may stop searching for it. Some studies, however, have not shown a strong relationship between language development and object permanence (Bates et al., 1979; Leonard, 1978), although it is included in many scales often administered to language-developing children (Merhabian & Williams, 1971; Uzgiris & Hunt, 1975).

Another cognitive skill thought to be related to the acquisition of language is the ability to appreciate the means–end relationship (Bates et al., 1979; Morehead & Morehead, 1974). The idea that a particular process is a means to accomplishing an end is similar to the use of language to affect the environment. Language is, in fact, a means to accomplish a variety of ends, such as regulating the environment, obtaining information, sharing information, and so on (Halliday, 1975). If the child does not have the basic means–end concept, it is doubtful that language will be used as a means to accomplish any purpose.

Functional object use has also been related to the development of communication (Steckol & Leonard, 1981). Using an object for its intended purpose (e.g., combing hair with a comb) requires the mental representation of both the object and its use. Also, when a child begins to talk about basic relations in the environment, utterances typically concern objects, their functions, and all the relationships an object enters into (Nelson, 1974). Steckol and Leonard (1981) found that training the functional use of objects resulted in an increase of protoimperative responses (nonverbally using adults to accomplish a task or manipulate objects) in nonverbal children.

Imitation and deferred (delayed) imitation have also been related to the development of language (Bates et al., 1979). Imitation requires mental representation of an act for a short time period, and deferred imitation requires holding onto an event for a longer duration. Both suggest an ability to represent reality for a length of time without depending on immediate stimulus support.

Finally, symbolic play (pretend behavior) is frequently regarded as evidence of a child's general symbolic capacity. One can think of symbolic play on a continuum from playing with exemplars of an object that are physically similar to the real object (e.g., a box representing a car), to playing with exemplars that are dissimilar to the real object (e.g., a comb for a car), and finally to playing with no object at all (pantomine) (Elder & Pederson, 1978). The use of one object to "stand for" another is similar to the way that words represent objects in the real world. A basic symbolic capacity must be present in order to use a symbolic play routine, and these routines should be noted in a child's behavior as a positive sign of increased symbolic capacity.

To this point, the cognitive attainments of object permanence, means–end, functional use of objects, imitation, deferred imitation, and symbolic play have been suggested as having some importance for the development of language. Of course, no one really knows how much each contributes, or even if each does actually contribute to the acquisition of language. They may only be correlated with language development (Newhoff & Leonard, 1983).

Piaget divided the sensorimotor period of cognitive development into six substages. Table 4.2 shows possible relations among cognitive attainments. Several investigators report that a child must have at least attained stage 4 to evidence gestural communication and stages 5 or 6 for expressive single and early multiword constructions. Again, children exhibit individual variability in this cognitive–linguistic correspondence, and this attests to a more general relationship between representational development and language acquisition. It is clear, though, that language development is related in very potent and complex ways to cognitive capacities.

There appears to be some agreement that most children are not typically using verbal language in a productive way prior to Piaget's sensorimotor stage 5. The present authors can find no report of a child in stage 3 or 4 using language normally. Thus, it appears that the diagnostician would find it useful to obtain at least a "ballpark" estimate of a child's level of development in the sensorimotor period. A primary reason to do an assessment of cognitive level is to confirm or deny a child's ability to represent reality and deal with symbols. As we mentioned in an earlier section, some of the specific behaviors that have been associated with language development are imitation, deferred imitation, means–end, functional use of objects, and symbolic play (pretend). These cognitive attainments are focused upon here because they are the behaviors included in cognitive test batteries and have been referred to most often as possibly being related to language development.

An important notion to keep in mind is that when we assess cognitive prerequisites, we watch a child's behavior and infer his conceptual holdings. As Lund and Duchan (1983) point out, it is often difficult to categorize a behavior as indicating knowledge of a concept since we have no history of how a child behaves. Lund and Duchan say, for example, that a child who tries to drink from an empty cup may not be exhibiting symbolic play by pretending to drink. Rather, the child may be *trying* to drink, which is a functional use of an object and not symbolic play. Thus, in cognitive assessment we can only make inferences about what a child knows and we must bear this in mind as the assessment is completed. We should obtain as much information as possible about the child's typical play routines and object use. The parent interview is invaluable here. The failure of a child to perform a task that we set up to evaluate a particular cognitive prerequisite is not necessarily evidence of a lack of the concept. A child can

Table 4.2 Piaget's Sensorimotor Stages

STAGE AND AGE (MONTHS)	GENERAL	IMITATION	OBJECT CONCEPT	CAUSALITY	MEANS–END
Stage 1 Birth–1	Reflexive Adaptive intelligence	Notion not present	No differentiation of self from objects	Egocentric	Notion not present
Stage 2 1–4	Primary circular reactions (self-repetitions) Coordination of sensory schema	Self-imitation of actions with unexpected results "Preimitation"	Object followed with eyes until out of view Change in perspective interpreted as change in object	No differentiation of self and moving objects	Notion not present Intentionality lacking
Stage 3 4–8	Secondary circular reactions Repetition of actions of others	Imitation of others' actions already in repertoire	Anticipation of position of moving objects; no manual search	Self as cause of all events	Repetition of events with unexpected outcomes; heightened interest in event outcome Intentionality follows initiation of behavior
Stage 4 8–12	Coordination of secondary schemata Known means applied to new problems	Imitation of behaviors different from those in repertoire Facial imitation	Manual search for object where last seen Object constancy	Some externalization of causality Realization that objects can cause action	Coordination and integration of schemata Establishment of goal prior to initiation of activity Anticipation of outcomes
Stage 5 12–18	Tertiary secondary schemata Experimentation	Imitation of behaviors markedly different from repertoire	Sequential displacements considered Awareness of object spatial relations	Realization that he/she is one of many objects in environment	New means through experimentation Tools used
Stage 6 18–24	New means through mental combination Representational thought	Deferred imitation	Representation of displacements Awareness of unseen movements	Representation of causality Able to predict cause-effect relationship	Language used to influence others Representation of outcome or end

"fail" a cognitive task due to inattention, disinterest, or some other reason that has nothing to do with her cognitive status.

With these admonitions in mind, how does one perform a cognitive assessment and what type of child undergoes the evaluation? We have found it productive to take note of cognitive prerequisites in children who are nonverbal and those who are at the single-word level. Those children who are currently using *productive* early multiword utterances are evidencing some representational ability and symbolic ability just by using language normally. It is not useful to routinely administer a lengthy and complex cognitive test battery initially. We recommend that the diagnostician move from general analyses to more specific ones. Figure 4.2 contains references for use in cognitive assessment.

The first level of analysis can be a lengthy behavioral observation of the child engaged in play. In our experience, children whose cognitive levels are lower will exhibit primitive play routines and perseverative use of objects. Westby (1980) outlines some useful stages to use in assessing the developmental relationship among cognitive development, language, and play. The clinician can set up a play situation and watch the child interact with objects and people. The examiner should be looking for behavior that suggests specific cognitive prerequisites. It is optimal to videotape the play interaction for later specific analysis (Lund & Duchan, 1988). The clinician must always view the specific behaviors in terms of the context in which they occurred. For instance, pretending that a block is a car can qualify as symbolic play only if the clinician did not demonstrate this activity earlier in the session. At any rate, it is important to view children's nonverbal play behaviors contextually and if possible, obtain some historical data on their play routines. Sometimes, there is a clear cognitive deficit as in the following example:

> Ralph was enrolled in a preschool handicapped classroom. He was two years old and nonverbal. He seemed to enjoy imitating the clinician when she put blocks into a coffee can. When presented with other toys, however, Ralph just persisted in putting the blocks in the can and dumping them out again. The cycle continued—putting the blocks in and dumping them out. The other toys were immediately mouthed and banged on the floor. No matter what other toys Ralph had

Figure 4.2 Measures of Cognitive Development

- The Ordinal Scales of Psychological Development (Uzgiris & Hunt, 1975)
- Albert Einstein Scales of Sensorimotor Development (Corman & Escalona, 1969)
- Infant Cognitive Development Scale (Merhabian & Williams, 1971)
- A Clinical and Educational Manual for Use with the Uzgiris and Hunt Scales of Psychological Development (Dunst, 1980)
- Beyond Sensorimotor Intelligence: Assessment of Symbolic Maturity Through Analysis of Pretend Play (Nicolich, 1977)
- The Symbolic Play Test (Lowe & Costello, 1976)
- Evaluation of Cognitive Behavior in Young Nonverbal Children (Chappel & Johnson, 1976)
- Assessment of Cognitive and Language Abilities Through Play (Westby, 1980)

access to, he would put them in his mouth and/or bang them on the floor. When the clinician attempted to provide a model of functional use of objects or more productive play routines, Ralph would persist with his limited repertoire.

Subsequent to observation of play routines, the clinician should note whether the quality of play exhibited indicates a cognitive delay. Sometimes the sophistication of the play routines observed will make it clear that there is no representational problem. Other times, as depicted in the previous example, behavior will occur that strongly suggests a rather primitive representational ability. Many cases fall between these two ends of the cognitive continuum, and these children may require further testing to determine which level of cognitive development they have attained. We recommend Westby (1980) for an account of "normal" play behavior. Sometimes, in dealing with so many disordered clients it is easy to forget that we must also be familiar with normal behavior. Students should actively observe and play with normal children to learn what kinds of things they typically do at various ages.

The second level of analysis can involve the administration of cognitive "screening scales" and specific tasks that more closely evaluate certain conceptual prerequisites. Chappel and Johnson (1976) and Merhabian and Williams (1971) have devised rather simple scales that help the clinician to arrive at a general level of cognitive development. These scales can be administered in a short time period and involve the clinician's setting up task situations to which the child responds. Again, we recommend proceeding to this second level of analysis primarily with children who are clearly not playing normally or who are "suspicious" to the clinician on behavioral observation. If the child performs at a delayed level of cognitive development on the screening scale, then further testing might be undertaken.

A final level of analysis is to administer a more detailed scale, such as that developed by Uzgiris and Hunt (1975). Dunst (1980) has developed some helpful procedures for use with the Uzgiris and Hunt scales that streamline the clinical administration of the tasks. Such lengthy measures should be administered to a child who is strongly suspected of exhibiting cognitive deficits.

The speech-language pathologist should guard against the perception by professionals or parents that this evaluation procedure is testing the child's intelligence. We should make no judgments about how "smart" a child is or even her potential for cognitive growth. Children whose play behavior and performance on cognitive scales indicate they are lacking cognitive prerequisites for language should be referred to other professionals (e.g., psychologist, special educator) for diagnosis of their mental ability and potential for learning. It should be emphasized that we examine cognitive prerequisites only because they appear to be related to the acquisition and use of abstract language systems. If we determine that a child does not possess the cognitive holdings for acquiring our normally abstract and arbitrary symbol system, we then can consider attempting to train cognitive prerequisites (Kahn, 1984) or a communication system that is less abstract, such as simple signs that code concrete and frequently occurring activities.

There are some significant alterations necessary to these procedures if the clinician is evaluating an older, severely handicapped client. Most measures of sensorimotor intelligence were pioneered on normally developing children, and there are some difficulties in applying them directly to older children or adults. Snyder-McLean, McLean, and Etter (1988) provide many useful suggestions in evaluating the cognitive status of older, severely involved clients.

Assessment of Communicative Intent and Function

Some authorities have indicated that a frequent manifestation of early language disorder in children is their different use of language (Fey, 1986; Lucas, 1980; Wetherby & Prutting, 1984). We can divide language use into a number of different levels of analysis (Chapman, 1981). As a child's MLU becomes longer, it is more difficult to discern a particular intent behind his utterance. Chapman (1981, p. 133) gives the example of a person saying, "Hey Jim, find the red ball, ok?" This, as Chapman points out, is a request for attention, a request for action, and a request for information about the listener's compliance. This same sentence could also be analyzed at the discourse level to determine the child's conversational competence.

We have found it useful to separate our thinking about the use of language into early language cases and older language cases. For instance, a child who is in the single-word stage or early multiword stage is most often reported to have difficulty with the number of uses he/she has for language. Frequently, these children are referred because they do not initiate language enough and only respond to communications. These children are typically not referred for being poor conversationalists. Indeed, Bloom, Roscissano, and Hood (1976) have reported that children at this level are not normally very "contingent" in their conversations. The point here is that when one considers disorders of communicative intent and language function, it is often helpful to think separately about early language cases and later language cases. The early ones need to have an inventory taken of why they use language; the later ones need to be examined for the quality of their conversational participation. This portion of the chapter will focus on the assessment of communicative intent in early language cases.

A prelinguistic or nonverbal child has no expressive language. This does not imply, however, that the child does not communicate. Any mother of a prelinguistic child will attest that these children communicate profusely about their desires, moods, and a variety of pleasing and noxious biological states. Bates (1976) studied the sensorimotor performatives of young children and determined that they have primitive forms of imperatives or commands in which they use adults to obtain access to objects in their environment. One can initially see the child physically manipulating the adult, as in putting the adult's hand on a jar to open it. Later, the child may use pointing coupled with vocalizations to indicate to the adult what she wants done. Bates also noted primitive forms of the declarative in which the child uses an object with the goal of gaining the adult's attention. There appears to be a progression that begins with the child showing and giving objects to adults. Ultimately, the child exhibits the declarative by pointing toward objects with alternating gaze between the adult and object. Bates et al. (1979) reported a "gestural complex" that, in part, may be related to language development. Thus, communication is taking place quite vividly in the preverbal child.

There are also preverbal evidences of the "functions" of language alluded to by Halliday (1975) and Dore (1975). That is, children use the greeting function nonverbally by waving, question by exhibiting a quizzical look, and regulate adults physically before they use language for these purposes. In preverbal children, the primary evidence for their communication ability is found in gestures, facial expressions, and/or vocalizations. These phenomena can be observed by a clinician in a diagnostic session or caretakers can be asked in an assessment interview about how the child makes his needs known at home and at school. A nonverbal child is also beginning to expand the phonetic inventory, and the clinician can transcribe phonetic elements present in the child's system.

A possible diagnostic variable found in prelinguistic children was contributed by Dore et al. (1976). Dore and his colleagues noted that a prelinguistic child is not simply uttering "jargon" vocalizations. At a certain point in development, Dore noted the presence of *phonetically consistent forms* (PCF), which he termed "transitional phenomena." Phonetically consistent forms are vocalizations that are stabilized around certain situations. They are not word approximations, but they are fairly stable phonetic productions typically consisting of vowel or consonant-vowel combinations. They are repeatedly associated with specific situations such as expressing affect (emotion), indicating or pointing to aspects of the environment, or expressing a desire to obtain an object or event. Dore observed that these PCFs seem to act as a transition to words where certain phonetic elements must be stabilized around a specific referent. Thus, it would be important in an evaluation of communicative function to determine not only which basic functions are present, but if they are realized on a gestural, vocal, or verbal level.

According to Chapman (1981), the clinician may adopt an existing classification scheme or change these available systems so that functions that are of interest can be coded. The two most famous systems referring to children's uses of language are the schemes developed by Halliday (1975) and Dore (1975). However, other systems might also be useful clinically (Coggins & Carpenter, 1978; Folger & Chapman, 1978; Lucas, 1980; Tough, 1977). From examining the categories in these systems, it is clear that many of the terms overlap regarding the functions they describe. McLean and Snyder-McLean (1978) have suggested that functions of language may be distilled down into two basic uses. One use is to influence joint attention and the other is to influence joint activity. These functions basically correspond to the imperative and the declarative in English. Thus, as Chapman (1981) suggests, it makes little difference exactly which system is used to assess function of language. The clinician should select a system, however, that at least contains some basic declarative and imperative operations so that the child's initiation of a response to communications can be coded.

The clinician using any system of coding a child's communicative intent should be aware that there are several issues to consider. First, there are very little data available on the reliability of the major coding schemes. Dale (1980) has found that clinicians can reliably code imperatives and declaratives; however, little information has appeared in the literature on the reliability of clinical judgments using the Dore or Halliday systems. Reliability should be checked routinely because functions that are unreliably assigned are not useful to the clinician. Chapman (1981) provides some questions for troubleshooting when reliability is low:

1. Is sufficient information about the context available so a decision can be made about what the child "intended"?
2. Are the categories used in the coding scheme overlapping and not clearly defined?
3. Are the categories too detailed for easy use by the clinician?
4. Are there too many categories?
5. Has the clinician practiced the system enough? Reliability is a function of practice.

Some additional general guidelines should be discussed. The assessment of communicative function should be carried out in a naturalistic situation. It is sometimes difficult to contrive situations in which a child will express a genuine communicative intent. The clinician should have a wide variety of toys and stimuli in the room to stimulate a number of different conversational possibilities and expressions of need or declarations. If there are other children or adults in the situation, the clinician must remember that the functions expressed by the child are inextricably related to the behavior and utterances of other conversational participants. Also, functions are only interpretable in light of the nonverbal context of communication. For instance, if a child points at a cow beside the highway and says "cow," we might assume the child is "labeling" or "commenting" about the animal. This would be suspected more strongly if the child's attention then went to something else. Another variable to bear in mind is the notion of sampling functions of communication in multiple settings. Our earlier example of how a child's use of language was dramatically different in the preschool setting as opposed to the clinic should illustrate the importance of multiple sampling. It would be a shame to target the regulatory function for training in the clinic when the child frequently regulates the behavior of people in other situations. It is not necessarily a communication disorder when a child does not regulate in the clinic.

Some authors have suggested using standard eliciting tasks for basic communicative functions. This has been done for imperatives and declaratives (Dale, 1980; Snyder, 1978, 1981; Staab, 1983) but not as widely for more specific functions of communication. Generally, declaratives seem to be elicited most effectively by presenting discrepant events and objects in the sampling situation. The child may then comment on the novel stimulus. Imperatives are more reliably obtained than declaratives, since the clinician can maintain control over the stimuli and activities in the sampling situation. The child will ask for access to toys, or ask the clinician to assist in certain operations (winding of toys, etc.). Chapman (1981) recommends that we assess functions in terms of how often they are verbally realized. Regulation, comment, greeting, and other functions may be expressed gesturally or behaviorally, and it would be important to determine if a child can use oral language to express these communications.

Wetherby et al. (1988) contributed research that practicing clinicians will find most helpful. These researchers studied normally developing children at the preverbal, single-word, and early multiword stages of development to describe their intentional communication. Rate of communicative acts increased predictably as the children increased in MLU. The communication acts were analyzed in categories of regulating behavior, social interaction, and referencing joint attention. The subjects exhibited acts in all categories and tended to initiate more than respond to communication. They tended to move from gestural modes in the prelinguistic stage to verbal modes in the early multiword stage. This report outlines specific procedures for structured and nonstructured sampling of communication acts and provides guidelines for use in discriminating poten- tially language-delayed clients from normally developing children. We have only preliminary normative data on the typical use of communicative functions in normally developing children, but we suspect that there is considerable variabil- ity in these functions as a product of individual children, differing contexts, and types of interactants. Wetherby, Yonclas, and Bryan (1989) used similar proce- dures on language-impaired, Down syndrome, and autistic children and found that some of these measures (e.g., rate of intentional communication) may be useful clinically to describe these populations.

So far in this portion of the chapter, we have not mentioned form/ structure of language. Earlier, we indicated that the process of language should not be fractionalized. The implication of this is that structure and function should be analyzed interactively. In cases where the child is nonverbal or at the single-word level, it is feasible to analyze functions and target communicative functions in treatment (Wilcox, 1984). For example, the clinician may want to increase the number of regulatory attempts in a particular child, or increase the verbal realizations of regulation in a client. When a child reaches the point of late single-word and early multiword utterances, however, we recommend anal- ysis of structure and function interactively, as indicated in the following section.

Assessment of Structure and Function in Early Utterances

So far, we have briefly sketched the development of cognitive and social prerequisites to language, as well as communicative intent and function. The present section deals with the formation of the linguistic code in communicative development. Our discussion will consider two general phases: single-word and early multiword. These stages are based on length of utterance, which up to about age four generally correlates with chronological age (Miller & Chapman, 1981) and linguistic attainment (Brown, 1973; Carrow-Woolfolk & Lynch,

1982; Lund & Duchan, 1988). Each stage has certain acquisitions associated with it that may indicate that the child is ready to make the transition into the next stage.

Single-Word Utterances. After a period of using no real words and becoming more consistent with the use of vocalizations accompanied by gestures, the child begins to use single words to code objects and events. The words are not adult productions, but typically CV or CVCV approximations of the correct production (Nelson, 1973). Nelson has found that children's early lexicons represent specific categories. These one-word utterances were formerly called *holophrases*—a single word referring to an entire thought (e.g., "cookie" may really mean "I want a cookie") (McNeil, 1970). Recent research has reported that subgroups of language-developing and language-disordered children are *referential* (word and object oriented) or *expressive* (social and conversation oriented). That is, the referential children use mostly nouns and refer to objects and events. They also like to play with objects and spend more time playing alone. The expressive children, on the other hand, enjoy talking to and being with people and use more personal-social words (Weiss et al., 1983). There are perhaps other ways to characterize early single-word productions, but the point is that children go through a period of talking, as Lois Bloom (1973) says, using "one word at a time." Toward the end of the single-word period, Nelson indicates that the child accrues an expressive lexicon of about 50 words and then begins to attempt word combinations.

Children in the single-word period can be examined for both the types of words they use and the apparent reasons they use them. The form of single-word utterances has been viewed in different ways by various authorities. Nelson (1973) categorized single words as members of the classes shown in Table 4.3. Other researchers have found similar results (Benedict, 1975). Bloom and Lahey (1978) and Lahey (1988) provide a lengthy discussion and examples of their system for early utterance analysis. Ideally, single words should be paired with functions such as those discussed by Chapman (1981). Parent checklists are especially useful in obtaining data on lexicon size and content. Bates et al. (1986) developed a list of over 400 words that parents can use to check items both comprehended and produced by their child. Clinicians can also keep an ongoing tally of lexical items produced in treatment as well as their functions.

Table 4.3 Percentage of First 50 Word Lexicon Accounted for by Grammatical Categories in Two Major Studies

CATEGORY	NELSON (1973)	BENEDICT (1975)	EXAMPLE
General Nominal	50	51	chair, kitty
Specific Nominal	11	14	person's name
Action Word	19	14	go, eat
Modifier	10	9	dirty, big
Personal-Social	10	9	hi, no, please
Function	0	4	that, for

Rice, Sell, and Hadley (1990) provide a system for online coding of children's verbal initiations and responses in natural classroom settings as a function of environmental and play variables. Although the system does not examine types of single words used, it documents whether the child is using single-word, multiword or gestural communications.

Prior to the first word combinations, Dore et al. (1976) noted another transitional phenomenon known as the *presyntactic device* (PSD). Dore stated that a syntactic utterance is one in which two words that have a meaning relationship are combined under the same intonational pattern (e.g., "mommy go"). A presyntactic device is the combination of two elements under an intonation contour that does not have a meaning relation because one element is not a real word, or because the word combination is reduplicated or a highly learned "rote production." Thus a child who says /WIKITI/ is combining a real word (KITI) with a nonword (WI) under an intonation contour. Other presyntactic transitional elements that have been reported are empty forms, which are consistently used productions that appear to be nonsense words (e.g., "wida," "gocking," etc.) (Bloom, 1973; Leonard, 1975). Bloom (1970) reports the use of two single words that have a meaning relationship with a pause inserted between the two elements (e.g., "car . . . go"). All of these presyntactic devices prepare a child to combine two meaningful language elements under an intonation pattern that is the essence of early multiword combinations.

Early Multiword Utterances. Perhaps the most researched and reported period of language acquisition is the time when children begin to combine lexical items to form meaning relationships (semantic relations). There has been a long history of interpreting these early utterances as traditional parts of speech (e.g., noun, verb), telegraphic speech (Brown & Fraser, 1963), pivot/open classes (Braine, 1963), and underlying structures of transformational grammar (McNeill, 1970). Currently, many authorities support a semantic view of early multiword utterances using a case grammar (Fillmore, 1968) and have rendered interpretations of early utterances using semantic relations (Bloom, 1970; Bloom & Lahey, 1978; Bowerman, 1974; Brown, 1973; Leonard, 1976; Schlessinger, 1974). Some of the basic early multiword constructions are composed of the semantic cases (Brown, 1973) in Figure 4.3. Note that these basic semantic relations code aspects of the world that the child has learned about during the sensorimotor period of cognitive development, and this is one reason that some authorities have indicated the strong cross-cultural similarities in early utterances (Brown, 1973). There are many more "fine grained" analyses of children's early multiword utterances (Bloom, Lightbrown, & Hood, 1975; Braine, 1976; Leonard, 1976) and the basic relation types in Figure 4.3 are included in these analyses along with some other more subtle distinctions. Semantic relations must always be interpreted in light of the nonverbal context surrounding the utterance. The main point here is that children begin to use word combinations that code various common relationships in their environments, and if we merely assign adult, syntactic categories (e.g., noun, verb) to the utterances we miss some of the skill that children have in coding rather subtle relations cognitively understood in the sensorimotor period.

Nomination + X	"This ball"
Recurrence + X	"More milk"
Nonexistence + X	"Allgone egg"
Agent + action	"Mommy run"
Action + object	"Hit ball"
Agent + object	"Mommy shoe"
Action + locative	"Go outside"
Entity + locative	"Ball kitchen"
Possessor + possession	"Mommy skirt"
Entity + attribute	"Ball red"
Agent + action + object	"Mommy hit ball"
Agent + action + locative	"Mommy run outside"

Figure 4.3   Semantic Relations Reported by Brown (1973)

This has been termed a "rich interpretation" by Brown (1973) and gives the child credit for being able to talk about various relationships that syntactic metrics do not. As in the single-word period, these semantic relations are used for various functions; that is, agent + action can be used as a comment/label (e.g., "mommy run"—when a child points to mother jogging) or as a regulatory statement (e.g., "mommy push"—when the child is trying to get mother to push the wagon). According to authorities, it is wise to always consider both the structure (form) and use (function) of early multiword utterances (Bloom & Lahey, 1978; McLean & Snyder-McLean, 1978). There is a more recent move toward not using a priori semantic relation categories and giving a child credit for a multiword relation only after he has demonstrated "productivity" of use (Lund & Duchan, 1988; Howe, 1976; Leonard, Steckol, & Panther, 1983).

    As mentioned previously, there are existing methods of viewing and analyzing early semantic relations in children's utterances (Bloom, 1973; Braine, 1976; Brown, 1973; Leonard, 1976). We have also discussed a number of systems for examining communicative functions in children (Dore, 1976; Halliday, 1975). However, few systems exist that interactively analyze structure and function in early utterances. Bloom and Lahey (1978) have described an analysis system that takes into account structure and function. The system suggests that the clinician transcribe the child's utterances, the adult's utterances, and the nonverbal communicative contextual events that are relevant to the communication. Bloom and Lahey (1978) and Lahey (1988) prefer the use of videotape in recording a sample for use in their analysis since all linguistic and contextual information can be preserved and reviewed. If videotape equipment is unavailable, they recommend using audiotape and transcribing the nonlinguistic context. Finally, Bloom and Lahey (1978) and Lahey (1988) recommend the use of hand transcription if it is not feasible to use instrumentation. They indicate that hand transcription is the least accurate of the three methods of recording because it must be done "online." Using notes is helpful in noisy situations where taping is not feasible. It is also possible to transcribe each third or fourth utterance instead of every one. Bloom and Lahey recommend that the beginning clinician begin by gaining practice with a particular coding taxonomy through carefully scoring videotaped sessions. When speed and reliability are increased, then hand transcriptions may be easier and more accurate.

At the very least, we recommend that the clinician observe the child in an interaction with caretakers, teachers, or children so he/she can transcribe the child's utterances and note the context of communication. We feel that the following assumptions are important in a basic early multiword assessment:

1. It is important to determine if there is a "basic" set of semantic relations or if there is a limited usage of just a few relations in a child's language (Lahey, 1988; McLean & Snyder-McLean, 1978).
2. A child should be able to verbally code many relationships and aspects of the environment.
3. The clinician should obtain an inventory of communicative functions (uses) used by a child to determine if there is a "basic set" of uses of language (Wetherby et al., 1988).
4. Structure and function should be viewed interactively (Bloom & Lahey, 1978; Lahey, 1988; Muma, 1978).
5. The clinician may find it valuable to get a feeling for the percent of time a child initiates language versus adult-initiated utterances (Bloom & Lahey, 1978; Wetherby et al., 1988).
6. The clinician must be able to analyze utterances between 1–4 words in length.
7. Early multiwords are analyzed differently from later syntax typically using semantic grammars (Bloom & Lahey, 1978; Bowerman, 1973; Brown, 1973; Leonard et al., 1983).
8. The clinician should be sensitive to later developing forms present with the early multiwords (e.g., word endings, function words) to project development into later stages (Lahey, 1988; Miller, 1981).

A number of taxonomies could be used in assigning semantic cases to early multiword utterances. Since neither function nor semantic relations can be assigned without taking into account the context in which they occur, the clinician must become quite familiar with the cases and functions in her coding system so she can immediately assign functions and cases to utterances as they occur. If the clinician is present in the context, this could save much time since nonverbal and verbal contributions of others need not be transcribed. The clinician can simply make an immediate judgment about structure and function based on a limited set of cases and uses. If a clinician is viewing videotape or listening to audiotape, notation about the nonlinguistic context should be made on the transcription sheet. Appendix C contains a suggested transcription sheet for use with the analysis. The clinician should first write down the child's utterance either phonetically or orthographically, then follow this with the immediate interpretation of a semantic relation and function. Thus, the first three columns can be filled out at the time of each utterance. This procedure could be used as a preliminary part of an assessment to find out basic semantic relations and functions in a child's communication (Taenzer, Harris, & Bass, 1975). It can also be carried forward as a means for monitoring treatment progress. From the data, later analysis can determine the percent of child-initiated versus adult-initiated utterances as well as the percent use of each function and semantic relation in the sample. The remaining columns (4–5) of the transcription sheet can be filled out by the clinician subsequent to the evaluation session and used to complete the summary sheet. A summary sheet is presented in Appendix D. Bloom and Lahey (1978) indicate that an immediate note-taking system is not necessarily the ideal way to analyze early multiword utterances for the busy clinician. Similarly, Lahey states:

> Thus, the use of handwritten notes as a method of recording behavior does offer possibilities to the overscheduled clinician who feels that tape-recorded observations are an extreme burden and therefore language samples are an impossible assessment procedure. Videotaped or audiotaped observations are the preferred methods of recording language samples, but a record of utterances and context provided by on site hand notes is better than no sample at all and is worthy of considerations if the limitations are fully recognized. (1988, p. 296)

The disadvantages of making handwritten notes are (1) the clinician must make an immediate decision about the form and function based on knowledge of the context. This is difficult at first but becomes easier as the clinician becomes familiar with the coding system. Many of the child's utterances will be quite clear in terms of form and function but a core of them will be more problematic. (2) The categories the clinician selects for form and use are determined a priori and may bias the view of the child's system (Leonard, Steckol, & Panther, 1983). This is true of any system approach. It is, however, better to use a system that looks at structure and function interactively rather than one that does not. Most often, the client enrolled in treatment for noninitiation of language (a problem with function) also has structural problems. In a child at the early multiword level, we do not often target for function alone, and it is not often that we concentrate only on structure to the exclusion of use. (3) The online method will necessarily miss some utterances and thus the clinician should realize that the data are incomplete. (4) As the child's MLU and volume of utterances increases, the utility of online transcription decreases and tape recordings must be used or the target of assessment narrowed severely to include only one or two specific forms (e.g., Belkin, 1975). When a child is leaving the early multiword period, he/she has reached a mean length of utterance of over 2.25. At this point, the acquisition of a variety of syntactic conventions begins to emerge.

Assessment of Children's Early Language Comprehension

Perhaps the area of children's linguistic assessment that has been the subject of the most test development has been language comprehension. A major reason behind the development of language comprehension tests is the longstanding belief that in language acquisition, reception precedes expression. The implication, then, is that one must understand language in order to adequately express it. Historically, programs for language training have been organized in terms of receptive or comprehension modules first, followed by expressive language training. Bloom (1974) discussed some basic differences between expression and reception of language. She brings up the important point that children's responses to language are multidetermined. That is, a child's correct response could be primarily in reaction to nonverbal contextual aspects of the situation. Following is a typical scenario:

> The mother says, "He can understand everything that we tell him. He just doesn't talk." The clinician leans forward and says, "Can you show me how you know he understands what you tell him?" The mother shifts uncomfortably in her chair and tells the child to "go turn off the light," as she points alternately between the light switch and the ceiling fixture. The child turns the light off and on several times. Later when the mother was told to provide only verbal stimuli, the child was not able to perform many one- and two-level commands if they were unaccompanied by gestures.

Thus, children and adults rely on the context in which language is used to aid in the interpretation of what was said. Young children, between the ages of two and six are especially dominated by perception and tend to understand things in terms of how they appear rather than by the language or logic that is used to explain events (Ginsburg & Opper, 1969).

In 1978, Chapman discussed the notion of *comprehension strategies* exhibited by children. According to Chapman, a comprehension strategy is

> a short cut, heuristic or algorithm for arriving at sentence meaning without full marshalling of the information in the sentence and one's linguistic knowledge. Thus, it sometimes yields the correct answer, although it may more usually give the appearance of understanding. (1978, p. 310)

Clinicians who attempt to assess early language comprehension should be wary of correct responses by children that could have been generated by attention to contextual stimuli or comprehension strategies. An example is that many children process the name of an object and then they act on the object in a habitual manner. This gives the appearance of knowing an entire sentence (e.g., "throw the ball") when in actuality, the child may understand only the word "ball" and simply throws it as he usually does. Chapman gives many other comprehension strategies and we encourage clinicians to become familiar with these patterns.

We have suggested that comprehension is difficult to test without contaminating influences from the context and comprehension strategies. Further, we have said that failure to perform well on a test of comprehension does not necessarily indicate the presence of a comprehension disorder. Based on the current literature, about all we can say with some conviction is that adequate performance on a standardized test of language comprehension probably means that the child is capable of comprehending some language in a highly artificial situation. This does not necessarily represent his/her comprehension in natural situations. Failure of a comprehension test, on the other hand, does not necessarily mean that the child is incapable of comprehending language in either the contrived testing situation or the natural environment. Understanding of single words in young children appears to us to be testable. If they direct their attention to or will retrieve the appropriate object when its name is uttered by an examiner (with appropriate controls for contextual cues), they probably recognize the lexical item. We begin to run into trouble when we try to test two-word utterances and longer sentences. Some attempts have been made to remove the effects of context by using anomalous commands in testing children (Duchan & Siegel, 1979; Kramer, 1977). This involves giving commands to children that are not likely to be expected from their past experience. A child may be told to "sit on the ball" or "kiss the phone." If the child performs, she is said to have comprehended both elements in the command. If the child does not perform (and this is where we run into the problem again) is it that she has not understood? Perhaps anomalous commands are "silly" to children and are disregarded. There may be a cognitive mismatch between the command and the child's knowledge of the object's typical use. At any rate, failure to perform an anomalous command may not really mean lack of comprehension. The clinician should also not avoid more naturalistic assessment methods such as engaging the child in play or conversation and evaluating the appropriateness of verbal and nonverbal responses.

Assessment of Utterances Using Length Measures

One of the most common measures recommended for use in a basic language evaluation is the mean length of utterance (MLU) (Miller, 1981). Length measures are not new in speech pathology and were used historically as a mainstay of our clinical armamentarium (Johnson, Darley, & Spriestersbach, 1963). There are several reasons that authorities have continued to recommend computing a length measure on utterances obtained in a language sample. First, there is a general correlation between the MLU and chronological age in many groups of children up to age four (Miller, 1981). Thus, the MLU may be used as a very gross indicator of language development in children up to that age, but the clinician cannot simply rely on length measures alone in an analysis. A second important reason for computing MLU on a child is that Brown (1973) has used this length measure to demarcate his five stages of language development. Allegedly, MLU is a much better predictor of language development than chronological age. Brown (1973) has postulated that if two children are matched on MLU, a clinician may predict that the constructional complexity of their language will be similar. Brown (1973) and Miller (1981) provide suggestions for the computation of MLU (Table 4.4 is from Brown). Miller (1981) recommends a distributional analysis to ensure that the MLU has a relatively normal distribution around an average length. The analysis is simply a listing of the number of utterances at each morpheme level (e.g., 1, 2, 3, 4). If the distributional analysis reveals an MLU with a small variation, perhaps an organic condition or sampling error has played a role in the length of utterance. Chapman and Miller (1981) report normative data for MLU (see Table 4.5) and research on temporal reliability on older children has been published (Chabon, Udolf, & Egolf, 1982). The latter investigators report that MLU has weak temporal reliability (stability over time) in older children and its use for prediction of language level may be less sensitive than previously thought.

There may be some difficulties with MLU as it is presently computed (Muma, 1983), and some investigators report stronger relationships between

Table 4.4   Rules for Calculating Mean Length of Utterance and Upper Bound

1. Start with the second page of the transcription unless that page involves a recitation of some kind. In this latter case start with the first recitation-free stretch. Count the first 100 utterances satisfying the following rules.

2. Only fully transcribed utterances are used; none with blanks. Portions of utterances, entered in parentheses to indicate doubtful transcription, are used.

3. Include all exact utterance repetitions (marked with a plus sign in records). Stuttering is marked as repeated efforts at a single word; count the word once in the most complete form produced. In the few cases where a word is produced for emphasis or the like (*no, no, no*) count each occurrence.

4. Do not count such fillers as *mm* or *oh*, but do count *no, yeah,* and *hi.*

5. All compound words (two or more free morphemes), proper names, and ritualized reduplications count as single words. Examples: *birthday, rackety-boom, choo-choo, quack-quack, night-night, pocketbook, see saw.* Justification is that no evidence that the constituent morphemes function as such for these children.

6. Count as one morpheme all irregular pasts of the verb (*got, did, went, saw*). Justification is that there is no evidence that the child relates these to present forms.

7. Count as one morpheme all diminutives (*doggie, mommie*) because these children at least do not seem to use the suffix productively. Diminutives are the standard forms used by the child.

8. Count as separate morphemes all auxiliaries (*is, have, will, can, must, would*). Also all catenatives: *gonna, wanna, hafta.* These latter counted as single morphemes rather than as *going to* or *want to* because evidence is that they function so for the children. Count as separate morphemes all inflections, for example, possessive {s}, plural {s}, third person singular {s}, regular past {d}, progressive {in}.

9. The range count follows the above rules but is always calculated for the total transcription rather than for 100 utterances.

From: Brown, R. (1973). *A First Language: The Early Stages,* Cambridge: Harvard University Press, Used with permission. © 1973 by the President and Fellows of Harvard College.

Table 4.5   Predicted MLU Ranges and Linguistic Stages of Children Within One Predicted Standard Deviation of Predicted Mean Length of Utterance

AGE ± 1 MO.	PREDICTED MLU[a]	PREDICTED SD[b]	PREDICTED MLU ± 1 SD (middle 68%)
18	1.31	0.325	0.99–1.64
21	1.62	0.386	1.23–2.01
24	1.92	0.448	1.47–2.37
27	2.23	0.510	1.72–2.74
30	2.54	0.571	1.97–3.11
33	2.85	0.633	2.22–3.48
36	3.16	0.694	2.47–3.85
39	3.47	0.756	2.71–4.23
42	3.78	0.817	2.96–4.60
45	4.09	0.879	3.21–4.97
48	4.40	0.940	3.46–5.34
51	4.71	1.002	3.71–5.71
54	5.02	1.064	3.96–6.08
57	5.32	1.125	4.20–6.45
60	5.63	1.187	4.44–6.82

[a]MLU is predicted from the equation MLU = $-0.548 + 0.103$ (AGE).
[b]SD is predicted from the equation SD MLU = $-0.446 + 0.0205$ (AGE).

From: Miller, J. and Chapman, R. (1981). Research note: The relation between age and mean length of utterance in morphemes. *Journal of Speech and Hearing Research,* 24, 154–161. Used with permission.

MLU and language ability if the measure is computed with single-word utterances removed (Klee & Fitzgerald, 1983). The norms for MLU are presently reported on a rather narrow population and further data gathering is necessary. The use of MLU may presently be in a state of transition, but until more conclusive data and viable alternatives are provided, we feel that MLU should be routinely calculated in a language evaluation of limited-language children.

Infant, Toddler, and Family Assessment

Public Law 99-457 mandates that the speech-language pathologist assess and treat children between the ages of three and five. Speech-language pathologists in many states are currently serving the birth to five population, and this will no doubt become the norm before the current decade is over. This section provides some references for SLPs faced with the assessment of infants and toddlers in hospital and clinical settings.

Many different infants and children are at risk for communication disorders. There are many syndromes (e.g., Turner's, 18Q, Down, Hurlers, Morquio, Goldenhar, Mohr, Treacher-Collins) with associated speech, language, and hearing problems (Clark, 1989). Also, communication disorders can result from a variety of other sources, such as environmental toxins (e.g., mercury, lead, cadmium, fetal alcohol exposure), infections prior to birth (e.g., syphilis, rubella, congenital cytomegaloviris, toxoplasmosis), or postnatally acquired infections (e.g., herpes, otitis, streptococcus infections). Premature infants and those suffering early respiratory distress or intracranial hemorrhages are also high risk for communication disorders. The SLP is more frequently involved than ever before on evaluation and intervention teams working with these high-risk infants and their families. Often, this population is intimidating to those without experience serving infants and toddlers.

Assessment of infants and toddlers must involve several components: (1) assessment of the infant; (2) assessment of the family situation; (3) assessment of the primary caregiver; and (4) assessment of caregiver-child interaction patterns.

Sparks (1989) provides some general guidelines for assessment of the infant. First, the SLP should become intimately familiar with the child's prenatal and perinatal history so that he/she can try to predict which types of communication disorders are likely to be associated with a particular syndrome or condition. This allows the SLP to take preventive measures against a variety of secondary impairments. Second, we should gain a general appreciation of the infant's ability to maintain homeostasis. This means learning how individual infants cope with handling, when they lose control, and how we need to help them maintain respiration, thermal control, and proper nutrition (Sparks, 1989). Frequently used measures for this are the *Neonatal Behavioral Assessment* (Brazelton, 1984) or the *Assessment of Preterm Infant Behavior* (Als et al., 1982). Third, the child's oral-motor behavior is an important skill to evaluate. Proctor (1989) provides an excellent description of vocal development and a detailed assessment protocol for use in evaluating infant oral-vocal skills. Finally, the infant's hospital environment should be examined in terms of available stimulation and opportunities for communication. Often, these children are in neonatal intensive care units (NICU) or in other hospital units, and these environments provide the only exposure to communication to which the child has access.

Some team member, perhaps the SLP if he/she is the case manager, will participate in a family strength and needs assessment. Bailey and Simeonsson (1988) provide procedures and suggestions for family assessment. With infants and toddlers, the assessments of family status and interaction patterns are as important or even more significant than evaluation of the child. Without an intact family that functions adequately as a system, the planning and implementation of intervention cannot take place. Also, PL 99-457 requires an Individualized Family Service Plan (IFSP), which specifies not only goals for the child, but objectives for the family as a unit. Thus, assessment of infants and toddlers typically involves a team approach with the SLP working closely with social workers, psychologists, medical professionals, early childhood special educators, and others.

In terms of evaluating caregiver-infant interactions, a number of potential schemes are available (Cole & St. Clair-Stokes, 1984; Duchan & Weitzner-Lin, 1987; Klein & Briggs, 1987; Lifter et al., 1988; McCollum & Stayton, 1985; Wetherby et al., 1988). We are also interested in more basic issues such as availability of the caregiver and caregiver expectations about communication. The actual analysis of caregiver-child interaction embodies many behaviors discussed earlier in this chapter. The reader should examine some of the references listed here for specific procedures.

Assessment of Special Populations

The nature of communication/language and the model that we subscribe to does not change with the client; therefore, the assessment of special populations should not be dramatically different from that of developmentally language-disordered children. That is, our goal is still to assess the integrity of the communication system (cognitive, linguistic, social, pragmatic) and this process should be in operation regardless of etiology. We feel, as Bloom and Lahey (1978) and Lahey (1988) have indicated, that the diagnostic group a child belongs to contributes little insight into his/her language impairment. Certainly, however, there are some characteristics that are important to consider in evaluating specific populations. Lahey (1988) provides an excellent summary of the research on communication skills associated with specific language-impaired, hearing-impaired, autistic, mentally retarded, acquired aphasia, learning-disabled, and blind populations. The clinician should be familiar with this research because it helps in parent counseling as well as in knowing what to expect in an evaluation session. It is our view that the basic assessment of the communication of any client should focus on the process from an integrative vantage point. Thus, whether the clinician is confronted with a mentally retarded, autistic, or hearing-impaired child, the major task remains to determine the child's linguistic structural capability, presence of cognitive/social/biological prerequisites to language, as well as exploring the child's use of language in the environment.

Dealing with special populations increases the probability of having to assess biological, social, and cognitive prerequisites to language. Clearly, a mentally retarded child is, by definition, cognitively impaired (Cosby & Ruder, 1983; Kamhi & Johnston, 1982; Rogers, 1977; Weisz & Zigler, 1979). The clinician must be certain that the child possesses the cognitive holdings necessary for learning a particular symbol system (objects, pictures, words, gestures, etc.). Autistic children have also been reported to have cognitive difficulties and the clinician should attempt to gain insight into this area in the evaluation (Clune, Paolella, & Foley, 1979; Curcio, 1978; Rutter, 1978). This is a difficult enterprise, at best. Autistic children are frequently reported to be socially withdrawn and their general nonverbal social interaction may have to be modified in treatment before they can be expected to use functional communication (Baltaxe & Simmons, 1975; Opitz, 1982).

While many autistic children are unusual, the domains assessed in children with autism are identical to those previously advocated for any language-impaired child (Prizant & Wetherby, 1988). Thus, one implication of special populations is that they may involve the clinician in more broad-based analysis of both precommunicative as well as communicative behaviors presented by the child.

Another aspect involved in dealing with a special population is that the clinician has an increased probability of prescribing a nonverbal/nonvocal response mode or prosthetic communication device. Recent research has shown that both mentally retarded and autistic children may benefit from training in gestural communication modes (Silverman, 1989). Thus, it may be incumbent on the diagnostician to determine the potential that a given client may have for learning a nonvocal system. Shane and Bashir (1980), Coleman, Cook, and Meyers (1980) and Owens and House (1984) provide some guidelines for considering a nonvocal communication system with severely involved clients. Clinicians who do formal evaluations in the area of augmentative communication should have specialized training and experience in this field prior to prescribing a nonvocal mode for a client.

Special populations, as a whole, generally have a poorer prognosis than language-impaired children without complicating difficulties. The prognosis worsens in proportion to the number of ancillary problems that the child exhibits (hearing impairment, neuromotor involvement, mental retardation, absent caretakers, etc.). Also, the existence of ancillary problems increases the likelihood that a larger multidisciplinary team will be involved in the evaluation. The assistance of special educators, audiologists, psychologists, and medical personnel is necessary and invaluable to the clinician in making treatment recommendations for children from special populations. As dictated by federal legislation (PL 94-142; PL 99-457), the speech pathologist has the opportunity to collaborate in staffings with other professionals to discuss assessment and treatment of language-disordered children. We have found this, in most cases, to be stimulating and in the best interest of all concerned (especially in early-language cases).

With certain types of children, the diagnostician should make an inventory of characteristic behaviors that may need to be modified in the treatment program. For instance, both autistic and mentally retarded children have been reported to engage in self-stimulatory behaviors (arm flapping, masturbation, rocking, etc.). Some authorities believe that new learning cannot effectively take place while the child is in a self-stimulatory state. Thus, one goal of treatment might be to reduce the occurrence of self-stimulation and these behaviors should be catalogued by the diagnostician. Alternatively, some self-stimulatory acts can even be used as reinforcers in more structured types of treatment. With autistic and other behavior-disordered children, self-abusive behaviors have been reported. These should also be noted by the clinician as potential treatment targets.

MEASURING CLINICAL EFFECTIVENESS

In the continuing process of evaluation of limited-language clients, there are a number of possible measurements that can be derived from research and clinical practice. The measure taken largely depends on the goals of the treatment program and can encompass cognitive, social, and communicative domains.

Cognitive Measures

In cases where the clinician is targeting conceptual goals for a limited-language child (e.g., nonverbal), a number of naturalistic measurements can be taken. For example, an ongoing goal for a cognitively delayed child might be to increase the number of objects he/she can use functionally while engaging in language treatment. Thus, the number of different episodes of functional object use can be plotted over time. Also, the percent of time during a session that a child spends in productive play (functional object use) can be plotted over time. This might be important for a child whose play is primitive (e.g., mouthing, banging, running around). If specific cognitive goals (e.g., means-end, object permanence) are targeted in treatment, some criterion-related measures such as the *Ordinal Scales of Psychological Development* (Uzgiris & Hunt, 1975) might be given on a pretest–posttest basis. There are also various scales for measuring levels of symbolic play (Nicolich, 1977) that could show gains in the quality and quantity of pretending with objects.

Social Measures

There are a host of different measurements on caretaker behaviors that could be applied to ongoing evaluation of a limited-language child. This would be especially applicable in cases where the caretaker was a major focus of treatment in terms of altering interactive behaviors. Specific percentages of caretaker language uses, such as requests for imitation, requests for action, label/comments, use of language stimulation techniques, or use of acknowledgments could be monitored over time to reflect the effects of parent counseling and training. If the focus of caretaker treatment was to modify joint referencing behaviors, these could be operationally defined and quantified. It may be desirable to train some caretakers to follow their child's lead more during interactions; thus, the relative percentage of adult- versus child-initiated play or interaction could be recorded over time.

In examining the child's social behaviors, a variety of different types of data could be kept. If a child did not engage in many social interactions with others, the frequency and duration spent in social interactions could be recorded and plotted over time. If initiation of interaction is a problem, data could be acquired on the number and types of child-initiated interactions during treatment and generalization sessions. The language functions mentioned earlier in the chapter could also be targeted in treatment and specific percentages of language uses plotted over time as each is specifically made the focus of therapy.

Linguistic Measures

Clearly, the goal for a nonverbal child would be to use single words in communicative interactions. We would want to expand the vocabulary of a nonverbal child and increase the use of verbal coding of communicative intents. It is assumed that if our goal is to increase verbal productions, that the child is exhibiting communicative intents through nonverbal means such as pointing and physical regulation of adults. Data could be gathered on the frequency and types of verbal responses and also their functions in communications. In this way the SLP could plot the occurrences over time and focus intervention on form, function, or both for a given child.

The goal for a single-word child would be to expand the size of the lexicon and/or to begin use of early multiword combinations. The types of word combinations used (semantic relations) and the variety of these multiword utterances would be important data for the SLP to gather. The functions used in multiword communication can also be monitored to ensure that the child is using a variety of word combinations for a spectrum of different communicative intents. The earlier section on analysis of multiword utterances would be helpful here.

Again, it can be seen that there is no one test that the SLP can use to monitor treatment progress. Naturalistic sampling is the best way for us to document real language usage in relevant environments and is the most potent testimony to our intervention efforts. Nevertheless, formal tests have their place in assessment and evaluation of limited-language children.

USE OF TESTS AND FORMAL PROCEDURES
WITH LIMITED-LANGUAGE CHILDREN

Only two decades ago, there were few assessment instruments available to the speech-language pathologist for use with children having limited language. This is not necessarily because speech-language pathologists were uninterested in preschool children—we have always dealt with youngsters of this age. There have been several recent influences on test development that have increased the construction of instruments appropriate for the preschool, or limited-language, population. First of all, PL 99-457 mandates that preschool children between the ages of three and five years will be dealt with by clinicians working in the public school setting. It is only a matter of time until the public school SLP will be responsible for children from birth onward. Indeed, in many states, SLPs are currently dealing with the birth to five population. With the enactment of federal legislation, test developers have increased their efforts in devising test instruments for preschoolers. The second influence on test development has been the significant strides that we have made in communication development research in the past 20 years. Much early research on language development focused on syntax and provided little information on the early stages of language learning. Most of the critical information about the integrative processes of cognitive, social, and linguistic acquisition has been produced since 1970. In light of the increased knowledge about early language development and the passage of federal legislation emphasizing preschoolers, there has been a recent proliferation of test instruments for this population. As we mentioned in Chapter 3 on psychometric considerations, the development of a plethora of tests does not necessarily mean that these instruments are superior to nonstandardized procedures for evaluating communication. In fact, most of the instruments mentioned in the following discussion do not do an adequate job of assessing cognitive, social, and linguistic parameters of communication. We would be remiss, however, if we did not mention some guidelines on the use of formal tests with limited-language children.

We can divide the preschool tests dealing with communication into several categories. First, there are large test batteries that include language or communication as one aspect of assessment. For example, a general test instrument often referred to is the *Battelle Developmental Inventory (BDI)* (see Table 4.6). This instrument is a standardized battery that includes sections on motor skill, cognition, personal-social behavior, adaptive behavior, and communication. The portion dealing with communication is necessarily incomplete and superficial since the entire battery must examine so many different domains. This general battery, however, could suggest that a child's communication development may be delayed in comparison to the norming sample, and herein lies the value of the test (problem–no problem issue). Certainly, the test could never tell a clinician specific aspects of communication that are delayed or suggest treatment objectives.

On a more specific level, there are tests that focus completely on language and communication. These instruments may be helpful to the speech-language pathologist in providing direction toward areas in need of probing through nonstandardized methods. Table 4.7 includes a selected list of instruments that could be applied to limited-language cases. Some of these are standardized, norm-referenced tests, and others may be criterion-referenced. The inclusion on this list does not suggest that the measures meet rigid psychometric standards; in most cases, the devices do not. It is the view of the present authors that the administration of *any* of these instruments is *never* a substitute for naturalistic assessment and should always be done *in addition to* nonstandardized

Table 4.6 General Developmental Measures

Battelle Developmental Inventory
    Publisher: DLM Teaching Resources

Brigance Diagnostic Inventory of Early Development
    Publisher: Curriculum Associates, Inc.

Denver Developmental Screening Test
    Publisher: University of Colorado Medical Center

Developmental Programming for Infants and Young Children
    Publisher: University of Michigan Press

Developmental Indicators for the Assessment of Learning (DIAL-R)
    Publisher: Childcraft Education Corporation

Hawaii Early Learning Profile
    Publisher: VORT Corporation

McCarthy Scales of Children's Abilities
    Publisher: The Psychological Corporation

Miller Assessment for Preschoolers
    Publisher: American Guidance Service

Minnesota Child Development Inventory
    Publisher: Behavior Science Systems, Inc.

Vineland Adaptive Behavior Scales
    Publisher: American Guidance Service

Table 4.7 Communication/Language Measures

Assessing Prelinguistic and Early Linguistic Behaviors in Developmentally Young Children
    Publisher: University of Washington Press

Birth to Three Assessment and Intervention System
    Publisher: DLM Teaching Resources

Bracken Basic Concept Scale
    Publisher: The Psychological Corporation

Cognitive, Linguistic and Social Communicative Scales
    Publisher: Modern Education Corporation

Cognitive Abilities Scale
    Publisher: Pro-Ed

Early Language Milestone Scale
    Publisher: Modern Education Corporation

Evaluating Acquired Skills in Communication (EASIC)
    Publisher: Communication Skill Builders

Individualized Assessment and Treatment for Autistic and Developmentally Disabled Children
    Publisher: Pro-Ed

Preschool Language Scale
    Publisher: The Psychological Corporation

Preverbal Assessment-Intervention Profile (PAIP)
    Publisher: ASIEP Education Co.

Program for the Acquisition of Language with the Severely Impaired (PALS)
    Publisher: Charles E. Merrill

Receptive-Expressive Emergent Language Scale (REEL)
    Publisher: Pro-Ed

evaluation tasks. These measures should satisfy any administrative requirements on obtaining scores in assessment imposed by work settings. They could also prove useful as a beginning point for naturalistic evaluation tasks.

CONSOLIDATING DATA AND ARRIVING AT TREATMENT RECOMMENDATIONS

To a certain degree, even if the diagnostician adheres to an integrative model of language, the assessment process tends to fragment the child and the information obtained in the evaluation. Before arriving at treatment recommendations, suggestions for further testing, and/or referral decisions, the clinician should pause and take stock of what has been done in the assessment process. We have found it useful and insightful to summarize the following areas (see Appendix D):

Data Obtained in the Evaluation.   This section refers to the actual behaviors observed and procedures administered to a child in the evaluation. It does not include the different analyses of the data. For instance, a spontaneous language sample can be subjected to a variety of analyses (MLU, form-function analysis, phonological analysis, etc.). Often, at the end of an evaluation, a clinician will be struck by the need for additional data that may be obtained in the initial phase of treatment. We sometimes wonder why we cannot make clinical judgments about certain aspects of a child's language, and then we find that we did not gather all of the data necessary to make these decisions. Appendix D provides a checklist for clinicians to use in summarizing the data collected. Where blanks are provided, specific measures should be filled in if applicable.

Analyses Performed on the Data.   This section allows the clinician to summarize the analysis procedures performed on the data collected. Each analysis procedure should be specified by name. On the surface, this procedure may appear to be rather simplistic; however, language has so many aspects that may be important to assess, and it is easy to forget to gather certain data or perform certain analyses.

Remarks on the Data.   This section is intended for the clinician to comment on any remarkable findings or difficulties in the data gathering. If the parents were hostile or the formal testing was considered unreliable due to fatigue, report such data here.

Synthesis of the Findings.   In this section, the clinician makes brief summary statements about each aspect of the assessment model. Any remarkable or normal aspects of the prerequisites to communication should be noted. By making a summary statement about portions of the language assessment model and the various stages of language development, the clinician is confronted with any omissions in the data gathering or analysis. If the clinician cannot make an adequate summary statement about a child's social abilities, then he/she must make further observations. By being forced to respond with a summation of each relevant area in the assessment model, a clinician can see areas of strength and weakness in a child's communication system and can be better prepared to make treatment recommendations and prognostic statements.

Areas of Concern and Strength.   By examining the summary statements about each area in the communicative process and language development stages, the clinician will be impressed with areas of normality, strength, and concern. The clinician should look for hierarchical patterns in the data that are revealed when a judgment must be made about the overall effectiveness of each area in the language model. For instance, a child may evidence summary statements in the biological prerequisite area that indicate concern over poor motor coordination and remarkable birth and developmental histories. The same child may have performed poorly on cognitive tasks and the clinician questions the child's conceptual basis for language development. Similarly, on social areas of the model, the child is not operating according to age level and is not exhibiting optimal social prerequisites for communication. Adaptive behavior scales show a delay in all areas of development. In the language development area, the child turns out to be nonverbal. When the clinician checks the areas of concern and strength, based on the summary statements, the child will get a minus $(-)$ for biological prerequisites and minuses for social and cognitive prerequisites as well. The child will also receive a minus for delayed language. If no clear-cut statement for concern or strength can be made, then the clinician should examine the data gathered and the analyses performed to determine if enough information has been accumulated. In most cases, an inability to make a general statement about areas of the model is due to insufficient information, poor quality information, or insufficient analysis.

Recommendations.   The areas that are covered in the recommendation section revolve around four topics. First, the child may require referral to other professionals to obtain further information. For instance, referral to a psychologist or special educator may be warranted to determine the child's mental ability and potential for learning. Audiometric referral may be another common need.

Second, the clinician may have been unable to perform certain tests or analyses due to time constraints or lack of cooperation from the child. Before specific treatment recommendations can be made, it may be that more data are required. By examining the sections on data obtained and analyses performed, the clinician can determine this need.

Third, if enough data were obtained and analyses performed, the clinician is in a position to make treatment recommendations. By examining the child's areas of strength and weakness, the clinician can consider intervention avenues that are the most appropriate. For instance, if a child is biologically, cognitively, and socially ready for communicative development, and the clinician has located the child in the language development process, an appropriate goal might be to begin concentrating on the language forms that develop next according to the acquisition literature and the child's need to communicate. If the child is normal in most respects and the major concern is intelligibility, then this carries with it a phonological treatment priority. If the child has cognitive and social problems in addition to language delay, then some of the treatment goals might revolve around these prerequisite areas (facilitating cognitive development, improving social nonverbal skills, etc.).

The areas of concern and strength also carry with them prognostic implications. To date, we really have no certain method of computing a given child's prognosis for success in language treatment. There are so many variables dealing with the child's capacities, skills, motivation, environment, caretaker participation, time in treatment, and other factors. One approach to prognosis that will probably reflect reality is to regard the child with fewer concerns in the major areas of the model as having a more favorable prognosis than one who has many deficiencies.

CONCLUSION

We have attempted to show that assessment of limited-language children is no simple matter. It requires the clinician to learn a multitude of skills and read a disparate literature in order to perform it competently. The diagnosis of language disorder requires more than just a single test or procedure. It demands that the clinician examine the communicative process differently for each type of child. There are high probability areas of investigation for certain types of cases, as we have tried to demonstrate. Finally, no chapter in a textbook can teach a clinician how to do a language assessment. The most we can do is to show the clinician some of the tools and procedures that authorities have indicated might be important in language diagnosis. The clinician must then read the primary sources we have cited, administer the measures to clients, and judge whether or not the information obtained is clinically useful.

BIBLIOGRAPHY

ALS, H., LESTER, B., TRONICK, E., & BRAZELTON, T. (1982). Toward a research instrument for the assessment of preterm infants' behavior (APIB). In H. Fitzgerald, B. Lester, & M. Yogman (Eds.), *Theory and research in behavioral pediatrics* (Vol. 1). New York: Plenum Press.

ALLEN, D., BLISS, L., & TIMMONS, J. (1981). Language evaluation: Science or art? *Journal of Speech and Hearing Disorders, 46,* 66–68.

ARAM, D., & NATION, J. (1975). Patterns of language behavior in children with developmental language disorders. *Journal of Speech and Hearing Research, 18,* 229–241.

ARAM, D., & NATION, J. (1982). *Child language disorders.* St. Louis, MO: C. V. Mosby Co.

BAILEY, D., & SIMEONSSON, R. (1988). Family assessment in early intervention. Columbus, OH: Merrill.

BALTAXE, C., & SIMMONS, J. (1975). Language in childhood psychosis: A review. *Journal of Speech and Hearing Disorders, 40,* 439–458.

BALTHAZAR, E. (1973). *Balthazar Scales of Adaptive Behavior II. Scales of social adaptation.* Palo Alto, CA: Consulting Psychologists Press.

BATES, E. (1976). *Language in context.* New York: Academic Press.

BATES, E., BENIGNI, L., BRETHERTON, I., CAMAIONI, L. & VOLTERRA, V. (1979). *The emergence of symbols: Cognition and communication in infancy.* New York: Academic Press.

BATES, E., BEEGHLY, M., BRETHERTON, I., HARRIS, C., MARCHMAN, V., MCNEW, S., OAKES, L., O'CONNELL, B., REZNICK, S., SHORE, C., SNYDER, L., THAL, D., VOLTERRA, V., & WHITESELL, K. (1986). *Language and gesture inventory.* Unpublished Vocabulary Checklist.

BEARD, R. (1969). *An outline of Piaget's developmental psychology for students and teachers.* New York: Basic Books.

BELKIN, A. (1975). *Investigation of the functions and forms of children's negative utterances.* Unpublished doctoral dissertation, Columbia University.

BENEDICT, H. (1975). Early lexical development: Comprehension and production. *Journal of Child Language, 6,* 183–200.

BLOOM, L. (1970). *Language development: Form and function in emerging grammars.* Cambridge, MA: MIT Press.

BLOOM, L. (1973). *One word at a time: The use of single word utterances before syntax.* The Hague: Mouton.

BLOOM, L. (1974). Talking, understanding and thinking. In R. Schiefelbusch & L. Lloyd (Eds.), *Language perspectives—Acquisition, retardation and intervention.* Baltimore: University Park Press.

BLOOM, L., & LAHEY, M. (1978). *Language development and language disorders.* New York: Wiley.

BLOOM, L., LIGHTBROWN, P., & HOOD, L. (1975). Structure and variation in child language. *Monographs of the Society for Research in Child Development, 40,* 1–41.

BLOOM, L., ROCISSANO, L., & HOOD, L. (1976). Adult-child discourse: Developmental interaction between information processing and linguistic knowledge. *Cognitive Psychology, 8,* 521–552.

BOWERMAN, M. (1973). Structural relationships in children's utterances: Syntactic or semantic? In T. Moore (Ed.), *Cognitive development and the acquisition of language.* New York: Academic Press.

BOWERMAN, M. (1974). Development of concepts underlying language. In R. Schiefelbusch & L. Lloyd (Eds.), *Language perspectives: Acquisition, retardation, and intervention,* Baltimore: University Park Press.

BRAINE, M. (1963). The ontogeny of English phrase structure: The first phrase. *Language, 39,* 1–14.

BRAINE, M. (1976). Children's first word combinations. *Monographs of the Society for Research in Child Development, 41,* 1–104.

BRAZELTON, T. (1984). *Neonatal behavior assessment scale.* Philadelphia: Lippincott.

BROWN, R. (1973). *A first language: The early stages.* Cambridge, MA: Harvard University Press.

BROWN, R., & FRASER, C. (1963). The acquisition of syntax. In C. Cofer & B. Musgrave (Eds.), *Verbal behavior and learning: Problems and processes.* New York: McGraw-Hill.

CARROW-WOOLFOLK, E., & LYNCH, J. (1982). *An integrative approach to language disorders in children.* New York: Grune & Stratton.

CHABON, S., UDOLF, L., & EGOLF, D. (1982). The temporal reliability of Brown's mean length of utterance measure with post stage V children. *Journal of Speech and Hearing Research, 25,* 124–128.

CHAPMAN, R. (1978). Comprehension strategies in children. In J. Kavanagh & W. Strange (Eds.), *Speech and language in the laboratory, school and clinic,* Cambridge, MA: MIT Press.

CHAPMAN, R. (1981). Exploring children's communicative intents. In J. Miller (Ed.), *Assessing language production in children: Experimental procedures.* Baltimore: University Park Press.

CHAPPEL, G., & JOHNSON, G. (1976). Evaluation of cognitive behavior in young nonverbal children. *Language, Speech and Hearing Services in Schools, 7,* 17–27.

CHOMSKY, N. (1957). *Syntactic structures.* The Hague: Mouton.

CLARK, D. (1989). Neonates and infants at risk for hearing and speech-language disorders. *Topics in Language Disorders, 10*(1), 1–12.

CLUNE, C., PAOLELLA, J., & FOLEY, J. (1979). Free play behavior of atypical children: An approach to assessment. *Journal of Autism and Developmental Disorders, 9,* 61–72.

COGGINS, T., & CARPENTER, R. (1978). *Categories for coding prespeech intentional communication.* Unpublished manuscript, University of Washington, Seattle.

COLE, E., & ST. CLAIR-STOKES, J. (1984). Caregiver-child interactive behavior: A videotape analysis procedure. *Volta Review, 86,* 200–217.

COLEMAN, D., COOK, A., & MEYERS, L. (1980). Assessing non-oral clients for assistive communication devices. *Journal of Speech and Hearing Disorders, 45,* 515–527.

CORMAN, H., & ESCALONA, S. (1969). Stages of sensorimotor development: A replication study. *Merrill Palmer Quarterly, 15,* 351–361.

COSBY, M., & RUDER, K. (1983). Symbolic play and early language development in normal and mentally retarded children. *Journal of Speech and Hearing Research, 25,* 404–411.

CURCIO, F. (1978). Sensorimotor functioning and communication in mute autistic children. *Journal of Autism and Childhood Schizophrenia, 8,* 281–292.

DALE, P. (1976). *Language development: Structure and function.* New York: Holt, Rinehart & Winston.

DALE, P. (1980). Is early pragmatic development measureable? *Journal of Child Language, 7,* 1–12.

DEVILLIERS, J., & DEVILLIERS, P. (1978). *Language acquisition.* Cambridge, MA: Harvard University Press.

DORE, J. (1975). Holophrases, speech acts and language universals. *Journal of Child Language, 2,* 21–40.

DORE, J., et al. (1976). Transitional phenomena in early language acquisition. *Journal of Child Language, 3,* 13–28.

DUCHAN, J., & SIEGEL, L. (1979). Incorrect responses to locative commands: A case study. *Language, Speech and Hearing Services in Schools, 10,* 99–103.

DUCHAN, J., & WEITZNER-LIN, B. (1987). Nurturant-naturalistic intervention for language impaired children: Implications for planning lessons and tracking progress. *Journal of the American Speech and Hearing Association, 29*(7), 45–49.

DUNST, C. (1980). *A clinical and educational manual for use with the Uzgiris and Hunt scales of infant psychological development.* Baltimore: University Park Press.

ELDER, J., & PEDERSON, D. (1978). Preschool children's use of objects in symbolic play. *Child Development, 49,* 500–504.

FEY, M. (1986). *Language intervention with young children.* San Diego, CA: College-Hill.

FILLMORE, C. (1968). The case for case. In E. Bach & R. Harms (Eds.), *Universals in linguistic theory.* New York: Holt, Rinehart & Winston.

FOLGER, J., & CHAPMAN, R. (1978). A pragmatic analysis of spontaneous imitations. *Journal of Child Language, 5,* 25–38.

GALLAGHER, T. (1983). Preassessment: A procedure for accommodating language use variability. In T. Gallagher & C. Prutting (Eds.), *Pragmatic assessment and intervention issues in language.* San Diego, CA: College-Hill.

GARNICA, O. (1974). *Some characteristics of prosodic input to young children.* Paper presented at the SSRC Conference on Language Input and Acquisition, Boston.

GINSBURG, H., & OPPER, S. (1969). *Piaget's theory of intellectual development: An introduction.* Englewood Cliffs, NJ: Prentice Hall.

GOPNIK, A., & MELTZOFF, A. (1987). The development of categorization in the second year, and its relation to other cognitive and linguistic developments. *Child Development, 58,* 1523–1531.

HALLIDAY, M. (1975). *Learning how to mean: Explorations in the development of language.* New York: Elsevier.

HAYNES, W., & SHULMAN, B. (1992). *Communication development: Foundations and clinical applications.* Englewood Cliffs, NJ: Prentice Hall.

HEDRICK, D., PRATHER, E., & TOBIN, A. (1975). *Sequenced inventory of communication development.* Seattle: University of Washington Press.

HOLLAND, A. (1975). Language therapy for children: Some thoughts on context and content. *Journal of Speech and Hearing Disorders, 40,* 514–523.

HOWE, C. (1976). The meanings of two word utterances in the speech of young children. *Journal of Child Language, 3,* 29–47.

HUBBELL, R. (1981). *Children's language disorders: An integrated approach.* Englewood Cliffs, NJ: Prentice Hall.

JOHNSON, W., DARLEY, F., & SPRIESTERSBACH, D. (1963). *Diagnostic methods in speech pathology.* New York: Harper & Row.

KAHN, J. (1984). Cognitive training and initial use of referential speech. *Topics in Language Disorders, 5,* 14–18.

KAMHI, A., & JOHNSTON, J. (1982). Towards an understanding of retarded children's linguistic deficiencies. *Journal of Speech and Hearing Research, 25,* 435–445.

KIRK, S. & KIRK, W. (1971). *Psycholinguistic Learning Disabilities,* Rev.-Ed, Urbana: University of Illinois Press.

KLEE, T., & FITZGERALD, M. (1983). *The relation between grammatical development and mean length of utterance in morphemes.* Paper presented at the convention of the American Speech and Hearing Association, Cincinnati, OH.

KLEIN, M., & BRIGGS, M. (1987). Facilitating mother infant communicative interactions in mothers of high risk infants. *Journal of Childhood Communication Disorders, 10*(2), 95–106.

KRAMER, P. (1977). Young children's free responses to anomalous commands. *Journal of Experimental Child Psychology, 24,* 219–234.

LAHEY, M. (1988). *Language disorders and language development.* New York: Macmillan.

LAMBERT, N., WINDMILLER, M., THARINGER, D., & COLE, L. (1981). *AAMD Adaptive Behavior Scale.* Monterey, CA: Publishers Test Service.

LEONARD, L. (1975). On differentiating syntactic and semantic features in emerging grammars: Evidence from empty form usage. *Journal of Psycholinguistic Research, 4,* 357–364.

LEONARD, L. (1976). *Meaning in child language: Issues in the study of early semantic development.* New York: Grune & Stratton.

LEONARD, L. (1978). Cognitive factors in early linguistic development. In R. Schiefelbusch (Ed.), *Bases of language intervention.* Baltimore: University Park Press.

LEONARD, L., STECKOL, K., & PANTHER, K. (1983). Returning meaning to semantic relations: Some clinical applications. *Journal of Speech and Hearing Disorders, 48,* 25–35.

LIFTER, K., & BLOOM, L. (1989). Object knowledge and the emergence of language. *Infant Behavior and Development, 12,* 395–423.

LIFTER, K., EDWARDS, G., AVERY, D., ANDERSON, S., & SULZER-AZAROFF, B. (1988). *Developmental assessment of children's play: Implications for intervention.* Paper presented at the convention of the American Speech-Language-Hearing Association, Boston.

LOWE, M., & COSTELLO, A. (1976). *The symbolic play test.* London: National Foundation for Educational Research Publishing.

LUCAS, E. (1980). *Semantic and pragmatic language disorders.* Rockville, MD: Aspen Systems Corporation.

LUND, N., & DUCHAN, J. (1988). *Assessing children's language in naturalistic contexts.* Englewood Cliffs, NJ: Prentice Hall.

MCCARTHY, D. (1935). *The language development of the preschool child.* University of Minnesota Institute of Child Welfare Monograph Series IV. Minneapolis, MN: University of Minnesota Press.

McCOLLUM, J., & STAYTON, V. (1985). Social interaction assessment/intervention. *Journal of the Division for Early Childhood, 9,* 125–135.

McLEAN, J., & SNYDER-McLEAN, L. (1978). *A transactional approach to early language training.* Columbus, OH: Merrill.

McNEILL, D. (1970). *The acquisition of language: The study of developmental psycholinguistics.* New York: Harper & Row.

MERHABIAN, A., & WILLIAMS, M. (1971). Piagetian measures of cognitive development for children up to age two. *Journal of Psycholinguistic Research, 1,* 113–125.

MILLEN, K., & PRUTTING, C. (1979). Consistencies across three language comprehension tests for specific grammatical features. *Language, Speech and Hearing Services in Schools, 10,* 162–170.

MILLER, J. (1981). *Assessing Language Production in Children: Experimental Procedures,* Baltimore: University Park Press.

MILLER, J., & CHAPMAN, R. (1981). The relation between age and mean length of utterance in morphemes. *Journal of Speech and Hearing Research, 24,* 154–161.

MOREHEAD, D., & MOREHEAD, A. (1974). From signal to sign. In R. Schiefelbusch and L. Lloyd (Eds.), *Language perspectives—Acquisition, retardation and intervention.* Baltimore: University Park Press.

MUMA, J. (1973). Language assessment: Some underlying assumptions. *Journal of the American Speech and Hearing Association, 15,* 331–338.

MUMA, J. (1978). *Language handbook: Concepts, assessment, intervention.* Englewood Cliffs, NJ: Prentice Hall.

MUMA, J. (1983). Speech language pathology: Emerging clinical expertise in language. In T. Gallagher & C. Prutting (Eds.), *Pragmatic assessment and intervention issues in language.* San Diego, CA: College-Hill Press.

NATION, J., & ARAM, D. (1982). *Diagnosis of Speech and Language Disorders.* St. Louis: C. V. Mosby.

NELSON, K. (1973). Structure and strategy in learning to talk. *Monographs of the Society for Research in Child Development, 38,* 11–56.

NELSON, K. (1974). Concept, word and sentence: Interrelations in acquisition and development. *Psychological Review, 81,* 267–285.

NEWHOFF, M., & LEONARD, L. (1983). Diagnosis of developmental language disorders. In I. Meitus & B. Weinberg (Eds.), *Diagnosis in speech-language pathology.* Baltimore: University Park Press.

NICOLICH, L. (1977). Beyond sensorimotor intelligence: Assessment of symbolic maturity through analysis of pretend play. *Merrill Palmer Quarterly, 23,* 89–101.

OPITZ, V. (1982). Pragmatic analysis of the communicative behavior of an autistic child. *Journal of Speech and Hearing Disorders, 47,* 99–108.

OWENS, R. (1988). *Language development: An introduction.* Columbus, OH: Merrill.

OWENS, R., & HOUSE, L. (1984). Decision making processes in augmentative communication. *Journal of Speech and Hearing Disorders, 49,* 18–25.

PRIZANT, B., & WETHERBY, A. (1988). Providing services to children with autism (ages 0 to 2 years) and their families. *Topics in Language Disorders, 9*(1), 1–23.

PROCTOR, A. (1989). Stages of normal noncry vocal development in infancy: A protocol for assessment. *Topics in Language Disorders, 10*(1), 26–42.

Project RHISE (1974). *Manual for administration of the Rockford Infant Developmental Evaluation Scales.* Bensenville, IL: Scholastic Testing Service.

REYNELL, J. (1969). *Reynell Developmental Language Scales.* Buckinghamshire, Eng.: National Foundation for Educational Research in England and Wales.

RICE, M., SELL, M., & HADLEY, P. (1990). The social interactive coding system (SICS): An on-line, clinically relevant descriptive tool. *Language, Speech and Hearing Services in Schools, 21,* 2–14.

ROGERS, S. (1977). Characteristics of the cognitive development of profoundly retarded children. *Child Development, 48,* 837–843.

RUDER, K., & SMITH, M. (1974). Issues in language training. In R. Schiefelbusch & L. Lloyd (Eds.), *Language perspectives—Acquisition, retardation and intervention.* Baltimore: University Park Press.

RUTTER, M. (1978). Diagnosis and definition of childhood autism. *Journal of Autism and Childhood Schizophrenia, 8,* 139–169.

SCHLESINGER, I. (1974). Relational concepts underlying language. In R. Schiefelbusch & L. Lloyd (Eds.), *Language perspectives—Acquisition, retardation and intervention.* Baltimore: University Park Press.

SHANE, H., & BASHIR, A. (1980). Election criteria for the adoption of an augmentative communication system: Preliminary considerations. *Journal of Speech and Hearing Disorders, 45,* 408–444.

SIEGEL, G. (1975). The use of language tests. *Language, Speech and Hearing Services in Schools, 6,* 211–217.

SILVERMAN, F. (1989). *Communication for the speechless.* Englewood Cliffs, NJ: Prentice Hall.

SNOW, C. (1972). Mother's speech to children learning language. *Child Development, 43,* 549–565.

SNOW, C. (1977). The development of conversation between mothers and babies. *Journal of Child Language, 4,* 1–22.

SNYDER, L. (1978). Communicative and cognitive disabilities in the sensorimotor period. *Merrill Palmer Quarterly, 24,* 161–180.

SNYDER, L. (1981). Assessing communicative abilities in the sensorimotor period: Content and context. *Topics in Language Disorders, 1,* 31–46.

SNYDER-McLEAN, L., McLEAN, J., & ETTER, R. (1988). Clinical assessment of sensorimotor knowledge in nonverbal, severely retarded clients. *Topics in Language Disorders, 8,* 1–22.

SPARKS, S. (1989). Assessment and intervention with at risk infants and toddlers: Guidelines for the speech-language pathologist. *Topics in Language Disorders, 10*(1), 43–56.

STAAB, C. (1983). Language functions elicited by meaningful activities: A new dimension in language programs. *Language, Speech, and Hearing Services in Schools, 14,* 164–170.

STECKOL, K., & LEONARD, L. (1981). Sensorimotor development and the use of prelinguistic performatives. *Journal of Speech and Hearing Research, 24,* 262–268.

TAENZER, S., HARRIS, L., & BASS, M. (1975). *Assessment in a natural context.* Paper presented at the American Speech and Hearing Association National Convention, Washington, DC.

TOFFLER, A. (1981). *The third wave.* New York: Bantam Books.

TOUGH, J. (1977). *The development of meaning.* New York: Halsted Press.

TRANTHAM, C., & PEDERSEN, J. (1976). *Normal language development.* Baltimore: Williams and Wilkins.

UZGIRIS, I., & HUNT, J. (1975). *Assessment in infancy.* Urbana, IL: University of Illinois Press.

WEISS, A., LEONARD, L., ROWAN, L., & CHAPMAN, K. (1983). Linguistic and nonlinguistic features of style in normal and language impaired children. *Journal of Speech and Hearing Disorders, 48,* 154–163.

WEISZ, J., & ZIGLER, E. (1979). Cognitive development in retarded and nonretarded persons: Piagetian tests of the similar sequence hypothesis. *Psychological Bulletin, 86,* 831–851.

WESTBY, C. (1980). Assessment of cognitive and language abilities through play. *Language, Speech, and Hearing Services in Schools, 11,* 154–168.

WETHERBY, A., CAIN, D., YONCLAS, D., & WALKER, V. (1988). Analysis of intentional communication of normal children from the prelinguistic to the multiword stage. *Journal of Speech and Hearing Research, 31,* 240–252.

WETHERBY, A., & PRUTTING, C. (1984). Profiles of communicative and cognitive-social abilities in autistic children. *Journal of Speech and Hearing Research, 27,* 364–377.

WETHERBY, A., YONCLAS, D., & BRYAN, A. (1989). Communicative profiles of preschool children with handicaps: Implications for early intervention. *Journal of Speech and Hearing Disorders, 54,* 148–158.

WILCOX, M. (1984). Developmental language disorders: Preschoolers. In A. Holland (Ed.), *Language disorders in children: Recent advances.* San Diego, CA: College-Hill.

WOLFUS, B., MOSCOVITCH, M., & KINSBOURNE, M. (1980). Subgroups of developmental language impairment. *Brain and Language, 10,* 152–171.

WOOD, B. (1981). *Children and communication: Verbal and nonverbal language development.* Englewood Cliffs, NJ: Prentice Hall.

ZIMMERMAN, I., STEINER, V., & EVATT, R. (1969). *Preschool language scale.* Columbus, OH: Merrill.

5

ASSESSMENT OF SCHOOL-AGE AND ADOLESCENT LANGUAGE DISORDERS

The diagnosis and evaluation of language abilities in school-age children and adolescents have become so specialized that it warrants consideration separate from early language assessment. The days are gone when a textbook could cover language assessment from birth through adolescence in the context of a single chapter. In the previous chapter on limited-language children, we dealt with assessment of communication through the early multiword level of development. The present chapter focuses on school-age and adolescent students speaking at the sentence level who may well have difficulty with syntactic rules, but may also have deficiencies in semantics, pragmatics, metalinguistics, morphology, reading, writing, cognitive abilities, and general language processing. Thus, the reader will find that the assessment targets, tasks, and measurements we discuss in the present chapter differ dramatically from those mentioned in Chapter 4.

Table 5.1 lists some common symptoms of language disorder in school-age and adolescent students. One can see that these symptoms span all areas of language and include comprehension as well as production impairments. There are also phonological disorders in these populations which are addressed in Chapter 6. It should be noted that some of the symptoms are rather gross linguistic errors that would be easily detected in conversation (e.g., syntactic rule violations), while some errors are rather subtle and discernible only with specialized communication sampling. We should reinforce the point here that standardized tests may not reveal a subtle linguistic impairment in a school-age child. It is not unusual for an elementary-level student to pass many of our formal language tests and yet exhibit a significant linguistically based communication disorder. Many

Table 5.1   Common Symptoms of Language Disorder in Older Students

Semantics

- word finding/retrieval deficits
- use of a large number of words in an attempt to explain a concept because the name escapes them (circumlocutions)
- overuse of limited vocabulary
- difficulty recalling names of items in categories (e.g., animals, foods)
- difficulty retrieving verbal opposites
- small vocabulary
- use of words lacking specificity (thing, junk, stuff, etc.)
- inappropriate use of words (selection of wrong word)
- difficulty defining words
- less comprehension of complex words
- failure to grasp double word meanings (e.g., can, file)

Syntax/Morphology

- use of grammatically incorrect sentence structures
- simple, as opposed to complex, sentences
- less comprehension of complex grammatical structures
- prolonged pauses while constructing sentences
- semantically empty placeholders (e.g., filled pauses, "uh," "er," "um")
- use of many stereotyped phrases that do not require much language skill
- use of "starters" (e.g., "you know . . .")

Pragmatics

- use of redundant expressions and information the listener has already heard
- use of nonspecific vocabulary (e.g., thing, stuff) and the listener cannot tell from prior conversation or physical context what is referred to
- less skill in giving explanations clearly to a listener (lack of detail)
- less skill in explaining something in a proper sequence
- less conversational control in terms of introducing, maintaining, and changing topics (may get off the track in conversation and introduce new topics awkwardly)
- rare use of clarification questions (e.g., "I don't understand," "You did what?")
- difficulty shifting conversational style in different social situations (e.g., peer vs. teacher; child vs. adult)
- difficulty grasping the "main idea" of a story or lecture (preoccupation with irrelevant details)
- trouble making inferences from material not explicitly stated (e.g., "Sally went outside. She had to put up her umbrella." Inference: It was raining.)

From: Haynes, W., Moran, M. & Pindzola, R. (1990) *Communication Disorders in the Classroom*, Dubuque, IA: Kendall-Hunt.

of these errors would only be seen in nonstandardized probing and conversational sampling.

USE OF STANDARDIZED TESTS WITH SYNTAX-LEVEL CHILDREN

As we indicated in Chapter 3, formal tests are best suited for comparing performance on some measure to that of same-age peers who took the test under similar conditions. Formal tests, as Muma (1973a) stated, address the issue of whether or not a problem exists. These measures are not particularly good at defining the nature of the problem or helping in the selection of treatment targets. Appendix E lists some instruments that are commonly available. The fact that we have compiled this list does not suggest that we are recommending these tests or even the notion of formal testing in general. In fact, many of these instruments are not psychometrically sound and are missing data on reliability and validity. We provide the list simply as an informational tool to demonstrate that there are many formal tests in the area of language disorders, and more become available each year. No doubt, by the time you are reading this chapter, there will be many new tests and some of the ones on our list will be out of print. Especially in the area of language, it is almost impossible to remain abreast of all recent test developments. Another problem, of course, is that no single individual, clinical setting, or training program can afford to purchase every test instrument that is published. Some of our information in Appendix E comes from examining the actual test instruments themselves; however, in other cases we had to rely on catalogues or flyers that advertise the tests. Thus, we make no attempt to critically analyze or detail these tests. Other sources provide substantial reviews and descriptions of many of these instruments (Aram & Nation, 1982; Conoley & Kramer, 1989; Darley, 1979; Peterson & Marquardt, 1990).

The reader will note that the tests are designed to tap a variety of language skills (expression, vocabulary, comprehension, imitation, cognition, pragmatics, syntax, etc.), are targeted for use with a wide spectrum of age ranges, and represent a number of different theoretical points of view. The older tests obviously do not take into account current advances in thinking about language acquisition or assessment. Clinicians who elect to use a formal test should consider the following: (1) the assumptions the test is based on; (2) the age, culture, and socioeconomic status of the population the test was normed on; (3) the validity and reliability data provided; (4) the quality of information the test will provide as it relates to treatment; and (5) the aspects of language that are tested. Owens et al. (1983) provide a summary of specific grammatical forms examined by a wide variety of tests. This information might be helpful to a clinician who wishes to probe only selected grammatical forms. Rarely, however, will formal tests include enough items to thoroughly evaluate a particular linguistic structure.

Most of the test instruments listed in Appendix E have been designed for children between the ages of three and adolescence and focus on structural aspects of language (syntax, semantics, literal meaning of sentences), although there are several that deal with other areas as well (e.g., pragmatics, metalinguistics, concepts). Some of these tests may well be used by the SLP to gain preliminary insights into selected aspects of language performance, and they certainly can fulfill institutional expectations for obtaining scores on formal instruments.

LANGUAGE SAMPLING:
A GENERAL LOOK AT THE PROCESS

A common thread that has woven its way through the text thus far has been the notion of ecological validity. When done appropriately, language sampling of a spontaneous conversation is perhaps the closest we come to evaluating real communication. As Miller (1981) says, we must broaden our definition of what sampling is to include the very young child who may be one-year-old, and not much of a conversationalist. We do, however, sample his/her communication. Perhaps a better name for this process would be *communication sampling* rather than *language sampling*. Spontaneous sampling is the only way to hold content, form, and use intact, so it is one of our most powerful tools.

Most speech-language pathologists have had the opportunity to sit in a small room with a child and attempt to fill a cassette with a representative sample of language. Most of us have also experienced the despair and humiliation (if observed) of harvesting a string of one-word utterances and elliptical responses. Faced with this, we begin to put pressure on the child for longer utterances and ask questions about the obvious. "What is in this picture?" we ask, when both the child and the clinician know the answer. "Tell me about what you did at school today," we cajole and the child shrugs his/her shoulders and says, "nuthin." A very wise observation was made by Hubbell (1981) after he studied spontaneous talking in young children. When children feel they are being interrogated and there is a great deal of pressure for them to talk, they tend to clam up. One of the worst liabilities the clinician can have is a mother who says to her child in the waiting room, "Now this person wants you to talk, so be sure you do." This is, in many cases, the "kiss of death" for a decent language sample. Children need to feel at ease and not pressured to talk. Clinicians should also try to resist the very strong urge to "interrogate" school-age children and, worst of all, to question them about the obvious. As we mentioned earlier, all communication is affected by the context in which it occurs, and language sampling is no different. Since each sampling session is a product of an individual student, clinician, and communicative environment, it is impossible to provide guidelines that will work with all cases. All we can do is play the probabilities and provide some suggestions that may facilitate spontaneous talking with most cases.

For detailed treatments of language sampling procedures, the reader is referred to the ample sources dealing with the topic (Barrie-Blackley, Musselwhite, & Rogister, 1978; Miller, 1981). Some general guidelines follow:

1. Always tape-record the sample. We tend to subjectively fill in utterances that are incomplete if we transcribe during the sample. Additionally, it is distracting

if we are attempting to carry on a legitimate conversation while scribbling on a yellow pad. Either we are engaging in a real conversation or we are not.

2. Use a good quality tape recorder and position it in such a way to promote optimal recording. This is one of the most often overlooked aspects of sampling language. It is a real disappointment when a clinician has done a masterful job of eliciting natural conversation from a child only to have it rendered unintelligible by a poor recording.

3. Minimize the use of yes/no questions. Remember, as soon as you ask these, you know the answer will be "yes," "no," or "I don't know." Beginning clinicians typically bombard the child with yes/no questions, and the sample may be so loaded with single-word utterances that the child's MLU is severely underestimated due to sampling error (see Miller, 1981).

4. An attempt should be made to minimize questions that can be answered with one word (e.g., "What color is your dog?"). Although you have to ask some of these in the normal course of conversation, they do elicit single-word responses.

5. Try to ask broad-based questions such as "What happened?," "What happened next?," "Tell me about . . . ," "Why?," "How?," and so on.

6. Do not be afraid to make contributions to the conversation. One of the most common errors that beginning clinicians make is that they want the child to do all the talking. This is not a natural conversational situation. Also, the child's utterances are typically in the role of responder. Think back to the last language sample you took and ask yourself if the child had opportunities to initiate conversation instead of merely responding to your interrogations. Also, ask yourself if you were a semitruthful conversational participant. Did you tell the child some of your feelings and experiences? Did you talk mostly about things that were obvious or trivial? As Hubbell (1981) states, a facilitator of conversation is a good conversational model. It has been our experience that as soon as we stop the barrage of questions and begin to make some observations about what is going on in the session and what we think about things, the child begins to make some contributions to the conversation.

7. As Miller (1981) says, try not to "play the fool" during a language sample, especially with an older child. We have heard clinicians say, "I don't know what's in this picture, can you tell me?" Another example is a clinician who says, "Tell me how to make a sandwich, I don't know how." Give the child credit for the intelligence to know that you could easily describe pictures or do simple, everyday tasks.

8. Learn to tolerate periods of silence or pauses. Beginning clinicians seem to feel that they have to fill up all the communicative space with verbalizations. Give the child an opportunity to initiate conversation.

9. Stay on a topic long enough to converse about it. Do not change topics after the child says one utterance on the issue. This encourages a series of "one liners" from children and the clinician is again placed in the position of having to interrogate. It also interferes with the clinician's ability to gather a sample that is appropriate for analyzing conversational mechanisms such as topic maintenance.

10. Finally, be aware of children's cognitive levels when you ask questions. The clinician should be aware that children have differing conceptual frameworks from adults and altered perspectives of time and space. We should not ask questions which are cognitively too complex for younger children. Conversely, we do not want to ask questions that are cognitively too simple for older students.

There are variables that appear to affect the length and complexity of language samples obtained by researchers and examiners. First, the racial backgrounds of the participants could have a potential influence on a child's conversation. Several studies have suggested that young black children may engage in style shifting or code switching when confronted with a white, adult examiner (Cazden, 1970; Labov, 1970). Cazden (1970) has stated that black children speak in a school register (for teachers and administrators) and a street register (for peers and family). Interestingly, the school register is different in content, has a shorter MLU, is less complex, and is more disfluent than the street register. Of course, everyone's style shifts to some degree when conversing with people from different social, cultural, educational, and economic backgrounds. This certainly has implications for language sampling. Clinicians should realize that the samples they obtain from young minority children may underestimate their linguistic abilities.

Verbalizations of the examiner may also affect language sampling. Lee (1974) suggests that the clinician attempt to speak with a variety of syntactic structures when sampling a child's language. The modeling literature has shown that children, in as little as a single session, can use language that is roughly similar in complexity to an adult model, whether the model uses extremely simple sentences or complex sentences involving embedding and conjoining (Haynes & Hood, 1978). Children are also sensitive to pragmatic aspects of a communicative situation. If they are placed in a play situation with younger children, their language will be simpler than when they talk to adults.

Presupposition may also play a role in the length and complexity of samples obtained from children. Like adults, children will elaborate linguistically about objects and events that are not present in the current communicative context (Strandberg & Griffith, 1969). If a child does not share visual access to the stimuli with the clinician, he/she will tend to elaborate linguistically to a greater degree (Haynes, Purcell, & Haynes, 1979).

Several studies have shown that children provide longer and more complex language samples if they are engaged in conversation as opposed to picture description tasks (Haynes, Purcell, & Haynes, 1979; Longhurst & File, 1977; Longhurst & Grubb, 1974). Picture description tends to lend itself to the naming of elements in a picture rather than linguistic elaboration about a topic unknown to the clinician. These are typically single-word responses or elliptical answers. Especially if the clinician views the picture with the child, the task becomes not one of conversation, but of naming aspects of pictures. Conversation, of course, carries with it an element of presupposition because the clinician does not know what the child will talk about, and there is no contextual support for things removed in time and space. Thus, the child is forced to linguistically elaborate since the clinician is not aware of the conversational aspects the child is attempting to convey. Picture description, however, is a viable method of sampling language for those children who will not readily engage in conversation, and picture description is needed to elicit some language for analysis (Atkins & Cartwright, 1982).

Several investigations have dealt with the difference between samples obtained at home versus in a clinical setting, as well as samples gathered by mothers versus speech-language pathologists. Kramer, James, and Saxman (1979) compared home and clinic samples and found that longer utterances were obtained in the home environment as compared to the clinical setting. They suggest that, if possible, samples from the home environment may be gathered prior to the evaluation in order not to underestimate a child's language ability. Olswang and Carpenter (1978) studied language samples collected by experienced clinicians and mothers of language-impaired children in a clinical setting. They found that the mothers elicited more language from their children in a given time period; however, the quality of the language elicited by the two adults was similar. That is, there was no significant difference in the lexical, semantic, or syntactic character of the child's language. This study suggests that speech-language pathologists should feel fairly confident that the samples they elicit from children are at least similar in quality to those samples elicited by mothers in a clinical setting.

Sometimes clinicians are interested in eliciting particular syntactic structures from a child as opposed to a general language sample. This occasion would arise if the clinician wanted to probe the child's use of certain constructions such as question forms in spontaneous speech. Mulac, Prutting, and Tomlinson (1978) suggest that a variety of tasks could be used to elicit a particular construction. They found that the most effective tasks for eliciting the "is interrogative" were those tasks that required intent and had contextual referents as well as some inherent structure to the activity. One example was a guessing game in which children had to guess what was in a bag (e.g., "Is it a _____?"). The notion of using several different informal elicitation tasks to evaluate certain syntactic structures has been supported by others as well (Leonard et al., 1978; Lund & Duchan, 1988; Musselwhite & Barrie-Blackley, 1980).

We have seen that obtaining a language sample is a critical part of doing a language evaluation. There are a host of variables that can affect the size and quality of the sample obtained by the examiner. These variables, and their effect on sample size, may play a major role in the clinician's interpretation of the student's language sample and must be considered when analyzing the client's communicative ability.

TESTING LANGUAGE COMPREHENSION

Bransford and Nitsch (1978) point out that comprehension involves a situation plus an input. A human organism is not a static system but has a history and background knowledge. A given input of language is placed in this situation along with the nonverbal context of communication. Many variables come to bear on the understanding of an input, not the least of which are the person's background and the linguistic and nonlinguistic contexts. Rees and Shulman (1978) have written an article in which they indicate that most tests of language comprehension measure only the literal meanings of utterances. For example, if asked to point to a picture of a boy running, the child can choose the correct picture and not point to one of a boy standing. Thus, the child understands the notions of "boy" and "run" and can discriminate them from other literal meanings such as "standing." Comprehension involves so much more than the literal meaning of utterances. For example, the skill of inferencing is used in almost every interaction and certainly many times during a school day. To fully comprehend an utterance such as "It's supposed to rain today, but I forgot my umbrella," one must infer that the person may get wet, although this is never specifically stated. Another broader notion of comprehension has to do with understanding the main point in a narrative, lecture, or conversation. If a child cannot do this, he/she has as much of a comprehension problem as one of not understanding literal meanings. Comprehension of figurative language such as idioms and metaphors involves more than just literal meaning. If a teacher says "This science project should really shine," the child should know that the teacher does not mean it requires lights (Simon, 1987). We must go past the idea of assessing only literal meanings when dealing with comprehension assessment.

Most comprehension tests are quite artificial when compared to the richness of language comprehension in a natural situation. The typical comprehension assessment situation involves presenting a child with test plates containing pictures. The child is asked to point to the picture that best represents some verbal stimulus uttered by the examiner. The pictures are often line drawings and the verbal stimuli are not discursively related to one another (in one case the child is asked to point to a "monkey," and in the next plate the topic is "shopping"). In these tests there is no temporal sequence of events that would allow a child to be able to predict what will be said, as in real language comprehension. Naturalistic situations also give the child the opportunity to ask for clarification or repetition in the face of information loss. The notion of comprehension monitoring implies that we are always scanning to determine if we are understanding someone's utterances; and if we do not, we initiate repair sequences that can clarify information we do not comprehend. We do not afford children this chance in comprehension testing. In fact, we are often forbidden by the examiner's manual from presenting a stimulus a second time, even if the child asks for a repetition! This discussion is meant to reinforce the notion that real language comprehension is a highly complex phenomenon and cannot be assessed easily.

Millen and Prutting (1979) studied three language comprehension tests for consistency of response on specific grammatical features. They found that on the *Northwestern Syntax Screening Test (NSST), Assessment of Children's Language Comprehension (ACLC),* and *Bellugi Comprehension Test,* there was general agreement in the overall scores generated by the measures. There were, however, significant differences among the tests for more than half of the specific grammatical features evaluated. The investigators logically suggest that the tests are not equivalent and not clinically sound for generating specific remediation targets. Other stimulus, task, and subject variables have been studied in comprehension tests. Haynes and McCallion (1981) found that children with a reflective cognitive tempo (long decision time) performed significantly better than impulsive (short decision time) children on the *Test of Auditory Comprehension of Language (TACL).* Further, these researchers reported that scores on the *TACL* improved significantly over standard administration when the subjects were given two stimulus presentations, or if the test was administered imitatively.

Thus, it appears that variables other than language comprehension enter into test performance, and failure to do well on a comprehension test could be explained by other factors. Attentional set, hearing impairment, ambiguous pictures, test administration procedures (Shorr, 1983), cognitive style, and unrelated stimuli—all could account for poor performance on a standardized test of language comprehension. Additionally, Gowie and Powers (1979) showed that a child's expectations about what a sentence was going to say significantly influenced his/her performance on a comprehension task. They say that ". . . knowing a word involves a set of expectations about the referents and about the types of messages in which the word is likely to occur" (p. 40).

We have suggested that comprehension is difficult to test without contaminating influences from the context and comprehension strategies. Further, we have said that failure to perform well on a test of comprehension does not necessarily indicate the presence of a comprehension disorder. Based on the current literature, about all we can say with some conviction is that adequate performance on a standardized test of language comprehension probably means that the child is capable of comprehending some language in a highly artificial situation. This does not necessarily represent comprehension ability in natural situations. Failure of a comprehension test, on the other hand, does not necessarily mean that the child is incapable of comprehending language either in the contrived testing situation or the natural environment.

Currently, language comprehension is tested in four ways by speech-language pathologists. First, there are a number of standardized tests of comprehension (see Appendix E). Second, some researchers have tested comprehension by having children act out certain commands (Leonard et al., 1978). Third, others have used a decision task where the child makes judgments such as "good or bad" or he/she engages in a preference task to say which of two sentences was better. Finally, similar to the standardized tests, clinicians have used pictures and/or objects and engaged children in an informal pointing task. Perhaps the "best" method of comprehension testing would be to examine it via several methods, both formal and informal. The clinician should utilize more naturalistic assessment methods such as engaging the child in play or conversation and evaluating the appropriateness of verbal and nonverbal responses. Observation in the classroom combined with teacher and parent interviews can provide valuable insight into comprehension in everyday situations. It should also be noted if the child uses requests for clarification or repetition in conversation. Research has shown that these clarification/repetition requests can be successfully elicited by the clinician using informal probes (Brinton & Fujiki, 1989).

ASSESSMENT OF SYNTAX USING ELICITED IMITATION

Elicited imitation has been used in psycholinguistic research on language development for decades (Slobin & Welsh, 1971). There is a correlation between age and the ability to imitate sentences of increasing length and complexity (Brown, 1973). Elicited imitation, as an assessment procedure, carries with it certain assumptions that the SLP user must believe to be true about language and linguistic processing. A basic assumption of imitative techniques is that children will repeat only those structures for which they have linguistic competence. If a child omits or misuses a syntactic element in a sentence imitation task, the examiner must suspect that the child does not have that element in his/her repertoire. Conversely, if the child does imitate an item, it is assumed that the youngster has that structure. This basic assumption of elicited imitation has been challenged during the last decade, and investigators have explored variables that affect the elicited imitation response other than linguistic competence.

One variable that has been recently explored is the use of a nonlinguistic context in conjunction with elicited imitation. Nelson and Weber-Olsen (1980) found greater mean length of imitative utterance and fewer errors when contextual support in the form of object manipulations was provided as compared to a no context condition. Similarly, Haniff and Siegel (1981) found significantly fewer errors in an imitation task that was accompanied by picture stimuli as compared to a no picture condition. These two studies suggest that imitation is improved when the clinician provides a context. A context may assist children in remembering elements presented in a model sentence or may allow them to focus on more obscure aspects of a sentence since the major subject-verb-object elements are depicted for them. One study, however, does not support the finding that context improves imitative performance (Connell & Myles-Zitzer, 1982).

Elicited imitation is also affected by stress patterns present in the model sentence (Blasdell & Jensen, 1970; Slobin & Welsh, 1971). If a child misses a syntactic element and the examiner stresses the element on the second trial, the probability of correct performance is increased. Clinicians must be aware of this if they use elicited imitation for pretest/posttest measures to evaluate treatment effects since they may inadvertently stress elements that were the targets of training.

Two studies have suggested a trial or practice effect in elicited imitation (Haynes & Haynes, 1979; Lang & Moore, 1977). Haynes and Haynes (1979) gave children a sentence imitation task two times separated by two days. They found that over 52 percent of the children's errors on the first trial had been corrected on the second trial. Interestingly, 22 percent of the children's errors remained the same, and 25 percent of the errors on the second trial were new ones that had not occurred at all on the first trial. Fujiki and Brinton (1983) reported that sampling reliability for elicited imitation may not stabilize until a syntactic structure is repeated over three trials. This certainly gives one pause when contemplating the administration of an elicited imitation test in a single trial and makes one wonder about what the clinician learns from the imitative task.

Elicited imitation tests are typically composed of a series of unrelated sentences. Imitation, because of its nature, violates a host of pragmatic conventions, and one of these is discursiveness. If sentences are unrelated, many of the linguistic forms are used inappropriately (e.g., pronouns, questions, demonstratives). Haynes and Haynes (1979) explored the use of discursively related sentences that made up a story versus imitation of the same sentences randomly arranged. It was found that there was no significant difference in the imitative performance of normal-language children in the related and unrelated sentence tasks. Thus, for normal children, the relatedness made little difference in performance; however, we do not presently know about this variable as it relates to language-impaired youngsters. On a subjective level, however, the experimenters noted that the normal children appeared to enjoy the task to a greater degree when the sentences were in a story format, and there were also fewer attentional lapses.

Bonvillian, Raeburn, and Horan (1979) studied the effects of rate, intonation, and length of children's elicited imitation. They found that there were significantly more errors on longer sentences as opposed to shorter ones. They also found a significant trend that indicated that the children made fewer errors when the stimuli they imitated were presented at a rate of about two words per second (wps), a rate similar to the children's own speech rate (1.8 wps). Finally, there was a significant relationship between length and intonation pattern. The children made fewer errors on the longer sentences when normal intonation patterns were used as compared to a monotone presentation. Perhaps intonation is a valuable cue used by children in decoding complex sentences.

Several investigators have expressed concern about the validity of elicited imitation being representative of spontaneous grammatical performance (Connell & Myles-Zitzer, 1982; Daily & Boxx, 1979; McDade, Simpson, & Larnt, 1982; Prutting, Gallagher, & Mulac, 1975; Werner & Kreseck, 1981). Bloom (1974) has reported a case of a child who was incapable of effectively imitating his own spontaneous utterances that were recorded and transcribed from a prior session. She attributed this performance decrement to a lack of context during the imitative task.

From this general review, it can be seen that performance on an elicited imitation task is affected by many variables. If this is true, then we cannot be certain what elicited imitation is measuring. Further, many studies have shown that elicited imitation performance can agree with or differ from spontaneous speech performance. As Prutting and Connolly so aptly state: "Elicited imitations alone may underestimate, overestimate, or accurately describe the child's language performance" (1976, p. 420). On a theoretical plane, elicited imitation violates the integrative model of language because it separates structure from function and uses unrelated utterances with no communicative intent.

There are several advantages to the use of elicited imitation, however. First, an imitative task can be administered in a short time, usually under 15 minutes. Second, with imitation, the clinician can assess specific structures instead of waiting for them to appear spontaneously in a language sample. Third, some tests (Carrow, 1974) include normative data for comparing children's performance in order to solve the problem–no problem issue. There are several tests that have been constructed in an elicited imitation format (Carrow, 1974; Zachman et al., (1978). The present authors feel that elicited imitation is a useful procedure, but clinicians should never rely solely on an imitative assessment. Treatment targets should only be selected from spontaneous language samples; and if imitative techniques are used, they should always be supplemented by spontaneous performance.

ASSESSMENT OF SYNTAX USING ANALYSIS PACKAGES

After the speech-language pathologist has obtained a language sample, judgments must be made regarding the syntactic development of the child. Analysis of syntax can be conceptualized on a continuum. On the left end of the continuum is the administration of formal tests. These measures can give the clinician some insight into general syntactic development. In the middle of the continuum, the clinician can analyze a language sample in accordance with specific packaged assessment procedures (Lee, 1974) and obtain more precise information than that available from standardized tests. Finally, on the right end, the clinician can analyze the sample using his/her own knowledge of linguistics and language development and not rely on a step-by-step package analysis procedure. The left end of the continuum requires less expertise than the right end in terms of clinician experience and training. It also takes less time but provides less clinically relevant information. Thus, the clinician must make a decision as to the time available for the analysis, as well as the training needed to develop expertise in linguistics, and the depth of information desired.

It is beyond the scope of the present chapter to instruct clinicians in performing an analysis of a child's syntax. The best way to learn an analysis system is to obtain a sample and follow the guidelines provided by authors of complexity analysis packages. Typically, the authors provide explicit instructions for obtaining a sample, segmentation, and analysis. Beginning clinicians should realize that any syntactic analysis method requires practice in order to be used effectively. The most widely known analysis procedures are listed in Figure 5.1.

Muma (1978) points out that descriptive procedures have greater power than normative ones because they help the clinician describe individual differences. Descriptive procedures also provide the clinician with more relevant intervention targets because they are based on spontaneous language samples and do not fracture the integrity of the content-form-use model as imitative

Figure 5.1 Selected Language Sample Analysis Procedures

- Assessing Children's Language in Naturalistic Contexts (Lund & Duchan, 1988)
- Assigning Structural Stage (Miller, 1981)
- Co-Occurring and Restricted Structures Analysis (Muma, 1973b)
- Developmental Sentence Analysis (Lee, 1974)
- Indiana Scale of Clausal Development (Denver & Bauman, 1974)
- Language Assessment, Remediation and Screening Procedure (Crystal, Fletcher, & Garman, 1976)
- Language Sampling, Analysis and Training (Tyack & Gottsleben, 1974)
- Length Complexity Index (Miner, 1969)
- Length of T-Unit or Communication Unit (Loban, 1976)
- Linguistic Analysis of Speech Samples (Engler, Hannah, & Longhurst, 1973)
- Mean Length of Utterance and Distributional Analysis (Miller, 1981)
- A Method for Assessing Use of Grammatical Structures (Kahn & James, 1980)
- Structural Complexity Score (McCarthy, 1930)

and standardized tests do. Thus, there are advantages to performing a descriptive analysis, and package systems provide the clinician with guidelines for completing such an analysis. We should, however, remember that each analysis procedure reflects the author's bias regarding language, and most systems look at a language sample in only limited ways.

Consumers who intend to use an analysis package should be aware that the procedures differ in important ways. These differences may determine whether or not a clinician finds it appropriate to use a particular package. We will use the *Developmental Sentence Analysis (DSS)* procedure in our examples since this methodology is widely known. Using this procedure in our discussion is not meant to be a criticism or an endorsement of this particular approach.

1. Some package systems recommend obtaining a specific sample size before subjecting the language to analysis. For instance, Lee (1974) recommends using 50 subject-verb utterances for computation of the *DSS*. A later study, however, stated that a sample of 150 utterances may be more appropriate for reliable scoring. If the clinician does not have a large enough sample, perhaps a different procedure would be more appropriate.

2. The analysis packages vary considerably in the time required for completion. This may be due to several influences. First, some procedures are quite detailed and lengthy (Bloom & Lahey, 1978; Crystal, Fletcher, & Garman, 1976). Other procedures use very specific terminologies and vocabulary or have complicated scoring systems (e.g. *DSS*) that require much time and practice in order for the clinician to use the procedure economically.

3. The procedures differ in terms of how they segment or separate utterances obtained in the sample. The *DSS*, for instance, analyzes subject-verb utterances and does not score sentence fragments. Some clinicians, however, feel that there is much useful information in sentence fragments (e.g., elliptical responses) that may be important to analyze.

4. Some systems are recommended by their authors as ideal for use with particular treatment approaches. Lee, Koenigsknect, and Mulhern (1975) use the *DSS* as an input to their interactive language teaching strategy and continue to monitor progress using the system.

5. Another way that evaluation systems differ is in terms of the structures they do or do not analyze. For example, the *DSS* does not specifically analyze certain forms (e.g., prepositions, articles) and accounts for their presence or absence by assigning a "sentence point" to an utterance if it is grammatical. Other systems specifically analyze most structural elements of English, even structures that may not be of interest to the clinician.

6. Analysis packages differ in their provision of normative data. The *DSS* has normative data, while some other packages are purely descriptive and make no attempt to cull numerical scores on normal and disordered children.

7. Finally, the analysis procedures are not uniform in applying the results to a normal language development progression. That is, some are designed to examine linguistic elements without locating the child on a language development

continuum. Lee (1974), Bloom and Lahey (1978), and Crystal, Fletcher, and Garman (1976) apply their results to developmental progressions.

Several investigations have shown that some of the package analysis procedures appear to be capable of documenting language changes in children, at least in a general way (Longhurst & Schrandt, 1973; Sharf, 1972). Further, any method that a clinician selects will require specific training and practice in order to use it effectively. It should be remembered that any method used depends to a significant degree on the quality of the sample obtained and typically analyzes only the structural elements of language independent of pragmatics. Thus, any analysis package procedure will take the clinician time and practice to learn and in the end will look at language only from a specific point of view (Miller, 1981). It is the preference of the present authors that if clinicians are going to spend time learning about analysis of the structural aspects of language, their time would be better spent learning linguistics and language acquisition instead of one specific analysis package that probably would not be appropriate for all clients. An analysis package could always be learned later to supplement the clinician's linguistic knowledge and would probably be learned more easily due to the experience with linguistics. A knowledge of linguistics would allow the clinician to analyze samples for structures that are present, absent, and inconsistent and still choose treatment targets that are relevant, instead of trying to find a package analysis procedure that is of "best fit" for the child. There are a number of fine textbooks that provide information on sentence structure and one of them should be a reference in the professional library of every speech-language pathologist (Hubbell, 1988; Quirk & Greenbaum, 1975). We feel that the clinician must ultimately determine (1) which structures the child appears to have acquired, (2) which structures are absent in obligatory contexts, (3) which structures are inconsistently used, and (4) which contexts seem to be associated with use and nonuse of the inconsistent structures. Muma (1973) and Kahn and James (1980) have advocated such descriptive procedures that focus on determining present, absent, and inconsistent syntactic elements and we view this as a commonsense approach to analysis that has direct clinical application. It also does not involve the clinician's commitment of time to learning one or two package procedures and their unique scoring systems.

Computer analyses of language samples have now become available. Software programs provide detailed information about a language sample; however, the clinician must remember that some time is typically invested in coding the transcript into the computer. In some cases, this may take more time than a paper and pencil analysis if the clinician merely wants to define treatment targets. Also, the computer analyses may provide the clinician with more information than is really needed. The output from these programs is truly phenomenal. For example, *Lingquest 1* performs a lexical analysis that includes specific assessment of nouns, verbs, modifiers, conjunctions, prepositions, negation, interjections, and WH words, as well as over 80 subcategories of parts of speech (Mordecai, Palin, & Palmer, 1982). A type-token ratio is also computed. In analyzing grammatical structure, various phrase and sentence types are identified and verb tense is analyzed. Mean length of utterance in words and morphemes is also computed. *Computerized Profiling* is a most useful program that does detailed phonological analysis, semantic analysis, *LARSP* (Crystal et al. 1976), *DSS* (Lee, 1974), conversational acts profile, prosodic analysis, single-word analysis, and early multiword analysis (Long & Fey, 1988). The outputs from this program are quite complex, and it is reasonably priced and user friendly. The *SALT: Systematic Analysis of Language Transcripts* program also provides analyses of specific grammatical classes and computes numerical indices similar to the other programs mentioned (Miller & Chapman, 1985). Additionally, it contains a very flexible search program that allows the user to address specific questions regarding specific words or constructions. These programs probably represent the most comprehensive and detailed applications to date, and there will no doubt be others in the near future.

The advantage of the computer would appear to lie in the multiple analyses that could be performed once the sample is inputted. That is, a clinician can take the same transcript and analyze it for insight into the child's semantic system, phonological system, syntactic system, and occurrence of speech acts (if appropriately coded). An important point to emphasize is that these programs are only as good as the coding of the language sample that they analyze. Some of the programs automatically classify lexical items or grammatical forms based on internal algorithms. Most programs allow the clinician to change these a priori classifications of transcript items if they are incorrect. That is, sometimes a program will not identify a word or grammatical construction correctly and the clinician needs to check how the computer has classified transcript items. There is no substitute for close clinician monitoring when using these programs. Even though the computer pumps out a profile or summary of a child's performance, the clinician needs to spot check the analysis for correctness. It is easy to be seduced into relying on complex summaries without checking on validity.

No doubt we will learn much in the next decade from these procedures about patterns of error and subtypes of language disorder. No single procedure can tell a clinician all he/she needs to know about a child's language. Again, ultimately it is the clinician's judgment that must be applied to a particular case, whether it is a decision to choose among several package analysis systems or a computer-assisted analysis, or to simply focus on a more specific descriptive linguistic analysis.

ASSESSMENT OF CONVERSATIONAL PRAGMATICS

Many reports exist in the literature that attest to pragmatic differences in language-impaired children. Some investigations report that language-impaired children have difficulty organizing narratives and staying on a topic (Johnston, 1982; Lucas, 1980). Fey and Leonard (1983) have hypothesized that there may be subgroups of language-impaired children exhibiting a variety of pragmatic problems. There have been reports of the language-disordered child having difficulty taking listener perspective into account (Muma, 1975). The problems

described here may or may not be significant for the speech-language pathologist to evaluate and/or treat. The research on the pragmatic performance of
language-impaired children has just begun, and there are methodological considerations that we must take into account when interpreting the investigations
(Fey & Leonard, 1983). There have been differences among pragmatic studies in
the composition of the research dyad (child-child; child-adult; normal child–
language-impaired child; language-impaired child–language-impaired child).
There have also been differences in the measures used in the studies as well
as age differences in the children investigated. Some of the studies have used
very small numbers of subjects (three dyads). Other reports are anecdotal and
present no empirical data (Lucas, 1980). Finally, since many of the studies used
language-disordered children whose linguistic structures were abnormal, it is
altogether possible that their pragmatics were abnormal partially due to structural differences. There is some evidence, however, that structure and use are
partially separate (Fey & Leonard, 1983). Whatever the extent of a child's pragmatic differences, however, the speech-language pathologist must be prepared
to evaluate conversational competence from a variety of perspectives. It is in
these kinds of analyses that the clinician can plumb communicative competence
(Hymes, 1971) and go beyond the basic evaluation of language structures.

Unfortunately, there are no tests that tap all relevant aspects of conversational pragmatics. While there are some formal measures that focus on limited facets of pragmatic ability (Blagden & McConnell, 1983; Shulman, 1986), it
would be difficult to develop a broader assessment device due to the many
aspects included under the rubric of pragmatics. Conversational abilities are
also difficult to tap using artificial tasks, limited samples, or contrived topics of
discourse. If the clinician is interested in conversational abilities, there is no
substitute for legitimate conversation. When the clinician focuses on conversation and discourse, it is necessary to obtain a sample of the child's conversational
performance and to transcribe both the utterances of the child and the inter-
locutor. This is a time-consuming task; however, if the clinician is to obtain data
on the child's conversational performance, the contributions of both participants cannot be ignored. There are several measures that the clinician might
elect to use to analyze conversation, depending on which aspects of the discourse are of interest. Some of these measures may overlap to a certain degree.

Prutting and Kirchner (1987) developed a pragmatic protocol that gives
an overall communicative index for children, adolescents, and adults. It includes
30 pragmatic aspects of language in the broad groupings of verbal, paralinguistic,
and nonverbal skills. There are specific definitions for each parameter used in the
system, and they provide preliminary data on both adults and children with normal and disordered language. One approach to evaluating a child's pragmatic
abilities is to begin with a general view of conversational performance to determine if certain types of errors are especially obvious to the clinician. Children's
conversation is rated by the clinician on the 30 parameters. The most inappropriate pragmatic parameters found in 42 language-impaired children involved turn-
taking, specificity/accuracy, cohesion, repair/revision, topic maintenance and
intelligibility. Use of this protocol at the very least forces the clinician to consider

the relevant parameters of pragmatics and make a judgment regarding each. Then more concentrated evaluation tasks can be applied to the case that might define the nature of the conversational errors more specifically.

Bloom, Rocissano, and Hood (1976) provide us with guidelines regarding the assessment of contingency, the evaluation of which is also recommended by Gallagher (1982). *Contingency* is the extent to which a speaker's contribution to a conversation reflects the effect of a previous utterance. Bloom, Rocissano, and Hood (1976) define three types of adjacent utterances: (1) contingent speech which shares the same topic with the preceding statement and adds new information, (2) imitative speech which shares the same topic but does not add new information, and (3) noncontingent utterances which do not share the same topic as prior utterances. Bloom, Rocissano, and Hood (1976) have shown that contingent speech increases between Brown's (1973) language development stages I and V while imitative and noncontingent speech decrease. Early in stage I, children are not particularly contingent and they become progressively more able to stay on a topic and make additional contributions. Obviously, a person cannot be contingent all of the time due to topic shifts. Children in stage V were contingent in their utterances about 50 percent of the time.

> Lamar, a 12-year-old boy, was referred for a language evaluation and was billed as "autisticlike." His clinician, teachers, and mother were interviewed, and they reported that he did not have much functional language, although he would frequently chant commercials and other routines he had memorized from television and radio. The clinician who accompanied Lamar "triggered" him on a commercial about a wrestling match to be held in a nearby city. He went on and on, repeating over and over, "Big time championship wrestling at the memorial auditorium at 8:00, . . ." We videotaped the evaluation in which we tried to engage Lamar in a variety of interactions and toward the end of the session we tried to extinguish some of his commercials. We decided to analyze the tape for the percent of Lamar's utterances that were contingent or related to another speaker's statement. We found that less than 10 percent of his utterances related to what someone else had said. At the subsequent staffing, we recommended that increasing contingent utterances and contextually relevant speech could be the treatment targets. The people from Lamar's school admitted that the commercials were a source of amusement and interest. Some school personnel mistakenly believed that these routines were "practice" in using language. Further discussion revealed that Lamar was frequently encouraged to say commercials for both entertainment and practice. They had not realized that so little of his communication was relevant and that they were playing a role in perpetuating his communication disorder.

Thus, one method of analyzing a child's conversational participation is to obtain a molar view of the contingency of the utterances. A child who is not capable of a reasonable degree of contingency will have trouble maintaining topics and perpetuating interactions with others.

Topic manipulation is another area that overlaps with contingency, but an analysis of topic may give the clinician slightly different information (Keenan & Schiefflin, 1976). Topics may use general knowledge shared by interactants, information physically present in the context, or previous discourse. According to Keenan and Schiefflin (1976), much conversational space is taken up by communicators to establish a topic. Once the topic is established, an interactant can use a turn to either maintain the topic (continuous discourse) or change the topic (discontinuous discourse). When speakers continue a discourse topic by collaborating a previous utterance with a related statement, or incorporating information in a prior utterance into their statement, the topic is maintained. A speaker discontinues a discourse topic by either introducing a topic that is unrelated to previous utterances or reintroducing a prior topic ("getting back to what we said about . . ."). Thus, topic maintaining utterances collaborate a prior statement or incorporate it into a new statement that is still on the topic. Developmentally, the length of continuous discourse increases with age.

In assessment, we need to determine how a child is able to secure the attention of a listener in order to initiate a topic (crying, yelling, gesturing, tugging, loudness, prosody, or an introduction such as "Know what?"). We can measure the length of the topic unit in terms of number of turns taken per topic. We also can measure the topic maintaining and shifting utterances used by a child. It is important in assessment to examine not only a child's ability to continue topics, but also to initiate them. In sampling, as mentioned previously, we may not often provide for this. Some of the most productive work on indepth analysis of topic manipulation has been done by Brinton and Fujiki (1984). Brinton and Fujiki (1989) provide detailed procedures for evaluation of all relevant aspects of topic manipulation in clinical work. We need further research to more specifically define the normal development of topic manipulation in both normal and language-impaired children. Some language-impaired children clearly have difficulty with these skills (Prutting & Kirchner, 1987), while other subgroups of children with linguistic impairment appear to manipulate topics normally (Edmonds & Haynes, 1988; Ehlers & Cirrin, 1983). We also need to know more about topic manipulation throughout the lifespan to determine changes in these skills in aging normal subjects since there is some evidence that differences exist among age groups (Stover & Haynes, 1989).

Another major category of measurement of conversational competence is the contingent query. A number of studies (Garvey, 1977a, 1977b) show that contingent queries are used by adults and children to achieve cohesion in conversation. Children as young as three years use contingent queries. Basically, the queries serve multiple functions in conversation, many of which have to do with repair procedures that allow the conversation to continue. For instance, a contingent query can be used to request a general repetition ("huh?"), a specific repetition ("a what?"), a confirmation ("a tape recorder?"), and an elaboration ("we have to go where?"). There are more complex aspects of contingent queries that are explained in the references cited. One can see, however, that these queries are important mechanisms of conversational competence and a child who does not know how to ask for clarification, for instance, will have difficulty continuing a particular topic with an interactant. The term *conversational repair* has been used most often in association with contingent queries. Clinically, it would be important to determine if a child can both respond to and produce requests for conversational repair (Brinton & Fujiki, 1989). For example, we would like to see if a child can adjust an utterance to a listener's request for repetition, clarification, or elaboration. On the other hand, we would like to determine if a child would ask for clarification if a clinician asks for a "ferbis" or makes a statement violating truth constraints in a particular context. Brinton and Fujiki (1989) provide many helpful suggestions for both assessment and intervention with conversational repair mechanisms.

Some children produce narratives or conversational turns that lack adequate cohesion. *Cohesion* is the relationship or tie between elements in discourse that are dependent upon one another (Halliday & Hasan, 1976). Stover and Haynes provide the following example:

> Wash the *dirty dishes* that are in the sink. Dry *them* and then put *them* in the cabinet. In the second sentence *them* refers directly back to the *dirty dishes* thus forming a cohesive tie. Of course, the cohesive marker may extend far beyond the immediately preceding sentence to an utterance produced earlier in the conversation. . . . In a complete tie, the referent to which a cohesive marker refers is easily found in a prior utterance with no ambiguity as in the above example. In an incomplete tie, a cohesive marker refers to something not mentioned in a prior utterance (e.g., I like ice cream. *He* does too.). In this example *he* cannot be associated with a particular person mentioned previously in the sentence. In an erroneous tie, there is ambiguity or error in interpreting who a referent is (e.g., Tom and Jerry live in the city. *He* likes it.). In this example, we do not know if *he* refers to Tom or Jerry. (1989, p. 40)

Liles (1985) provides specific procedures for cohesion analysis. One can readily see that this type of analysis would be useful in cases that are not taking into account the listener's perspective in discourse and are not aware of the requirements of conversational rules (Grice, 1975).

Another measure that has been used to describe the performance of language-impaired children is *back channel responding* (Fey & Leonard, 1983; Sheppard, 1980; Stein, 1976; Watson, 1977). Back channel responses are sentence completions, requests for clarification, and affirmations (e.g., "yeah," "uh-huh"). Back channel responding is typically associated with communicative nonassertiveness because the response is a way to keep the conversation going without adding much content. The child can take a turn without making more detailed conversational contributions. Not all researchers have noted back channel responding in all language-impaired children. Thus, there could be subgroups of cases that vary in their conversational assertiveness (Edmonds & Haynes, 1988; Fey, 1986). An analysis of this behavior could be an important part of evaluating a child's conversational competence, especially if it is noted that the child is reticent to participate in discourse.

Damico (1980, 1985) has taken a different approach and advocated the analysis of specific discourse errors in children's language. He provides a listing of nine discourse errors that can be detected in conversation and computed into a percent of utterances containing pragmatic difficulties. He recommends obtaining 180 utterances over two sessions in conversational interaction about home and school activities. The goal of the analysis is to describe specific discourse errors that exist in the interaction. Damico has gathered data on many normal and language-disordered children and proposes some error percentage ranges for determining very generally the existence and severity of a discourse problem.

EVALUATION OF METALINGUISTIC ABILITY
AND SCHOOL CURRICULUM

There are several groups of youngsters who are at high risk to develop a language disorder during the school years. A series of longitudinal investigations has shown that children with a history of preschool language delay are likely to experience subtle language disturbances throughout their school years and be at risk for academic problems (Aram & Nation, 1980; Bashir et al., 1983; Hall & Tomblin, 1978; King, Jones, & Lasky, 1982; Strominger & Bashir, 1977). These children were often dismissed from language treatment and then later rediagnosed as reading- or learning-disabled. Most exhibited low academic achievement throughout school because the curricular demands increase significantly in terms of language and communicative expectations while the child's linguistic abilities may not improve to meet these challenges. A second group of children who are likely to demonstrate subtle language impairments includes those diagnosed as reading- or learning-disabled. Wiig and Semel (1976) have suggested that between 75 percent and 85 percent of learning-disabled students have experienced language delays and that some of these continue into adulthood. Finally, children who are considered to be "academically at risk" due to poor school performance are also likely to have gaps in their ability to perform linguistic tasks (Simon, 1989).

The speech-language pathologist should carefully evaluate youngsters from these groups, especially when they are referred by classroom teachers. Many of the specific language symptoms likely to be seen in these groups were listed in Table 5.1. A variety of formal tests and nonstandardized assessment procedures have been discussed in this chapter and should serve well in appraising the communication abilities in these children. One aspect that has not been emphasized, however, is specifically examining the types of language and communication abilities that are important for classroom success.

If a school-age child has some subtle language impairments and shows poor academic performance, part of a thorough evaluation should include (1) assessment of the child's knowledge of successful strategies to perform well in the school culture; (2) an evaluation of the teacher's communication while instructing the child; and (3) an assessment of the curriculum and materials that the child is expected to learn. You may wonder why an SLP would be interested in assessing these factors when they are peripheral to the child's abilities. A school-age child is part of a complex system that is constantly changing its expectations for academic performance. The child may have to deal with differing types of educational content and a variety of teaching styles throughout the school day. The school-age child must use language in both comprehension and production for a variety of academic tasks that often involve complex metalinguistic abilities and abstract concepts presented verbally by a teacher. Teachers and SLPs should remember that metalinguistic abilities appear to be acquired in a general developmental order (Table 5.2). Additionally, the child must be aware of the expectations of the school culture and know how to study, memorize, and effectively learn classroom material upon which he/she will be thoroughly tested. If the child has no effective study skills or strategies for remembering and understanding information, failure will occur. The child's teacher could talk at a rapid rate during instruction or use figurative language and complex

Table 5.2 Development of Metalinguistic Abilities

Stage One (Ages 1½ to 2):
- Distinguishes print from nonprint
- Knows how to interact with books: right side up, page turning from left to right
- Recognizes some printed symbols, e.g., TV character's name, brand names, signs

Stage Two (Ages 2 to 5½ or 6):
- Ascertains word boundaries in spoken sentences
- Ascertains word boundaries in printed sequences
- Engages in word substitution play
- Plays with the sounds of language
- Begins to talk about talking (speech acts)
- Corrects own speech/language to help the listener understand the message (spontaneously or in response to listener request)
- Self-monitors own speech and makes changes to more closely approximate the adult model; phonological first; lexical and semantic speech style last
- Believes that a word is an integral part of the object to which it refers (word realism)
- Able to separate words into syllables
- Inability to consider that one word could have two different meanings

Stage Three (Ages 6 to 10):
- Begins to take listener perspective and use language form to match
- Understands verbal humor involving linguistic ambiguity, e.g., riddles
- Able to resolve ambiguity: lexical first, as in homophones; deep structures next, as in ambiguous phrases ("Will you join me in a bowl of soup?"); phonological or morphemic next (Q: "What do you have if you put three ducks in a box?" A: "A box of quackers.")
- Able to understand that words can have two meanings, one literal and the other nonconventional or idiomatic, e.g., adjectives used to describe personality characteristics such as *hard, sweet, bitter*
- Able to resequence language elements, as in pig Latin
- Able to segment syllables into phonemes
- Finds it difficult to appreciate figurative forms other than idioms

Stage Four (Ages 10 +):
- Able to extend language meaning into hypothetical realm (e.g., to understand figurative language such as metaphors, similes, parodies, analogies)
- Able to manipulate various speech styles to fit a variety of contexts and listeners

Wallach, G., & Miller, L. (1988). *Language Intervention and Academic Success.* Boston: College-Hill Press, p. 33.

sentence types. The teacher could be quite adept at using audio and visual media as aids to instruction or rely exclusively on the lecture modality. The reading curriculum could have a heavy emphasis on phonics or other metalinguistic tasks that may make the learning of reading extremely difficult or impossible for a child with metalinguistic problems. In some cases, an alternative approach could help a child learn a particular skill. What we are saying here is that the diagnostician cannot fully understand the language-impaired child unless he/she is familiar with the child's learning environment. Sometimes, the most potent treatment recommendations include curricular, instructional, and learning strategy modifications. Without examining these areas in a thorough assessment, a clinician cannot hope to make effective suggestions for remediation.

Some useful measures that focus on classroom communication abilities and/or metalinguistics in older students (e.g., upper elementary through junior high) are *Evaluating Communicative Competence (ECC)* (Simon, 1987), *Classroom Communication Screening Procedure for Early Assessment (CCSPEA)* (Simon, 1989), and *Analysis of the Language of Learning (ALL)* (Blodgett & Cooper, 1987). These procedures will provide insight into a child's ability to perform classroomlike tasks and pinpoint specific difficulties. The clinician can also experiment with any facilitating procedures that make difficult tasks more easily accomplished and mention these in the examination report for teacher use.

A FINAL NOTE ON MULTICULTURAL VARIATION

Brown (1973) has noted that there are striking cross-cultural similarities in children's language acquisition. That is, children from a variety of cultures tend to develop the same types of early word combinations, presumably because these semantic relations rest on concepts developed in the sensorimotor period of cognitive development. Although we may not find differences in word combinations across cultures, there may certainly be variations in prelinguistic and single-word development in various groups. Research on this issue has yet to be completed. In older children, however, there have been dramatic differences reported in the development of grammatical morphemes, vocabulary, specific sentence types, and pragmatics (Cole & Deal, 1991; Dillard, 1972; Taylor, 1986a, 1986b; Williams & Wolfram, 1977). We are only beginning to understand the specifics of multicultural variation in later language development, but we are certain that these differences exist. Especially when assessing school-age and adolescent students, it is of paramount importance that the SLP consider cultural differences in pragmatics and syntax. It is beyond the scope of the present chapter to outline all the possible linguistic variations produced by the various cultural groups in the United States (e.g., African-American, Native American, Hispanic, Asian). The references previously cited will provide a good beginning for the clinician in learning about cultural influences on language. It is the responsibility of each SLP to at least become familiar with the dialects spoken locally. Dialectal differences *must* be considered in making judgments about the existence of a disorder, in selecting test instruments, and in recommending treatment goals. It is our ethical responsibility to take multicultural influences into account.

CONCLUSION

One can easily see that the diagnosis and evaluation of school-age and adolescent clients is a complex activity. The speech-language pathologist must work closely with teachers, parents, and other professionals in successfully dealing with these cases. The interplay between linguistic, metalinguistic, conversational, and academic areas is great and the work of the SLP can potentially reap benefits in a child's educational performance.

BIBLIOGRAPHY

ARAM, D., & NATION, J. (1980). Preschool language disorders and subsequent language and academic difficulties. *Journal of Communication Disorders, 13,* 159–170.

ARAM, D., & NATION, J. (1982). *Child language disorders.* St. Louis, MO: C. V. Mosby Co.

ATKINS, C., & CARTWRIGHT, L. (1982). An investigation of the effectiveness of three language elicitation procedures on Headstart children. *Language, Speech and Hearing Services in Schools, 13,* 33–36.

BARRIE-BLACKLEY, S., MUSSELWHITE, C., & ROGISTER, S. (1978). *Clinical oral language sampling.* Danville, IL: Interstate.

BASHIR, A., KUBAN, K., KLEINMAN, S., & SCAVUZZO, A. (1983). Issues in language disorders: Considerations of cause, maintenance and change. In J. Miller, D. Yoder, R. Schiefelbusch (Eds.), *ASHA Report No. 12,* 92–106.

BATTLE, D., ALDES, M., GRANTHAM, R., HALFOND, M., HARRIS, G., MORGENSTERN-LOPEZ, N., SMITH, G., TERRELL, S., & COLE, L. (1983). Position paper on social dialects. *Journal of the American Speech-Language-Hearing Association, 25,* 23–24.

BLAGDEN, C., & MCCONNELL, N. (1983). *Interpersonal language skills assessment.* Moline, IL: Linguisystems.

BLASDELL, R., & JENSEN, P. (1970). Stress and word position determinants of imitation in first language learners. *Journal of Speech and Hearing Research, 13,* 193–202.

BLODGETT, E., & COOPER, E. (1987). *Analysis of the language of learning: The practical test of metalinguistics.* Moline, IL: Linguisystems.

BLOOM, L. (1974). Talking, understanding and thinking. In R. Schiefelbusch & L. Lloyd (Eds.), *Language Perspectives—Acquisition, Retardation and Intervention.* Baltimore: University Park Press.

BLOOM, L., & LAHEY, M. (1978). *Language development and language disorders.* New York: John Wiley.

BLOOM, L., ROCISSANO, L., & HOOD, L. (1976). Adult-child discourse: Developmental interaction between information processing and linguistic knowledge. *Cognitive Psychology, 8,* 521–552.

BONVILLIAN, J., RAEBURN, V., & HORAN, E. (1979). Talking to children: The effects of rate, intonation and length on children's sentence imitation. *Journal of Child Language, 3,* 459–467.

BRANSFORD, J., & NITSCH, K. (1978). Coming to understand things we could not previously understand. In J. Kavanagh & W. Strange (Eds.), *Speech and language in the laboratory, school and clinic.* Cambridge, MA: MIT Press.

BRINTON, B., & FUJIKI, M. (1984). Development of topic manipulation skills in discourse. *Journal of Speech and Hearing Research, 27,* 350–358.

BRINTON, B., & FUJIKI, M. (1989). *Conversational management with language-impaired children.* Rockville, MD: Aspen.

BROWN, R. (1973). *A first language: The early stages.* Cambridge, MA: Harvard University Press.

CARROW, E. (1974). *Carrow elicited language inventory.* Austin, TX: Learning Concepts.

CAZDEN, C. (1970). The neglected situation of child language research and education. In F. Williams (Ed.), *Language and poverty: Perspectives on a theme.* Chicago: Rand-McNally.

COLE, L., & DEAL, V. (1991). *Communication disorders in multicultural populations.* Rockville, MD: American Speech-Language-Hearing Association.

CONNELL, P., & MYLES-ZITZER, C. (1982). An analysis of elicited imitation as a language evaluation procedure. *Journal of Speech and Hearing Disorders, 47,* 390–396.

CONOLEY, J., & KRAMER, J. (1989). *Tenth mental measurements yearbook.* Buros Institute of Mental Measurements. Lincoln, NE: University of Nebraska.

CRYSTAL, D., FLETCHER, P., & GARMAN, M. (1976). *The grammatical analysis of language disability: A procedure for assessment and remediation.* London: Edward Arnold.

DAILY, K., & BOXX, J. (1979). A comparison of three imitative tests of expressive language and a spontaneous language sample. *Language, Speech and Hearing Services in Schools, 10,* 6–13.

DAMICO, J. (1980). *Clinical discourse analysis.* Miniseminar presented at the convention of the American Speech-Language-Hearing Association, Detroit.

DAMICO, J. (1985). Clinical discourse analysis: A functional approach to language assessment. In C. Simon (Ed.), *Communication skills and classroom success: Assessment of language-learning disabled students.* San Diego, CA: College-Hill.

DARLEY, F. (1979). *Evaluation of appraisal techniques in speech and language pathology.* Reading, MA: Addison-Wesley.

DEVER, R., & BAUMAN, P. (1974). Scale of children's clausal development. In T. Longhurst (Ed.), *Linguistic analysis of children's speech.* New York: MSS Information Corp.

DILLARD, J. (1972). *Black English.* New York: Random House.

EDMONDS, P., & HAYNES, W. (1988). Topic manipulation and conversational participation as a function of familiarity in school-age language-impaired and normal language peers. *Journal of Communication Disorders, 21,* 209–228.

EHLERS, P., & CIRRIN, F. (1983). *Topic relevancy abilities of language-impaired children.* Paper presented at the annual convention of the American Speech-Language-Hearing Association, Cincinnati, OH.

ENGLER, L., HANNAH, E., & LONGHURST, T. (1973). Linguistic analysis of speech samples: A practical guide for clinicians. *Journal of Speech and Hearing Disorders, 38,* 192–204.

FEY, M. (1986). *Language intervention with young children.* San Diego, CA: College-Hill.

FEY, M., & LEONARD, L. (1983). Pragmatic skills of children with specific language impairment. In T. Gallagher & C. Prutting (Eds.), *Pragmatic assessment and intervention issues in language.* San Diego, CA: College-Hill.

FUJIKI, M., & BRINTON, B. (1983). Sampling reliability in elicited imitation. *Journal of Speech and Hearing Disorders, 48,* 85–89.

GALLAGHER, T. (1982). *Pragmatics.* Workshop presented at Auburn University, Alabama.

GARVEY, C. (1977a). The contingent query: A dependent act in conversation. In M. Lewis & L. Rosenblum (Eds.), *Interaction, conversation, and the development of language* (Vol. 5). New York: Wiley.

GARVEY, C. (1977b). Play with language and speech. In S. Ervin-Tripp & C. Mitchell-Kernan (Eds.), *Child discourse.* New York: Academic Press.

GOWIE, C., & POWERS, J. (1979). Relations among cognitive, semantic and syntactic variables in children's comprehension of the minimal distance principle: A two year developmental study. *Journal of Psycholinguistic Research, 8,* 29–41.

GRICE, H. (1975). Logic and conversation. In P. Cole & J. Morgan (Eds.), *Studies in syntax, semantics and speech acts* (Vol. 3). New York: Academic Press.

HALL, P., & TOMBLIN, J. (1978). A follow-up study of children with articulation and language disorders, *Journal of Speech and Hearing Disorders, 43,* 227–241.

HALLIDAY, M., & HASAN, R. (1976). *Cohesion in English.* London: Longman.

HANIFF, M., & SIEGEL, G. (1981). The effect of context on verbal elicited imitation. *Journal of Speech and Hearing Disorders, 46,* 27–30.

HAYNES, W., & HAYNES, M. (1979). Pragmatics and elicited imitation: Children's performance on discursively related and discursively unrelated sentences. *Journal of Communication Disorders, 12,* 471–479.

HAYNES, W., & HOOD, S. (1978). Disfluency changes in children as a function of the systematic modification of linguistic complexity. *Journal of Communication Disorders, 11,* 79–93.

HAYNES, W., & McCALLION, M. (1981). Language comprehension testing: The influence of cognitive tempo and three modes of test administration. *Language, Speech and Hearing Services in Schools, 12,* 74–81.

HAYNES, W., PURCELL, E., & HAYNES, M. (1979). A pragmatic aspect of language sampling. *Language, Speech and Hearing Services in Schools, 10,* 104–110.

HUBBELL, R. (1981). *Children's language disorders: An integrated approach.* Englewood Cliffs, NJ: Prentice Hall.

HUBBELL, R. (1988). *A handbook of English grammar and language sampling.* Englewood Cliffs, NJ: Prentice Hall.

HYMES, D. (1971). Competence and performance in linguistic theory. In R. Huxley & E. Ingram (Eds.), *Language acquisition: Models and methods.* New York: Academic Press.

JOHNSTON, J. (1982). Narrative: A new look at communication problems in older language-disordered children. *Language, Speech and Hearing Services in Schools, 13,* 144–155.

KAHN, L., & JAMES, S. (1980). A method for assessing the use of grammatical structures in language-disordered children. *Language, Speech and Hearing Services in Schools, 11,* 188–197.

KEENAN, E., & SCHIEFFLIN, B. (1976). Topic as a discourse notion: A study of topic in the conversations of children and adults. In C. Li (Ed.), *Subject and topic.* New York: Academic Press.

KING, R., JONES, C., & LASKY, E. (1982). In retrospect: A fifteen year follow-up report of speech-language disorders in children. *Language, Speech and Hearing Services in Schools, 13,* 24–32.

KRAMER, C., JAMES, S., & SAXMAN, J. (1979). A comparison of language samples elicited at home and in the clinic. *Journal of Speech and Hearing Disorders, 44,* 321–330.

LABOV, W. (1970). The logic on nonstandard English. In F. Williams (Ed.), *Language and poverty: Perspectives on a theme.* Chicago: Rand-McNally.

LANG, M., & MOORE, W. (1977). *Some variables affecting sentence imitation of normal children.* Unpublished research, Auburn University, Alabama.

LEE, L. (1974). *Developmental sentence analysis.* Evanston, IL: Northwestern University Press.

LEE, L., KOENIGSKNECHT, R., & MULHERN, S. (1975). *Interactive language development teaching.* Evanston, IL: Northwestern University Press.

LEONARD, L., PRUTTING, C., PEROZZI, C., & BERKLEY, R. (1978). Nonstandardized approaches to the assessment of language behaviors. *Journal of the American Speech and Hearing Association,* May, *20,* 371–379.

LILES, B. (1985). Cohesion in the narratives of normal and language disordered children. *Journal of Speech and Hearing Research, 28,* 123–133.

LOBAN, W. (1976). *Language Development.* Champaign, IL: National Council of Teachers of English.

LONG, S., & FEY, M. (1988). *Computerized Profiling.* P.O. Box 1139, Arcata, CA, 95521.

LONGHURST, T., & FILE, J. (1977). A comparison of developmental sentence scores for Headstart children in four conditions. *Language, Speech and Hearing Services in Schools, 8,* 54–64.

LONGHURST, T., & GRUBB, S. (1974). A comparison of language samples collected in four situations. *Language, Speech and Hearing Services in Schools, 5,* 71–78.

LONGHURST, T., & SCHRANDT, T. (1973). Linguistic analysis of children's speech: A comparison of four procedures. *Journal of Speech and Hearing Disorders, 38,* 240–249.

LUCAS, E. (1980). *Semantic and pragmatic language disorders.* Rockville, MD: Aspen Systems Corporation.

LUND, N., & DUCHAN, J. (1988). *Assessing children's language in naturalistic contexts.* Englewood Cliffs, NJ: Prentice Hall.

MCCARTHY, D. (1930). The language development of the preschool child. *Child Welfare Monographs,* No. 4, Minneapolis: University of Minnesota Press.

MCDADE, H., SIMPSON, M., & LARNT, D. (1982). The use of elicited imitation as a measure of expressive grammar: A question of validity. *Journal of Speech and Hearing Disorders, 47,* 19–24.

MILLEN, K., & PRUTTING, C. (1979). Consistencies across three language comprehension tests for specific grammatical features. *Language, Speech and Hearing Services in Schools, 10,* 162–170.

MILLER, J. (1981). *Assessing language production in children: Experimental procedures.* Baltimore: University Park Press.

MILLER, J., & CHAPMAN, R. (1985). *SALT: Systematic analysis of language transcripts.* Madison, WI: Language Analysis Laboratory, University of Wisconsin.

MINER, L. (1969). Scoring procedures for the length-complexity index: A preliminary report. *Journal of Communication Disorders, 2,* 224–240.

MORDECAI, D., PALIN, M., & PALMER, C. (1982). *Lingquest 1.* Napa, CA: Lingquest Software.

MULAC, A., PRUTTING, C., & TOMLINSON, C. (1978). Testing for a specific syntactic structure. *Journal of Communication Disorders, 11,* 335–347.

MUMA, J. (1973a). Language assessment: Some underlying assumptions. *Journal of the American Speech and Hearing Association, 15,* 331–338.

MUMA, J. (1973b). Language assessment: The co-occurring and restricted structure procedure. *Acta Symbolica, 4,* 12–29.

MUMA, J. (1975). The communication game: Dump and play. *Journal of Speech and Hearing Disorders, 40,* 296–309.

MUMA, J. (1978). *Language handbook: Concepts, assessment, intervention.* Englewood Cliffs, NJ: Prentice Hall.

MUSSELWHITE, C., & BARRIE-BLACKLEY, S. (1980). Three variations of the imperative format of language sample elicitation. *Language, Speech and Hearing Services in Schools, 11,* 56–67.

NELSON, L., & WEBER-OLSEN, M. (1980). The elicited language inventory and the influence of contextual cues. *Journal of Speech and Hearing Disorders, 45,* 549–563.

OLSWANG, L., & CARPENTER, R. (1978). Elicitor effects on the language obtained from young language-impaired children. *Journal of Speech and Hearing Disorders, 43,* 76–86.

OWENS, R., HANEY, M., GRIESOW, V., DOOLEY, L., & KELLY, R. (1983). Language test content: A comparative study. *Language, Speech and Hearing Services in Schools, 14,* 7–21.

PETERSON, H., MARQUARDT, T. (1990). *Appraisal and diagnosis of speech and language disorders.* Englewood Cliffs, NJ: Prentice Hall.

PRUTTING, C., & CONNOLLY, J. (1976). Imitation: A closer look. *Journal of Speech and Hearing Disorders, 41,* 412–422.

PRUTTING, C., GALLAGHER, T., & MULAC, A. (1975). The expressive portion of the NSST compared to a spontaneous language sample. *Journal of Speech and Hearing Disorders, 40,* 40–48.

PRUTTING, C., & KIRCHNER, D. (1987). A clinical appraisal of the pragmatic aspects of language. *Journal of Speech and Hearing Disorders, 52,* 105–119.

QUIRK, R., & GREENBAUM, S. (1975). *A concise grammar of contemporary English.* San Diego, CA: Harcourt Brace Jovanovich.

REES, N., & SHULMAN, M. (1978). I don't understand what you mean by comprehension. *Journal of Speech and Hearing Disorders, 43,* 208–219.

SHARF, D. (1972). Some relationships between measures of early language development. *Journal of Speech and Hearing Disorders, 37,* 64–74.

SHEPPARD, A. (1980). *Monologue and dialogue of speech and language-impaired children in clinic and home settings: Semantic, conversational and syntactic characteristics.* Master's thesis, University of Western Ontario.

SHORR, D. (1983). Grammatical comprehension assessment: The picture avoidance strategy. *Journal of Speech and Hearing Disorders, 48,* 89–92.

SHULMAN, B. (1986). *Test of pragmatic skills—Revised.* Tucson, AZ: Communication Skill Builders.

SIMON, C. (1987). Out of the broom closet and into the classroom: The emerging SLP. *Journal of Childhood Communication Disorders, 11,* 41–66.

SIMON, C. (1989). *Classroom communication screening procedure for early adolescents (CCSPEA).* Tempe, AZ: Communi-Cog Publications.

SLOBIN, D., & WELSH, C. (1971). Elicited imitation as a research tool in developmental psycholinguistics. In C. Lavatelli (Ed.), *Language training in early childhood education.* Urbana, IL: University of Illinois Press.

STEIN, A. (1976). *A comparison of mothers' and fathers' language to normal and language deficient children.* Unpublished doctoral dissertation, Boston University.

STOVER, S., & HAYNES, W. (1989). Topic manipulation and cohesive adequacy in conversations of normal adults between the ages of 30 and 90. *Clinical Linguistics and Phonetics, 3,* 137–149.

STRANDBERG, T., & GRIFFITH, J. (1969). A study of the effects of training in visual literacy on verbal language behavior. *Journal of Communication Disorders, 2,* 252–263.

STROMINGER, A., & BASHIR, A. (1977). *A nine year follow-up of language-delayed children.* Paper presented at the convention of the American Speech-Language-Hearing Association, Chicago.

TAYLOR, O. (1986a). *Nature of communication disorders in culturally and linguistically diverse populations.* San Diego: College-Hill.

TAYLOR, O. (1986b). *Treatment of communication disorders in culturally and linguistically diverse populations.* San Diego: College-Hill.

TYACK, D., & GOTTSLEBEN, R. (1974). *Language sampling, analysis and training: A handbook for teachers and clinicians.* Palo Alto, CA: Consulting Psychologists Press.

WATSON, L. (1977). *Conversational participation by language deficient and normal children.* Paper presented at the convention of the American Speech and Hearing Association, Chicago.

WERNER, E., & KRESECK, J. (1981). Variability in scores, structures and errors on three measures of expressive language. *Language, Speech and Hearing Services in Schools, 12,* 82–89.

WIIG, E., & SEMEL, E. (1976). *Language disabilities in children and adolescents.* Columbus, OH: Merrill.

WILLIAMS, R., & WOLFRAM, W. (1977). *Social differences vs. disorders.* Washington, DC: American Speech and Hearing Association.

ZACHMAN, L., HULSINGH, R., JORGENSEN, C., & BARRETT, M. (1978). *Oral language sentence imitation test.* Moline, IL: Linguisystems.

chapter

6

ASSESSMENT OF PHONOLOGICAL DISORDERS

THE ARTICULATORY PROCESS

In the early portion of this century, articulation was conceptualized by most clinicians as primarily a motor act. The sensorimotor aspect of articulation was studied and trained in therapy. It was not uncommon for articulation treatment to emphasize almost exclusively the movements of the oral musculature through diagrams, models, and motoric drills (Scripture & Jackson, 1927). During this period, speech-language pathologists were content to call deviations of the sound system by the generic term *articulation disorders*. Many practicing clinicians today continue to use this term to refer to children and adults who exhibit omissions, substitutions, and distortions in their speech. With the advent of greater attention to language in the 1950s, however, it was noted that articulation had more components than simply motoric activity. In the mid 1970s, speech-language pathologists became highly interested in the work of linguists (e.g., Ingram, 1976) who examined sound production differences from the perspective of phonological theory. It is now well accepted that linguistic activity contributes to the articulatory process (Bernthal & Bankson, 1988; Schwartz, 1983; Shelton & McReynolds, 1979; Shriberg & Kwiatkowski, 1982a, 1982b).

Many events occur prior to the actual motor act of articulating. First, there is a biological component to articulation. The speaker must have a vocal tract and intact sensory and motor systems. Second, there is a cognitive-linguistic component in which the speaker conceives of something to say. The thought then undergoes linguistic processing in which semantic elements are selected, words are arranged in proper syntactic order, and the utterance is appropriately tailored to the communicative situation by the speaker, taking pragmatics into consideration. Finally, the selection of phonemic elements and their order is accomplished by applying the phonological rules of our language. The details of linguistic processing of an utterance are not yet fully understood. It is enough to say, however, that linguistic processing involving semantic, syntactic, pragmatic, and phonological areas must be necessary at some point in expressing an utterance. Subsequent to language processing, motor commands of some sort must be sent to the articulators in order to make them produce the sequence of sounds dictated by phonological programming. Much research has been directed toward determining the basic unit of articulatory motor programming, and we do not presently know its size or identity. Motor production in the vocal tract then gives rise to acoustic vibrations that travel through a medium of air and arrive at the ears of our listeners.

This brief sketch of the processes that result in articulatory production is highly simplified. It is possible to divide this process into at least three major areas. First, the biological component provides the basic structures for articulation. The vocal tract, the articulators, and the intact nervous system allow us to perform the sensory (auditory, tactile, kinesthetic, proprioceptive) and motor functions necessary for controlled movement. Second, there is a cognitive-linguistic component that includes the thought, semantic-syntactic-pragmatic processing and the application of phonological rules. Third, there is a sensori-motor-acoustic component that includes motor programming and motor learning of actual sequences of physical movement in a wide variety of phonetic contexts.

It is the view of the present authors that this gross division of the articulatory process into biological, cognitive-linguistic, and sensorimotor components carries with it several important implications. First, the diagnostician must be prepared to assess and treat any or all aspects of the process in a given client. For example, some authorities (Bernthal & Bankson, 1988) differentiate articulation disorders from *phonological disorders*. Bernthal and Bankson indicate that articulation disorders can be "motorically based errors (the ability to produce a target sound is not within the person's repertoire of motor skills) . . . or cognitively or linguistically based (the client can produce a sound but does not use the sound in appropriate contexts)" (1988, p. 3). They further state that differentiating a motoric from a linguistically based disorder is not always an easy task. If the client primarily exhibits a linguistically based problem (e.g., a phonological simplification such as deletion of certain final consonants), we should be able to examine a sample of speech for patterns of errors that represent these phonological reductions. Oral-peripheral, motoric, audiological, and ultimately medical/neurological evaluation procedures can pinpoint difficulties with the biological/sensorimotor foundations of articulation. The implication, then, is that a client can have difficulties with one or several parts of the process and the diagnostician should be equipped to assess these (Grunwell, 1988).

There are several ways of categorizing misarticulations. Historically, speech pathologists have used the traditional classifications of (1) substitution of one sound for another ("thoup" for "soup"); (2) omission of a sound ("kool" for "school"); (3) distortion of a sound (nonstandard production of a sound); and (4) addition of a sound ("puhlease" for "please"). These historical classifications have persisted because they do describe most articulatory deviations. If there is any fault with the categories, it is that they are not specific enough. The diagnostician must say more than "the child has substitutions and omissions." We need to know which sounds are substituted for others, how often, and in what contexts. The same could be said for distortions, omissions, and additions. Another example of the superficiality of the historical categories is that they do not imply what part of the articulatory process is affected. That is, we cannot discern from the category of "substitution" whether the error is related to deficiencies in the client's sensorimotor or linguistic/phonological systems. The traditional classifications, however, are a good place to begin the articulatory assessment. We can then assess further and attempt to determine variability of performance in specific phonetic contexts, as well as in utterances of different linguistic complexities.

Articulatory errors can also be divided into two categories: *organic* (some physical cause for the misarticulatation) and *functional* (no demonstrable organic cause). The latter term has come under criticism for quite some time. Powers (1971) calls the term *functional* a "diagnosis by default." This is because the diagnosis of organic requires some positive proof of organicity while the diagnosis of functional requires no positive evidence. The classification of functional is made only when a lack of evidence or organicity exists. Functional articulation errors are usually attributed to faulty learning patterns, resulting in an established habit. Thus, although the classification of functional has been justifiably criticized, it is still widely held that the vast majority of articulation disorders have no significant, maintaining organic basis and the treatment is behavioral in nature. However, future research may yet uncover subtle organic or behavioral differences in these individuals (Bernthal & Bankson, 1988). Assessment of organically based articulation disorders such as dysarthria and apraxia will be dealt with in our chapter on motor speech disorders. The present chapter focuses on misarticulations that have no obvious organic component. For the remainder of the chapter, we will use the term *phonological disorder* to refer to those functional cases that involve multiple phoneme errors. The term *articulation disorder* will be reserved for clients who misarticulate only one or two phonemes.

A second implication of a multicomponent conception of articulation is that no single measure is presently capable of adequately examining all parts of this complex process. It is naive to believe that administration of a traditional articulation test and an oral-peripheral examination are all that are necessary to perform a complete assessment of articulatory behavior. The articulatory process is just too complex and the disordered population too heterogeneous to rely on one or two standard tests. In this chapter, we are emphasizing the importance of knowing "where to go" and "what to do" to gain insight into aspects of articulation that are revealed to be problematic by the initial testing. As with any disorder area, no single chapter can possibly tell a student how to do everything well. Our goal is simply to make clinicians aware of the possibilities in articulatory assessment and refer the reader to the appropriate literature.

SEVEN IMPORTANT FACTORS IN THE EVALUATION OF PHONOLOGICAL DISORDERS

Before we discuss assessment of phonological disorders, there are several areas with which the clinician should be familiar. In actuality, there are more areas that could be considered, but these seven seem to us to be critical prerequisites to performing a diagnostic evaluation.

1. *Knowledge of the Anatomy and Physiology of the Speech Mechanism:* Before attempting to deal with an articulatory evaluation, the clinician should be fully familiar with the normal oral mechanism. Most students obtain this knowledge in their undergraduate training, and many textbooks provide this information (Daniloff, Schuckers, & Feth, 1980; Dickson & Maue-Dickson, 1982; Kahane & Folkins, 1984; Palmer, 1984; Zemlin, 1988).

2. *Knowledge of Phonetics:* It is one thing to know about the anatomy and physiology of the vocal mechanism, but it is quite another to be aware of how that apparatus actually produces the variety of consonant and vowel sounds in English. References have described sound productions and articulatory movements associated with them (Carrell & Tiffany, 1960; Shriberg & Kent, 1982; Van Riper & Smith, 1979). Aside from knowing articulatory phonetics, the clinician must have well-developed skills in phonetic transcription. This is important in order to record a client's productions accurately for later analysis. Reliable phonetic transcription abilities are especially important in order to accomplish phonological analyses (Shriberg & Kwiatkowski, 1980).

3. *Knowledge of Phonological Development:* A major goal in diagnosis is to compare a child's articulatory performance to the behavior of normal children in the same age range. In this way we can tell if a child's misarticulations are developmental in nature or clinically significant. There are at least three interpretations of articulatory development the clinician should be familiar with prior to doing an assessment.

The most abundant normative data available are the traditional studies of children's production of words with the target sound in the initial, medial, and final positions (Poole, 1934; Templin, 1957; Wellman et al., 1931). Although their procedures and criteria for acquisition differ (Smit, 1986), they provide ages at which children master phonemes. More recent data (Irwin & Wong, 1983; Prather, Hendrick, & Kern, 1975; Sander, 1972) suggest earlier development of speech sounds and provide age ranges for both "customary production" (two or three word positions) and mastery. The data provided by Irwin and Wong (1983) deal with sound production in connected spontaneous speech as opposed to the typical single-word responses reported in other traditional studies. Figure 6.1 provides an example of normative consonant development data. Most misarticulations in phonologically disordered children involve consonants, so only consonant

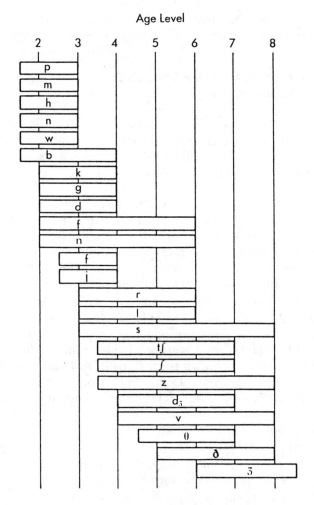

Figure 6.1 Average Age Estimates and Upper Age Limits of Customary Consonant Production. The Solid Bar Corresponding to Each Sound Starts at the Median Age of Customary Articulation; it Stops at the Age Level at Which 90 Percent of All Children Are Customarily Producing the Sound. (Sander, 1972: 62; © 1972, the American Speech-Language-Hearing Association, Rockville, Maryland.)

development data are presented here. Vowels are typically developed by age three (Bernthal & Bankson, 1988). This does not mean that vowels are never involved in phonological disorders (Hodson, 1980) or that vowels are easily acquired; in fact, their development is quite complicated (Davis & MacNeilage, 1990).

A second type of developmental data involves distinctive feature acquisition. Several sources report a developmental order in distinctive feature acquisition (Blache, 1978; Singh, 1976). These data could be used when analyzing a child's distinctive feature system as opposed to more traditional norms.

Finally, data are available regarding the occurrence of phonological reduction processes or patterns of error in normally developing children (Ingram, 1976; Shriberg & Kwiatkowski, 1980). These provide some general age cutoffs for certain phonological processes and give the SLP a view of a child's error pattern not found in traditional norms. If a clinician sees a child who is deleting final consonants, for instance, traditional norms cannot be used to determine when this tendency diminishes in normal children. Most studies have focused on children's phonological development between the ages of three and eight years. More recent investigations have concentrated on children from one to three years in response to the emphasis on early intervention and increased interest in early normal development (Dyson, 1988; Grunwell, 1988; Kahn & Lewis, 1986; Stoel-Gammon, 1987). Figure 6.2 provides an example of normative data developed within the phonological process perspective.

Bernthal and Bankson (1988) point out that there are very little longitudinal developmental data and most of the information was gleaned from cross-sectional investigations. No doubt, as in other aspects of development, a variety of articulatory acquisition strategies will eventually be found. A major point we wish to make here is that the clinician can look at an articulatory sample from a variety of perspectives. Traditional as well as distinctive feature and phonological norms provide a reference point to use in assessment and treatment.

4. *Knowledge of Factors Related to Phonological Disorders:* Whenever a clinician undertakes a phonological evaluation, it can be expected that parents will often ask questions regarding the etiology of the problem. The clinician, then, must be familiar with the pertinent literature dealing with research on etiological factors, as well as skills and abilities of articulation-disordered children. Questions may be asked about language development, reading, spelling, educational performance, dentition, oral structures, gross and fine motor skills, intelligence, auditory abilities, and much more. Several sources summarize this research and should assist clinicians in answering any questions (Bernthal & Bankson, 1988; Powers, 1971; Winitz, 1969).

5. *Knowledge of Dialectal Variation:* Many sources have reported articulatory differences as a product of regional dialect (Carrell & Tiffany, 1960; Van Riper & Smith, 1979). Other authorities report phonological differences in minority populations (Dillard, 1972; Stoller, 1975; Taylor, 1986). According to the American Speech-Language-Hearing Association, the clinician performing an articulatory evaluation must be able to differentiate a communication disorder from a dialectal variation (Battle et al., 1983). Since there are so few tests that take dialect into account, the clinician must become familiar with this material and routinely consider it when evaluating misarticulations.

6. *Coarticulation:* For at least 30 years, researchers have known that speech is produced in a parallel fashion as opposed to a serial, discrete manner (Winitz, 1975). This means that speech sounds are not isolated entities, but they overlap motorically and acoustically in time. Put simply, sounds are influenced

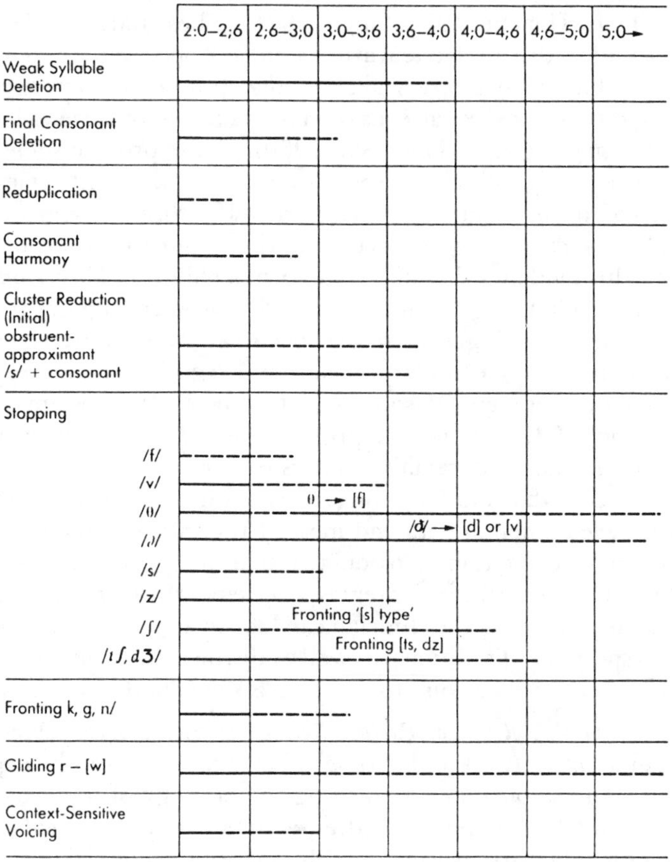

	2;0–2;6	2;6–3;0	3;0–3;6	3;6–4;0	4;0–4;6	4;6–5;0	5;0→
Weak Syllable Deletion	———	———	———	– – –			
Final Consonant Deletion	———	– –	–				
Reduplication	– – –						
Consonant Harmony	– –	– –					
Cluster Reduction (Initial) obstruent-approximant	———	– – –	– – –	———			
/s/ + consonant	———	– – –	– –	———			
Stopping							
/f/	– – –	– –	·				
/v/		– – –	– – –				
/θ/			θ → [f]				
/ð/				/ð/ → [d] or [v]		– – –	– –
/s/	———	– – –	– ·				
/z/	———	– – –	–				
/ʃ/	Fronting '[s] type'						
/tʃ, dʒ/	Fronting [ts, dz]						
Fronting k, g, n/	———	– – –	– ·				
Gliding r – [w]	———	– – –	– – –	———			
Context-Sensitive Voicing	– ·	– – –					

SOURCE: Adapted by permission from P. Grunwell, "The Development of Phonology: A Descriptive Profile." *First Language*, 2 (1981) pp. 161–191. Used with permission. © 1987 The William & Wilkins Co., Baltimore, MD.

Figure 6.2 Chronology of Phonological Processes

by other phonemes that surround them. This influence of one sound on another is called *coarticulation* and is one of the most basic facts about the articulatory process. The surrounding phonetic environment or phonetic context of a phoneme influences its production. There are two major types of coarticulation that can be described in terms of the direction of the influence of one sound on another. Left-to-right coarticulation refers to a preceding sound's having an affect on a following sound (the "t" in "boots" is produced with some lip rounding because of the rounding /u/ vowel that precedes it). This type of coarticulation is perceived by some to be a type of overflow of movement from the first sound to the second. Thus, the left-to-right coarticulation is thought to be primarily the result of mechanical-inertial factors. The other type of coarticulation is right-to-left. This means that a sound that occurs later in the speech sequence affects a sound earlier in the stream of speech. For example, the "t" sound in the word "tea" is produced differently from the "t" in the word "too." The difference in the two situations is that in the word "tea," the sound is followed by a vowel that is not produced with rounded lips. But the "t" sound in "too" might be produced with lip rounding because the following vowel is rounded. Note that in both of these cases, the sound that influences the "t" occurs after the "t" has been uttered. Researchers and theorists have suggested that the right-to-left influence is probably the result of articulatory preprogramming. That is, early sounds in a sequence are produced differently in anticipation of sounds that are yet to be said. This implies some sort of motor planning. There are many studies of coarticulation that have used cinefluorography, electromyography, and spectrographic analyses. These investigations have shown conclusively that coarticulation does, in fact, occur in speech sequences. Since it is a fact that coarticulation will be present in any utterance, it is a phenomenon that the speech pathologist can choose to use as a tool in assessment and treatment. Whether we use coarticulatory influences in assessment and treatment to increase the efficiency of our clinical work or not, the effects will still occur. Most authorities feel that as long as coarticulation exists, we might as well use it in the best interest of our client.

The implications of the existence of coarticulation for articulatory assessment are significant. One implication is that testing sounds in isolation is an unrealistic and artificial enterprise. What a child can do with a sound in isolation may be totally different from what is done with the same phoneme in connected speech. A second implication has to do with single-word testing. When we speak, we typically do not put oral pauses or "spaces" between our words. The speech stream has been called an "unsegmentable whole" (Kent & Minifie, 1977). Research on coarticulation has shown that the effects of one sound on another can cross both word and syllable boundaries and extend up to five phonemes (Amerman, Daniloff, & Moll, 1970; Daniloff & Moll, 1968; McClean, 1973; Moll & Daniloff, 1971). Thus, sounds located in two adjacent words can have an affect on one another. This means that testing sound production on the single-word level may not be representative of sound production in spontaneous speech, because connected words may provide different coarticulatory effects as compared to single words alone (Faircloth & Faircloth, 1970). We have known for some time that some specific phonemes are misarticulated less often in consonant cluster contexts as opposed to CV environments (Gallagher & Shriner, 1975; McCauley & Skenes, 1987). The final implication has to do with possible facilitating and sabotaging effects of phonemes surrounding a particular target sound. For instance, a misarticulated /r/ sound may be produced correctly by a child if it is preceded by a /k/ (e.g., /kraek/), perhaps because both sounds require grossly similar positioning of the tongue in the vocal tract (Hoffman, Schuckers, & Ratusnik, 1977). Conversely, an /r/ might be misarticulated as a /w/ if words surrounding the target sound contain a lip-rounded phoneme (e.g., /row/) (Winitz, 1975). Therefore, the effects of coarticulation can be either positive or negative, facilitating or sabotaging, and this is especially important for the clinician to consider in assessment and treatment. Perhaps the most important implication of coarticulation is in accounting for articulatory inconsistency. Most misarticulations are notoriously inconsistent, but if the clinician analyzes these productions in terms of context, commonalities may become evident. Phonetic context is often the common denominator among errors that appear inconsistent on the surface. We need not only think of phonetic context as a purely motoric phenomenon. In performing linguistic phonological analyses, a consideration of context is critical. For instance, in evaluating assimilation processes (e.g., nasal assimilation), the clinician may note that nonnasal sounds in the initial position are changed to nasals *only* when there is a nasal phoneme in the final or medial position of the words. This is most likely not related to a motoric difficulty and is linguistically based.

7. *The Linguistic-Articulatory Connection:* An important postulate in discussing articulatory assessment is the intimate relationship between language and articulation. This connection has been shown in several ways in the literature.

a. Theoretically, phonology has been considered a classical component of language models. Chomsky (1957), for instance, includes phonological rules in his model of transformational grammar along with semantics and syntax.

b. Many bound morphemes (e.g., -ed, plural -s, possessive -s) are realized through a rule-governed system in speech as single phonemes. The -ed in the word "walked" is really pronounced as a /t/ sound in a consonant blend at the end of the word /wɔkt/. Thus, a single sound can make a difference in word meaning and that same single unit is also a grammatical morpheme. A sound, therefore, can be much more than merely a phonetic unit; it makes a difference in word meaning and carries linguistic value.

c. Several studies have shown that misarticulations are affected by linguistic complexity (Haynes, Haynes, & Jackson, 1982; Panagos, Quine, & Klich, 1979; Schmauch, Panagos, & Klich, 1978). That is, more misarticulations will occur as syntactic complexity increases. This demonstrates a clear relationship between articulation and language.

d. Shriberg and Kwiatkowski (1980) have suggested that even the type of word or syntactic class of a word affects sound productions. They found, for instance, that blends may be reduced differently in verbs as compared to the same blend in nouns. In early language development, there appear to be more misarticulations on action words as opposed to object words in the first lexicon. This has been shown with normally developing as well as phonologically delayed children (Camarata & Schwartz, 1985).

e. Pragmatics has also been implicated as affecting sound productions in several investigations (Campbell & Shriberg, 1982; Leonard, 1971; Weiner & Ostrowski, 1979). That is, children may produce sounds more correctly in conditions of increased information load and misarticulate more frequently when the communicative value is lessened. This means that when there is a greater chance of being misunderstood the child may articulate more correctly.

f. A relationship between language and articulation can be inferred from the high co-occurrence of the two disorders in children. Generally, children who have articulation problems are at high risk for language disorders and vice versa. Somewhere between 75 to 85 percent of children with phonological problems have concomitant language disorders (Shriberg et al., 1986; Shriberg & Kwiatkowski, 1988).

g. Another connection was shown in a study of treatment effects by Matheny and Panagos (1978). These investigators examined children with both articulation and language disorders and demonstrated that the subjects trained only on language tended to improve their articulation skills and others trained on articulation only improved their language abilities.

The implications of these connections between articulation and language are significant for assessment. First, routine assessment of articulation with an exclusive sensorimotor orientation is not appropriate. Language and articulation are intimately intertwined when a person speaks spontaneously (Locke, 1983). Second, when the SLP is looking for sources of inconsistency, the significant effects of semantic, syntactic, or pragmatic variables could be investigated. Phonetic context, then, is not the only source of inconsistent productions. A final implication is that an articulatory deviation can be due more to linguistic influences of the child's phonological system than to sensorimotor difficulties. The clinician can see that a more productive view would be to consider both sensorimotor and linguistic components in the assessment repertoire (Schwartz, 1983).

SCREENING FOR PHONOLOGICAL DISORDERS

Speech-language pathologists in private practice may screen daycare facilities or private schools to detect children with phonological problems. Although many clinicians in the public schools may rely exclusively on referrals for case detection, screening is sometimes warranted depending on school system policies or special circumstances. The purpose of screening is to select children with significant communication problems by assessing a total population with a brief but discriminating testing procedure. The objective, then, is detection, not description of persons with disordered speech.

A screening test must be swift, yet discerning. The examiner must be able to detect individuals with impaired speech while rapidly passing over all the normal speakers. Although brief, the detection process should provide a sufficient sample of each person's oral communication to permit critical judgment of articulation, as well as voice, fluency, and language abilities. Since screening procedures and materials differ with various age groups, we shall briefly describe methods for various target populations.

1. *Preschool and Early Elementary Children:*   There are essentially five ways to screen the speech of a young child. In cases of very young children, it is quite possible that they will not talk to the clinician at all, especially if they are taken to a strange setting with an unfamiliar adult. With children who simply will not speak, it is prudent to recommend a rescreening or a diagnostic evaluation after all attempts at obtaining direct and indirect samples have failed. One way to obtain information about the communication of a reluctant child is to interview the parents or teachers, if they are available. Much important information can be provided by people who interact with the child day after day. They can provide "ballpark" data on the child's mean length of utterance, types of word combinations, fluency, vocal quality, and intelligibility, and they can summarize the occasions when the child communicates most. This interview process is no substitute for observing the child's communication firsthand, but it certainly can pinpoint significant problems in any area and can be the basis for recommending a diagnostic evaluation.

A second way of obtaining information about a young child is to observe play, perhaps with other children. This procedure is very effective, but time-consuming. One advantage of this process is that the child is not removed from the normal environment and isolated with a strange adult. The clinician can also interact with the child during free play and more structured tasks and involve other children to stimulate diverse interactions.

A third method of screening young children is to obtain a short sample of conversational speech. Research has found that screening judgments made by an experienced clinician from a two- to three-minute sample were as good or better than formal measures (Eveleigh & Warr-Leeper, 1983). This is similar to the high correspondence between formal and informal measures in language assessment (Allen, Bliss, & Timmons, 1981).

Another method of screening is to have the child repeat words, phrases, or sentences. However, the examiner's model may tend to influence the child's speech, which may not then be a fully representative sample. Stimulation tends to increase correct productions (Winitz, 1969). If the clinician must screen large numbers of children rapidly, then, an imitative protocol may be the most expedient method of obtaining the information in the shortest amount of time.

A fifth technique to use in screening is to have the child name colors, count, and identify pictures or objects. This is a common method used since it is easy and takes little time, and children seem to respond well to the task. However, it would be best to include a sample of conversational speech to avoid missing children with problems.

Many of the published diagnostic inventories cited later in this chapter include portions designed to serve as screening tests for children. For example, the first 50 items of the *Templin-Darley Tests of Articulation* (Templin & Darley, 1969) are a useful screening device; the authors provide tables of norms that permit comparison of an individual child's score with that of same-age peers. Hodson (1980) includes a screening portion in her *Analysis of Phonological Processes (APP)*. There are several other tests designed specifically as screening instruments (Bryant & Bryant, 1983; Fluharty, 1974; Monsees & Berman, 1968; Riley, 1971; Rogers, 1972).

2. *Later Elementary Children:*   Speech-language pathologists may use reading passages and conversation to screen children in grades four through eight who are typically referred by classroom teachers. The clinician may choose from among several published reading passages for later elementary children (Avant & Hutton, 1962; Eisenson & Ogilvie, 1977; Irwin, 1965).

To obtain a sample of spontaneous speech, questions about favorite hobbies and interests are useful. Actually, later elementary children are often rather engaging conversationalists; they are sufficiently mature to enjoy relating to a new adult, but not old enough to resent being scrutinized. The clinician should remember that conversationally inept children may have pragmatic difficulties that may need further evaluation. Also, a child of this age group with the problem of stuttering is sufficiently astute to avoid talking in some conversational situations.

3. *Older Groups:*   Reading passages, sentences loaded with consonant sounds most frequently defective, and conversations are commonly used to

obtain speech samples in screening programs for older individuals. The clinician can construct a reading passage or use any of the several published versions, which include "My Grandfather" (Van Riper, 1963); "Arthur the Young Rat" (Johnson, Darley, & Spriestersbach, 1963); "The Rainbow Passage" (Fairbanks, 1960); and "Directions" (Anderson & Newby, 1973). In addition to an oral reading, some questions are asked to elicit a sample of spontaneous speech. Queries such as "What are you majoring in and how did you select that field?" or "If I were to come to your home area as a tourist, what are some things I might want to see?" are good examples of starters.

Predictive Screening

A significant number of children entering kindergarten and first grade will not have acquired the normal complement of consonant sounds. This places the clinician in a dilemma: Some of the children's speech differences are merely the result of late maturation and do not require treatment, but how do you separate the normal speakers from the potentially permanent misarticulators? Some clinicians select certain children and not others on an ad hoc basis. They then find it difficult to explain their selection criteria to teachers, parents, and administrators. The opposite extreme is to work with all first-grade children who present articulation errors, which is not efficient and can be criticized ethically.

In an effort to provide some "objective" means of determining which children should be enrolled in treatment, several test instruments have been developed that attempt to identify those children who are high risk for articulation disorders (McDonald, 1968; Templin & Darley, 1969; Van Riper & Erickson, 1969). These tests vary in terms of whether they are administered imitatively or spontaneously, and they differ in the distribution of phonemes tested. Ritterman et al. (1982) compared the *Screening Deep Test of Articulation (SDTA), The Templin-Darley Screening Test (TDST),* and *The Predictive Screening Test of Articulation (PSTA)* in terms of the pass/fail judgments indicated on 91 first-grade children and found that there was a "poor correspondence among the tests as to the individuals failed. That is, only three subjects were failed by more than a single test" (p. 432). The three instruments evaluate either consistency of sound production (McDonald) or the total number of correctly produced spontaneous or imitative productions (Templin, *PSTA*). Certainly, a child who is dramatically delayed in articulatory development would fail all three of these tests, but this type of child is not particularly problematic to the clinician. It is the child on the borderline who presents a dilemma. Clinicians should not rely exclusively on such measures to determine if a child requires enrollment in treatment. Ultimately, it comes down to a clinical judgment for each case, based upon normative data; and although a formal screening test might be considered in concert with other variables, it cannot be the sole determiner of enrollment. Ritterman et al. (1982) state that

> Research has indicated that each of the underlying variables on which the *Templin-Darley Screening Test of Articulation, The Predictive Screening Test of Articulation* and *The Screening Deep Test of Articulation* are based have some degree of merit as pass/fail selection criteria. The results of the present study,

however, would seem to indicate that these variables are not well correlated in that different children failed for different reasons on the three tests. (p. 432)

A later test is the *Coarticulation Assessment in Meaningful Language (CAML)* (Kenney & Prather, 1984). This test uses meaningful sentences in a delayed imitation paradigm with pictures to obtain responses (e.g., "Look, the mouse fell and the cup fell. What happened here?"). The *CAML* and the *SDTA* were compared in kindergarten subjects, and the two tests were found to be similar in terms of general results; however, the former yielded a greater total number of errors (Prather & Kenney, 1986). Westman and Broen (1989) developed a screening procedure that took phonological content into account in testing phonemes and contexts thought to be "predictive errors" (e.g., deletions, manner changes, fronting, and velar deviations). They found that testing using the predictive errors was more related to eventual therapy placement than using total errors as a criterion.

Other variables that might enter into decision-making in screening for a particular case might be (1) the child's self-perception as a communicator, (2) parents' and teachers' perceptions and desires, (3) presence of concomitant disorders (e.g., language), and (4) existence of characteristically resistant articulatory deviations (e.g., lateral sibilants, vocalic /r/ distortions, omissions of consonants).

TRADITIONAL ASSESSMENT PROCEDURES

Subsequent to failure of an articulatory screening, a child may be scheduled for a complete assessment of phonological ability. There are a variety of articulatory assessments that differ in their theoretical assumptions, method of sample elicitation, type of information obtained, and therapeutic implications. Perhaps the most common type of assessment is what we will call *traditional*. The theoretical orientation of traditional testing is that each English phoneme must be evaluated in the initial, medial, and final positions of words. These words are typically elicited from the client by means of pictures, word lists, sentences, and/or conversational sampling. Even though the data for the analysis might range from words to connected speech, the orientation of the clinician is to determine omissions, substitutions, and distortions of phonemes in differing word positions. Many tests are available for use in traditional assessment (Bryant & Bryant, 1983; Edmonson, 1969; Fisher & Logemann, 1971; Fudala, 1970; Goldman & Fristoe, 1986; Hejna, 1963; Ingram, 1971; Pendergast et al., 1984; Templin & Darley, 1969). Some of these inventories include stimulus pictures for testing children and structured sentences for older clients to read. Several provide norms against which a child may be compared and one (Fudala, 1970) features a method of scaling the degree of articulatory defectiveness.

Traditional diagnostic procedures have in common other basic operations. Most traditional assessments accrue a phonetic inventory from the client. This is a listing of all phonemes produced in the sample. One reason for obtaining a phonetic inventory is to compare the sounds produced correctly by a given client to normative data on articulatory development. As mentioned earlier, most normative studies are based on traditional notions and report phoneme productions of sounds in the three word positions (Poole, 1934; Prather, Hedrick, & Kern, 1975; Sander, 1972; Templin, 1957; Wellman et al., 1931).

Another traditional procedure is the testing of a client's stimulability or his/her response to stimulation. In other words, we evaluate the impact that the examiner's model has upon the client's production. Is there some modification in the direction of normalcy or is there no change in the articulatory behavior? Testing for stimulability (Milisen et al., 1954) is a useful diagnostic procedure. If a client can produce the error sound correctly by imitating a standard model, either in isolation, in nonsense syllables, or in words, then there may be no serious organic obstacles that would prevent the eventual acquisition of the sound (Darley, 1964). Stimulability may also be useful in determining the level on which to start the treatment process. Research also suggests that clients with low stimulability scores will benefit to a greater degree from treatment as compared to those with high scores (Diedrich, 1983; Madison, 1979). In fact, stimulability has been implicated as a potential predicter of children who may develop normal speech through maturation (Farquhar, 1961) and may not require extensive treatment.

Stimulability is frequently given "short shrift" by students in training. Sometimes it is totally omitted. Often, we see students hurry through the stimulability testing, frequently giving inadequate instructions and rather imprecise models to the client. The spirit of stimulability testing is to see how the client performs under maximal, multimodality stimulation. This is why most tests recommend that the model be presented two or three times after the client has been given a strong attentional set. Students sometimes indicate that the client was not stimulable for error phonemes after rather cursory testing. Subsequent stimulability trials, done more intensively and systematically in a variety of contexts, may reveal that the client, in fact, can produce the target sound. Prior to making negative stimulability statements in a clinical report, the clinician should be certain that the stimulation tasks were administered effectively.

It is our contention that traditional testing is a good starting point in an articulatory assessment. In many cases, a traditional assessment may be all that is needed, especially when the client has only a few articulatory errors and is stimulable. In cases like this, the clinician knows what the errors are and how often they occur in a test and in spontaneous speech. Further, the clinician has a place to start production of the target sound, if the client can make it correctly with stimulation. In the majority of cases, however, traditional testing does not go far enough. For instance, our discussion of coarticulation suggested that sounds will be produced differently in different phonetic environments. Most traditional tests examine only a limited number of these phonetic contexts. If a child or adult is not stimulable, the clinician may want to rely on experimentation with different coarticulatory transitions to determine if there is a facilitating context. Most traditional tests are just not equipped to do this. Another example is that traditional testing procedures are not directed toward detecting patterns of error in a client's speech. In order to define patterns of error, a phonological analysis is the most efficient method to use. Traditional analyses do not systematically examine the effects of stress, syllable complexity (Panagos, Quine, & Klich, 1979), linguistic complexity, and pragmatics on misarticulation. Only spontaneous sampling and specific probing can do this. Finally, traditional analyses do not focus on certain parameters that may be relevant to certain cases such as distinctive feature acquisition and use. In short, no one method can do everything, and so it is with the traditional approach. The traditional test, however, is a viable instrument to use generically. If other analyses are required, they should be done as appropriate.

It is far easier to describe phonological testing than it is to administer a test. A student's first attempt is generally a confusing situation that requires careful listening, attention to visual cues, recording the client's responses appropriately, and maintaining a positive client-clinician relationship. We recommend that the beginning clinician listen for only one sound at a time. If the client is very difficult to understand, the use of toys and pictures will help the clinician decipher utterances. When possible, have the child repeat the test words a number of times. Tape-record, or better yet, videotape the child's responses on high-quality equipment to assist in later scoring of the test. Experienced speech pathologists are able to save time by testing more than one sound simultaneously (Fristoe & Goldman, 1968).

It is especially true with phonological assessment that the clinician is really the "test." Commercial tests are nothing more than stacks of pictures bound together by metal or plastic. Since articulatory responses are so transient and fleeting, clinicians must listen carefully, practice frequently, and above all, check their reliability. Studies have shown that speech pathologists are fairly reliable when the judgments they make are rather molar, such as "correct" or "incorrect" (Winitz, 1969). When judgments become more "fine grained," as in determining the nature of specific substitutions in certain word positions, our reliability tends to deteriorate. One can easily see that very complex analysis procedures such as those used in distinctive features and generative phonology are even more susceptible to misjudgments on the part of the clinician. Clinicians must always strive to improve their reliability through practice and rechecking their results. Our evaluation results are only as good as our ability to perceive the reality of the client's responses. No one, as an old professor said, has immaculate perception. Chapter 3 discussed interjudge reliability and provided a formula for its calculation.

TEST PROCEDURES THAT EVALUATE PHONETIC CONTEXT EFFECTS

Subsequent to a traditional assessment, a client may be judged not stimulable. Especially in cases where the client has only a few phoneme errors (i.e., an articulation disorder, not a phonological disorder), procedures need to be initiated to determine if a facilitating phonetic context can be found. Although we are also interested in phonetic contexts in describing phonological disorders, this interest is based more on determining effects of linguistic reduction rules than in attempting to define phonetic contexts that facilitate motoric productions. The present section focuses on the latter goal. As we mentioned in the section on coarticulation, phonemes are significantly influenced by other sounds that surround them. This phenomenon results in the existence of facilitating contexts that can encourage the correct production of a target consonant. The concept that certain phonetic environments can facilitate correct production was suggested in the early writings of Van Riper and Irwin (1958) where they indicated there were "key words" in which a phoneme could be produced more effectively. If certain key words were discovered for a nonstimulable client, then treatment could commence in these contexts. McDonald devised the *Deep Test of Articulation,* which, among other things, is based on the idea that phonemes will be produced differently depending on the sounds that precede and follow them. Through systematically permuting a variety of consonants before and after a specific phoneme, the contexts in which correct production is observed can be noted by the clinician and can serve as a starting point for treatment. In the *Deep Test,* each phoneme can be observed 40 or more times as the initiating or terminating sound in a syllable. Here is a part of a session in which the examiner is administering the /s/ portion of the *Deep Test* to a second-grade boy with a lateralized /s/:

CLINICIAN: Okay, Tony, you understand now that you are to make a funny "big word" from the names of the objects on the two pictures, like we did in the example "tubvase," without stopping between the words? Fine! Here we go:

1.	housepipe	no change
2.	housebell	no change
3.	housetie	improvement
4.	housedog	improvement
5.	housecow	no change
6.	housegun	no change

Note that the word "house," with a final /s/, is tested as it precedes other consonant phonemes. The examiner listens carefully to identify any changes in the child's misarticulations. Then, the examiner reverses the procedure so that /s/ follows other phonemes (e.g., cupsun, tubsun, kitesun). For older clients, McDonald has prepared a series of sentences to be read aloud that are constructed for the same purpose.

The *McDonald Deep Test* has certain limitations. For instance, when we combine two lexical items into one nonsense word, we are no longer dealing with sound production in real linguistic units. Also, as the test progresses, some children find the big words neither funny nor interesting. Some children also experience considerable difficulty blending the two test items into one large word (Goda, 1970). If there is a pause between the two words, the purpose of the test is defeated (McDonald, 1964). Finally, depending on the child's pattern of misarticulation, many of the intended phonetic contexts are altered (e.g., "housecow" becomes "housetow"). This changes the ability of the instrument to really evaluate all the contexts it is designed to elicit. We prefer to use the test during the initial stages of treatment, exploring the loci of improved, or at least altered, sound production. Additionally, researchers find the *Deep Test* valuable for charting improvement during the course of treatment because it deals with many contexts.

The evaluation of a variety of phonetic contexts provides an interesting contrast to the limited number of environments evaluated by traditional measures. Schissell and James (1979) compared the evaluation of articulatory abilities in children using a more traditional test, the *Arizona*, and the *McDonald Deep Test (MDT)*. It was found that the traditional test missed some of the children who did not have consistent control of certain sounds, and it was also noted that the traditional test failed children on certain sounds when in actuality they performed the sound productions well in a significant number of contexts on the *MDT*. One interpretation of the disparity in results between these two measures is that the traditional test evaluated a limited number of phonetic contexts, and for some children these happened to be facilitative and for others they were not. The implication, of course, is that the more phonetic contexts examined, the more realistic the picture of the clients' articulatory performance. Testing a variety of phonetic contexts also increases the probability of finding inconsistencies in production. These inconsistencies are invaluable aids in the selection of initial treatment targets.

Another way to examine phonetic context effects in children and adults is the use of sound-in-context sentences (Haynes, Haynes, & Jackson, 1982; Mazza, Schuckers, & Daniloff, 1979). These sentences can be read spontaneously by adults or imitated by children. Most of the work with these sentences has been done in research projects directed toward finding facilitating contexts for particular target consonants (mainly the /s/ and /r/ phonemes). The use of these sentence stimuli has shown that there are, in fact, facilitating contexts for /r/ and /s/ that occur for many clients. The essence of these sentences is that a clinician can have the client say any number of utterances that are constructed to determine phonetic context effects. For instance, if the clinician wants to evaluate the effects on /s/ production of a preceding /k/ sound and a following /p/ sound (e.g., /KSP/), a sentence can be constructed such as "The dress had a black spot". Also, phrases may be used instead of sentences. The clinician, then, can use knowledge of coarticulation and devise stimuli to probe phonetic context effects on a given client's articulation. Finally, Kent (1982) urges continued experimentation with phonetic context effects in clinical and research settings because there is much we do not yet understand about this phenomenon:

> The selection of so-called facilitating contexts involves decisions regarding stress, word position, expected or permissible allophonic variation, frequency of occurrence and the influence of neighboring sounds. . . . The final selection of a facilitating context also should recognize as precisely as possible the nature of the articulation error. It should not be assumed, for example, that the same context will facilitate correct production of /s/ in children who distort the sound by dentalization, lateralization and palatalization. (p. 75)

With a knowledge of the effects of coarticulation, the clinician may construct a variety of utterance types for a particular client and need not rely solely on instruments devised by others. A thorough assessment could provide significant information that could be used at the outset of treatment if more attention were paid to ferreting out sources of error inconsistency attributable to phonetic context. The clinician should also be willing to experiment with a variety of segmental, suprasegmental, and linguistic complexity variables in the search for sources of inconsistency (Shriberg & Kwiatkowski, 1980).

THE PHONETIC AND PHONEMIC INVENTORIES

A most important source of information about a phonologically disordered client is the phonetic inventory. After gathering a representative speech sample, one of the first operations a clinician should perform is to inventory the client's sound system in several ways. The *phonetic inventory* is a summary of sounds the client has produced either correctly or incorrectly in the sample and represents the sounds that can be physically produced by the person. That is, if the client produces a glottal stop, this is part of the phonetic inventory. If the client produces a Θ/s substitution and never produces the [Θ] correctly when it is required, the [Θ] is still included in the phonetic inventory. The *phonemic inventory,* on the other hand, includes sounds that are used contrastively and are implemented to make a meaning difference in the client's language. Thus, although a [t] may be a part of the child's phonetic repertoire in that it is occasionally produced, it may not be part of the phonemic system because it is never used to differentiate meaning. As we will mention later, an examination of the phonetic and phonemic inventories is a critical part of assessing a child's possession and use of distinctive features of English phonemes.

There are also some other ways to analyze data from a child's phonetic and phonemic inventories. Some authorities (Elbert & Gierut, 1986; Maxwell & Rockman, 1984) have recommended searching for various types of rules that may or may not be operating in a child's system and the phonetic/phonemic inventories are an important part of these analyses. For instance, static rules called *phonotactic constraints* (Dinnsen, 1984) may be operating to restrict the occurrence of certain sounds or phoneme combinations. Three types of phonotactic constraints have been reported. Positional constraints are rules that allow the production of a sound in only certain contexts or word positions (e.g., production in initial but not final positions). Inventory constraints reduce the production of particular sounds because the phonemes are not included in the phonetic inventory. Finally, sequence constraints are rules that may not permit the child to produce sounds in particular combinations (e.g., the child can produce the phoneme as a singleton, but not in a cluster). One can see that examination of the phonetic and phonemic inventory is an important part of arriving at an appreciation of a client's phonotactic rule system.

There are a variety of systems for reporting a client's phonetic inventory. Some approaches not only reflect sensorimotor production of a sound, but also provide some indication of appropriate or phonemic use of the element.

The phonetic inventory could also indicate failure to sample certain sounds so the clinician does not assume the client cannot produce them. Several examples show variations in the style of phonetic inventories. Shriberg and Kwiatkowski (1980) complete a phonetic inventory which differentiates among phonemes which were correct, appear in the sample, were glossed, and were never glossed. This can tell the clinician if the phonetic element is correct anywhere, whether it is used as a substitution for another sound (appears anywhere), whether it should have been in a word (glossed) but was not, or whether the sound was never expected to be produced in the sample. Other systems simply list the phones in the phonetic inventory from left to right in terms of place of articulation in the vocal tract (left = front, right = back) (Maxwell & Rockman, 1984, p. 83). Another way to consider a child's phonetic/phonemic inventory might be to array the phonemes on the continuum of phonological knowledge discussed later in the present chapter.

Whatever way the clinician decides to examine a client's phonological system, a phonetic/phonemic inventory is a good starting point because it can give significant insights into phonotactic rules (e.g., inventory constraints) and the client's overall knowledge of the sound system.

DISTINCTIVE FEATURE ANALYSIS

As we mentioned previously, neither traditional analyses nor appraisals of phonetic context effects examine all pertinent aspects of a child's articulatory system. Researchers indicate that the most basic unit that speech can be distilled into is the distinctive feature and the reality of features has been demonstrated both acoustically and physiologically (Singh, 1976). That is, as humans, we seem to pay attention to certain aspects of the speech signal in both perception and production. Phonemes are evidently made up of bundles of distinctive features that combine to produce a variety of different consonant and vowel sounds in a language. Singh (1976) states, "Children do not acquire phonemes one by one; rather, they acquire a feature that provides them with a basis for manifesting a number of phonemes distinctively in speech production and discrimination tasks" (p. 229). Features, then, are prerequisite to phonemes, because without the knowledge of and ability to produce a given feature of language, certain sounds containing that feature will not be produced. For instance, if a child does not learn that the feature of voicelessness is important in differentiating certain sounds from each other, the phonemes with the −voice feature will not be produced (e.g., /s, f, p, k/). Distinctive feature theory attempts to specify the characteristics of phonemes according to the presence (+) or absence (−) of each feature that distinguishes or contrasts one speech sound from another.

Several investigations have suggested that there are at least two different types of distinctive feature problems exhibited by children (McReynolds & Huston, 1971; Pollack & Rees, 1972; Ruder & Bunce, 1981). One type of distinctive feature difficulty is exemplified by a child who has not acquired the use of a feature at all. The child is not aware of the importance of the feature to differentiate English sounds and has difficulty producing the feature. The child might have one aspect or one-half of the feature (+ voicing), but not the other half (−voicing). Features are rather like light switches; they are only useful when you know about both turning them on and turning them off. Thus, a child has not really acquired the feature of voice until both voiced and voiceless sounds can be produced appropriately and contrastively (Grunwell, 1988). If a child's phonetic inventory does not include voiceless phonemes used correctly or incorrectly, the child cannot have contrastive use of the voice feature.

A second type of distinctive feature error is shown in a child who has acquired the feature but does not use it appropriately. Control of features, like many things, is on a continuum. One child may be aware of the importance of a feature and be capable of producing both aspects (+ and −) of it; yet, there might be several specific contexts in which the feature is not used appropriately. On the other hand, another child may be able to produce the feature aspects in only a few limited contexts.

Several approaches have been suggested for distinctive feature analysis. McReynolds and Engmann (1975) have prepared a manual featuring detailed clinical worksheets to guide the diagnostician in performing a distinctive feature analysis. This approach is quite time-consuming and has been criticized for procedural as well as theoretical shortcomings (Carney, 1979; Grunwell, 1988). Sommers (1983) has suggested a less formal shortcut method of analyzing distinctive features from a sample of speech. He indicates that the briefer method yields similar results at a considerable savings of analysis time. Currently, many authorities recommend the examination of distinctive features as part of the larger process of phonological analysis. That is, when we write phonological rules for a disordered child's system, we can use distinctive features to make our descriptions more specific and look for commonalities across different sound errors. Table 6.1 gives an example of how six individual sound errors can be construed as basically a problem with one aspect of a distinctive feature (+continuant). A phonological process analysis of the same errors would reveal a "stopping" rule, which is essentially a misuse of + continuant. It would be important to determine if the child ever produced the + continuant feature in the speech sample. One can easily see that using distinctive features is just another way to look at a client's misarticulations and can add some specificity to our descriptions, as well as allow us to see relationships among individual sound errors.

It was mentioned earlier that a major decision we must make in a distinctive feature analysis is whether a child is a feature misuser or has not yet acquired the feature. This decision is typically quite easy for a clinician to make after looking at the child's phonetic inventory to see if whole classes of sounds and features are missing. In many cases, this may be enough information to determine whether the treatment should be directed toward establishing a feature in a child's repertoire or altering the use of a feature that has already been acquired but is being used inconsistently.

What are the advantages of considering distinctive features in our analysis of misarticulations? We see four: (1) It provides a model for understanding

Table 6.1 Example of Distinctive Feature Approach to Analyzing Articulation Errors*

ERROR	FEATURES USED CORRECTLY	FEATURES IN ERROR	
Substitution/Target		Target Phoneme	Substitution
d/s	vocalic, consonantal, high, back, low, nasal	−voice +continuant +strident	+voice −continuant −strident
d/z	vocalic, consonantal, high, back, low, nasal	+continuant +strident	−continuant −strident
d/sh	vocalic, consonantal, high, back, low, nasal	−voice +continuant +strident	+voice −continuant −strident
b/f	vocalic, consonantal, high, back, low, nasal	−voice +continuant +strident	+voice −continuant −strident
b/v	vocalic, consonantal, high, back, low, nasal	+continuant +strident	−continuant −strident
d/th (*th*ink)	vocalic, consonantal, high, back, low, nasal	−voice +continuant	+voice −continuant
d/th (*th*at)	vocalic, consonantal, high, back, low, nasal	+continuant	−continuant

*The features associated with phonemes are from Chomsky and Halle (1968). Compare the feature bundles of the target and error phonemes to determine features misused. One can easily see the most misused features are the voicing, continuancy and stridency elements.

errors in many clients. An error on a given feature (e.g., voicing) that is shared by more than one phoneme accounts for the misarticulation of many phonemes, reducing the seemingly random errors to a simpler pattern. (2) It enables us to write phonological rules that are even more specific and economical. For example, a final position rule written this way:

$$C (+continuant, +voice) \rightarrow C (+continuant, -voice)$$

is more parsimonious than writing a rule containing all voiced continuants and their voiceless counterparts listed individually. (3) It may provide a basis for the selection of a target sound for treatment; the clinician can select a target phoneme that shares features with many other misarticulated sounds and then probe for generalization as treatment progresses. (4) It may provide a basis for more efficient therapy (Costello & Onstine, 1976; Ritterman & Freeman, 1974) by facilitating generalization to sounds not being directly treated.

Despite the many advantages, however, there are a number of factors that may limit the application of distinctive feature theory to clinical problems. First of all, some procedures for assessment (e.g., McReynolds & Engmann, 1975) are quite time-consuming; the clinician has to weigh this factor against the purported increase in efficiency. The second limiting factor is the obvious complexity of the system of analysis. Another drawback is that, on a phonetic level, the distinctive features advocated by Chomsky and Halle may have no conceptual reality (LaRiviere et al., 1974). By that we mean that there may be no one-to-one relationship between distinctive features (an acoustic classification) and articulatory production (a physiological level) (Parker, 1976). The physical act of articulation clearly is not a binary function that is either present (+) or absent (−), but it is multivaried. According to Walsh (1974), the categories employed in distinctive feature analysis are overgeneralized and may encompass too great a phonetic space to be of clinical value. Leonard (1973) points out that "articulation therapy involves giving phonetic instructions. Therefore, the features we deal with must have a specific physical interpretation" (pp. 141–142). A formal distinctive feature analysis may not be as important as consideration of the basic notion of distinctive features themselves, as indicated by Grunwell:

> The last few paragraphs have seriously thrown into question the clinical value of a formalized distinctive feature analysis procedure. This implication is intentional. None the less, the CONCEPTS of distinctive feature contrasts and natural classes are of major importance and considerable clinical applicability. The concept that phonemes are differentiated by their "content" of contrastive features enables the clinician to focus on the contrastive/distinctive feature that is in "error" and also to recognize similar "errors" in different phonemes, that is, patterns in disordered speech. (1988, p. 157)

PHONOLOGICAL ANALYSIS

Another approach to analyzing a child's articulatory behavior is to perform a phonological analysis. In 1976, a landmark book by David Ingram entitled *Phonological Disability in Children* sparked an interest in a more linguistic approach to misarticulation analysis. Ingram cited many early sources that reported common patterns of articulatory simplification in children's speech (Compton, 1970, 1976; Oller et al., 1972; Smith, 1973; Stampe, 1969). That is, most children develop the ability to articulate gradually and prior to perfecting an adult production, they reduce the complexity of words in characteristic ways. Space in the present chapter does not permit us to provide examples of each phonological pattern reported in the extant literature. Furthermore, most training programs now include extensive exposure to phonological processes in coursework. Readers are referred to any of the previously cited sources and the assessment measures mentioned later in this section for myriad examples of phonological processes.

A phonological approach rests on certain assumptions. First, phonologists assume that there is a structure to every child's sound system and that even in the most unintelligible child, there is a pattern of phonemic production. Sounds do not occur in random combinations. Second, a phonological approach assumes an underlying system that gives rise to the observable sound combinations that we hear from children. The implication is that a phonological error may be a product of the underlying system that organizes the overt sound combinations. Earlier in this chapter, we indicated that there can be both linguistically based and sensorimotor based misarticulations. The linguistically generated errors could be construed as products of rules generated by the child's underlying phonological system. Rules, to a certain degree, imply patterns of performance and phonological rules can be written to simply describe these patterns. Phonological rules, then, are descriptive of the way a child uses classes of phonemes.

Many investigators have reported that in development, it is commonly observed that children tend to simplify their word productions in comparison to the adult model. The simplifications are typically in the direction of producing physiologically easier sounds for more difficult ones. For reasons not presently known, some children appear to persist in using these simplification strategies, and if enough of them are retained, the child is likely to be quite unintelligible. Most authorities report that many of the patterns of error found in disordered children are those observed in normally developing youngsters at earlier ages (Ingram, 1976; Shriberg & Kwiatkowski, 1980). Ingram (1976), however, also points out that deviant rules not typically found in normally developing children may appear in phonologically disordered youngsters. Phonological rules can describe these simplification techniques, and each rule implies a change in the use of distinctive features. That is, a child who substitutes stops for continuants is altering an important distinctive feature of the target phonemes, as in the following example:

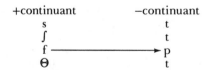

The clinician wishing to gain insight into phonological processes has at least two levels of analysis to choose from. First, there are instruments available that are targeted toward discovering phonological processes in children (Compton & Hutton, 1978; Hodson, 1980; Kahn & Lewis, 1986; Lowe, 1986; Steed & Haynes, 1988; Weiner, 1979). These measures provide picture or object stimuli and ask the child to give a single-word or connected speech response. These responses are analyzed by the clinician for particular phonological simplifications. Table 6.2 summarizes some of the specific phonological processes examined by the instruments discussed. The reader should consult these references for examples and guidelines in defining the processes. Table

Table 6.2 Phonological Processes Examined by Selected Evaluation Procedures

		PPA	APP	C-H	EASE	K-L	NPA	PPACL	PACS	ALPHA
FEATURE CONTRAST	STRIDENCY DELETION									×
	LABIALIZATION								×	×
	APICALIZATION								×	×
	DEPALITALIZATION		×						×	
	PALATALIZATION		×							
	DEAFFRICATION	×	×			×			×	×
	BACKING		×			×				×
	NEUTRALIZATION	×	×							
	DENASALIZATION	×	×				×			
	VOCALIZATION	×			×	×		×	×	×
	GLIDING	×	×	×	×	×		×	×	×
	FRICATIVE FRONTING	×	×	×	×	×	×	×	×	×
	VELAR FRONTING	×	×	×	×	×	×	×	×	×
	AFFRICATION	×	×	×	×					×
	STOPPING	×	×	×	×	×	×	×	×	×
HARMONY	METATHESIS		×							
	COALESCENCE		×							
	DEVOICING	×	×	×		×			×	×
	PREVOCALIC VOICING	×	×			×	×		×	×
	NASAL ASSIMILATION		×			×	×	×	×	
	VELAR ASSIMILATION	×	×			×	×	×	×	
	ALVEOLAR ASSIMILATION	×	×			×	×	×		
	LABIAL ASSIMILATION	×	×			×	×	×	×	
SYLLABLE STRUCTURE	EPENTHESIS		×							
	INITIAL CONSONANT DELETION		×			×	×		×	
	REDUPLICATION	×					×	×		
	CONSONANT CLUSTER RED	×	×	×	×	×	×	×	×	×
	UNSTRESSED SYLLABLE DELETION	×	×		×	×	×	×	×	×
	FINAL CONSONANT DELETION	×	×	×	×	×	×	×	×	×
	GLOTTAL REPLACEMENT	×	×			×			×	

6.3 outlines some selected stimulus and task variables in both traditional and phonologically oriented procedures.

The *Phonological Process Analysis (PPA)* (Weiner, 1979) is a descriptive procedure that is not sound specific and focuses on patterns. The *PPA* uses delayed imitation and is directed toward children between the ages of two and five. It uses action pictures that sample single words and sentence phrases. The stimulus items are organized by phonological process rather than the traditional grouping by phoneme or age of development of sounds.

Another measure is the *Compton-Hutton Phonological Assessment* (Compton & Hutton, 1978). The *Compton-Hutton* uses 50 picture stimuli to elicit consonants in initial and final positions of words. The test is aimed at children between the ages of three and seven, and each word is elicited two times to evaluate the consistency of productions. Two phonemes are examined in each word sampled. Phonological rules are provided on the scoring sheet to assist the clinician in defining common error patterns.

The *Assessment of Phonological Processes (APP)* (Hodson, 1980) is an additional measure. The *APP* elicits and requires transcription of 55 utterances. Toys are used instead of pictures, and the child spontaneously names each object while the examiner transcribes the responses. All consonants are assessed a minimum of two times pre- and postvocalically. Thirty-one consonant clusters are assessed. The *APP* assesses 42 phonological processes and "articulatory shifts."

The *Elicited Articulatory System Evaluation (EASE)* (Steed & Haynes, 1988) is an imitation sentence test composed of several short stories the child retells to the examiner. The *EASE* provides both a traditional and phonological analysis of 337 consonant productions and 10 phonological processes.

The *Assessment Link between Phonology and Articulation (ALPHA)* (Lowe, 1986) is a delayed imitation procedure that also provides a traditional as well as phonological process analysis of a child's responses to 50 target words embedded in sentences. Sixteen processes are specifically targeted and the test was standardized on over 1,300 normal subjects between the ages of three and nine years.

The *Kahn-Lewis Phonological Analysis* (Kahn & Lewis, 1986) utilizes the 44 words from the *Goldman-Fristoe Tests of Articulation* (Goldman & Fristoe, 1986) to examine 15 phonological processes. Norms for process occurrence are provided for children between the ages of two and six years.

Several other authors have advocated using all available phonemes found in single-word items on traditional articulation tests as did Kahn and Lewis. Preliminary research suggests that traditional test stimuli can be used to aid the clinician in a gross analysis of phonological process use (Garber, 1986; Garn-Nunn, 1986; Klein, 1984; Lowe, 1986). The measures mentioned can be administered in a reasonable time period (under one hour), and the scoring time will vary with the clinician's experience using the test and the severity of the phonological disorder under evaluation. The measures, however, do not evaluate spontaneous connected speech, and therefore the phonological rules obtained may only approximate those typically used by the child in conversation (Klein, 1984). Some research, however, suggests more similarities than differences between single-word and connected speech productions. Andrews and

Table 6.3 Stimulus and Task Variables in Traditional (T) and Phonologically (P) Oriented Evaluation Procedures

PROCEDURE	TYPE	SAMPLE TYPE		TASK		MATERIALS		NORMS
		Word	Connected Speech	Spontaneous	Imitation	Picture/Object	L. Sample	
TDTA	T	X		X		X		Y
GFTA	T	X		X		X		Y
FLTAC	T	X	X	X		X	X	N
ARIZONA	T	X		X		X		Y
PAT	T	X	X	X		X		Y
APP	P	X		X	X	X		N
PPA	P	X	X			X		N
NPA	P		X	X			X	N
K-L	P	X		X		X		Y
C-H	P	X		X		X		N
PPACL	P	X	X	X				N
PACS	TP	X	X	X			X	N
EASE	TP		X		X		X	N
TAP-D	T	X	X	X	X	X		N
ALPHA	TP		X		X	X		Y

179

Fey (1986) evoked the words from the *APP* in single-word and connected speech contexts and found that most phonological errors, severity ratings, and clinical recommendations would be similar for either response mode.

A second level of phonological analysis is to gather a spontaneous speech sample, transcribe it in the International Phonetic Alphabet, and attempt to discern patterns of error (processes) in the data. This is obviously more time-consuming than the measures already mentioned, but it is also more valid because the clinician is examining actual utterances that were generated by the client's cognitive-linguistic system. The analysis of a spontaneous speech sample is recommended by Shriberg and Kwiatkowski (1980) in the *Natural Process Analysis (NPA)*. This procedure specifically targets eight processes for analysis and provides a unique and useful phonetic inventory. The *NPA* can provide valuable information for the practitioner and represents a well-planned procedure.

Ingram (1981) developed *Procedures for the Phonological Analysis of Children's Language (PPACL)*, which includes a phonetic analysis, homonym analysis, substitution analysis, and phonological process analysis. Twenty-seven specific processes are targeted; however, Ingram stated that the analysis is "open ended" and can continue "until all the substitutions in a child's speech have been explained" (p. 7).

Grunwell (1985) developed the *Phonological Assessment of Child Speech (PACS)*, which provides a description of analysis procedures for a preferably spontaneous connected speech sample of over 200 words. The procedure results in phonetic analysis, contrastive analysis to determine which phones are used to make meaning differences, and a phonological process analysis. The *PACS* also provides a developmental framework, which is missing in many phonological analysis techniques.

There appears to be some agreement that certain processes are "high risk" in phonologically disordered children. Different authorities implicate specific phonological processes as being more "important" than others, at least in terms of focusing on them for assessment targets. Table 6.2 included the processes thought to be significant enough to test in formal evaluation procedures. Some preliminary evidence exists that suggests that similar phonological processes are detected whether one uses more involved, lengthy procedures (NPA, PPACL) or shorter tasks (APP) (Paden & Moss, 1985). This, of course, does not indicate that in-depth phonological analyses and shorter procedures are equivalent, just that both can identify basic phonological processes. Although there is considerable variation among the assessment techniques in the number of processes examined, there is also a high degree of agreement regarding processes that seem to be most at risk in unintelligible children. The actual number of processes targeted in an evaluation would seem to be related to the clinician's goals in the analysis (Ingram, 1981). If the clinician wanted to write a relatively complete generative phonology for a client, it would obviously contain a larger number of rules than if the clinician's goal were to determine which major processes interfered most with intelligibility. In the latter case, the clinician may find that six phonological processes account for over 90 percent of the child's misarticulations, and treatment targets might be selected from the processes having the most impact on intelligibility. For instance, if a child is exhibiting unstressed syllable deletion, final consonant deletion, and stopping, these will be initial treatment targets. Rules such as epenthesis, vocalization, gliding, and so forth, which may have less effect on intelligibility, will not be of immediate concern. It should be noted that most of the evaluation techniques discussed allow for the assessment of other processes, as discovered by the examiner, even though the process may not be specifically evaluated.

If a clinician wishes to write phonological rules from a child's conversational sample, there are certain basic issues common to most procedures. Let us cite some of them here.

1. *Glossing and Segmentation:* The clinician must interpret the child's utterances and provide adult interpretations or *glosses* of what the child was trying to say. One cannot arrive at a phonological rule system unless the child's intended utterance is known. This is one advantage of single-word procedures that utilize picture or object stimuli since the clinician knows the intended utterance (Hodson, 1980). Several methods of segmenting or arranging the data have been reported. One method is to arrange correct and incorrect child productions and glosses word-by-word in phonetic transcription:

Child's Production	Adult Gloss
/ki/	/ki/
/bækI/	/bæskIt/
/pæ/	/fæn/
/go/	/go/

This allows the clinician the opportunity to compare productions with the adult model and hypothesize a phonological reduction pattern (e.g., final consonant deletion in the words "basket" and "fan"). Another method of segmentation is to retain spontaneous connected speech intact and divide the sample into utterances:

Child's Production	Adult Gloss
/tidəgɔgi/	/siðədɔgi/

This method of segmentation can sometimes help the clinician account for certain phonological reductions (e.g., assimilations) in a word that are influenced by sounds in previous words. Different authors (Ingram, 1981; Shriberg & Kwiatkowski, 1980) recommend a variety of methods for organizing segments once they have been glossed (alphabetically, by syllable shape, by consonant, etc.). The purpose of these varied organizational schemes is to aid in the retrieval and comparison of individual words and sounds when attempting to prove the existence of a phonological rule.

2. *Hypothesizing a Natural Process:* After arranging the data from a sample, the clinician attempts to account for errors by hypothesizing a phonological reduction pattern. For instance, when comparing a child's production of a word to the adult gloss, it may be noted that there is a deletion of the final consonant. The clinician may hypothesize the process of final consonant deletion. The high-risk

processes listed in Table 6.2 should be ruled out before any deviant (idiosyncratic) processes are suspected.

3. *Finding Support for Hypothesized Rules:* It is not enough to simply postulate that final consonant deletion has occurred in a child's sample. Evidence must be obtained from the utterances to determine whether the process has, in fact, occurred and to what degree. For instance, the child may have deleted the final consonant in a CVC word. The clinician should examine all other words in the sample that end in singleton consonants to determine the frequency of occurrence of the hypothesized phonological reduction. If there is widespread support for the occurrence of final consonant deletion, then the clinician may write the rule. If only certain final consonants are deleted consistently while others are produced normally, then the clinician must change the hypothesis to a rule that specifies particular kinds of final consonant deletion (e.g., stop and nasal deletion). This is where the use of distinctive features is helpful.

4. *Specification of Frequency of Occurrence:* Authorities differ in their methods of specifying the frequency of occurrence of certain phonological rules. Some processes appear to be obligatory (occur virtually all the time) and others seem to be optional. In specifying optionality of a phonological rule, some authors recommend the three stage system of "always," "sometimes," and "never" (Shriberg & Kwiatkowski, 1980). Other authorities (Ingram, 1981) recommend the use of percentage ranges such as 0–20, 21–40, 41–60, 61–80, and 81–100. Whatever method is used, the important variable is to indicate how often the process is occurring.

5. *Writing the Rule:* After the clinician has gathered support for a rule from the transcript, the rule is written specifying the target phonemes, how they are changed, what context they are changed in, and how often the rule occurs. A phonological rule for final stop consonant deletion may look like this:

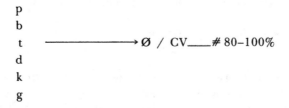

This rule says that the consonants p, b, t, d, k, and g are deleted in the context of the CVC word when the target sound is at the end. The slash stands for "in the context of," the blank represents the location of the target sound and the # refers to a word boundary. Note that the percentage of occurrence is indicated after the rule.

6. *Hypothesize an Idiosyncratic Rule and Recycle Steps 1–5:* As each rule is written and proof is gathered for each phonological reduction, the clinician repeats the process of examining the errors, hypothesizing a phonological process, looking for data to support the rule, and writing the rule. Soon, the clinician can account for the majority of the errors in the child's transcript with the

exception of a small residue of words that the rules do not describe. At this point, the clinician may wish to hypothesize a phonological rule that is not normally seen in children's articulatory development. For instance, the child may delete initial consonants of certain types. The procedure, however, is still the same. The clinician must hypothesize the rule and find support for it before it can be written.

The detection of phonological simplification patterns can be a powerful tool in the hands of the clinician. A sample of speech that appears to have many unrelated misarticulations can be reduced to only a few phonological reduction patterns. The clinical implication of these processes is that the child does not need to work on a single sound but may need to focus on the pattern of error. The assumption is that the observable error pattern is generated by an underlying rule; and if the rule is to be altered, then some of the segments it affects should be targeted (Compton, 1976; Hodson & Paden, 1983; Ingram, 1976). Again, the only way to discover these patterns of misarticulation is to search for them through a phonological analysis technique. Traditional tests are not constructed for this purpose, although they certainly could be suggestive for further analyses and provide hints for the clinician as to error patterns.

There are several cautions we might offer regarding phonological analysis of a child's misarticulations. First, a phonological approach requires that a clinician transcribe words and/or sentences of spontaneous speech. Although most speech-language clinicians have completed courses in phonetics during their undergraduate education, some of these courses may not have offered students the opportunity to transcribe disordered speech from a variety of male, female, adult, and child speakers. Some clinicians may not have adequate experience to reliably transcribe connected speech. One clinician of our acquaintance remarked that "the only thing I have used my phonetics for in the past 10 years is to fill in the little blocks on the *Goldman-Fristoe* score sheet." It may be quite a leap, then, for some clinicians to transcribe words or connected speech in practice. Second, if our reliability is low in scoring phoneme errors, then we can only assume that reliability is even more of an issue in phonological transcription and analysis because we must construct rules from the data (Shriberg & Kwiatkowski, 1977). A third concern is the compelling and captivating nature of phonological analysis. It makes an articulatory assessment rather like an interesting puzzle. When the clinician reaches the "solution" and divines the phonological rules, it is tempting to view the child's problem exclusively from a linguistic-phonological perspective. It is then quite easy to logically apply a phonologically based treatment. Children of various etiological groups will demonstrate phonological regularities in their speech. Even if the disorder has a sensorimotor basis, phonological rules can be written and the child perceived as a phonological-linguistic case. Shriberg and Kwiatkowski (1982a) suggest that the clinician must examine linguistic, sensorimotor, and psychosocial aspects of a child's behavior and select appropriate treatment goals. Clinicians should not assume a linguistically oriented treatment simply because the child exhibits a systematic phonology. The treatment of choice for each child may require different emphases, and these could include focusing on sensorimotor aspects of articulation. There is no doubt that phonological analyses are useful and a major innovation in articulatory assessment, but the clinician must be cautious to check reliability and not apply a phonological linguistic interpretation to all errors without examining sensorimotor and psychosocial aspects as well.

ASSESSMENT OF PHONOLOGICAL KNOWLEDGE

Some researchers have considered the notion of *phonological knowledge* in misarticulating children (Elbert & Gierut, 1986; Gierut, Elbert, & Dinnsen, 1987; Maxwell & Rockman, 1984). A basic question revolves around whether a child's phonological organization is similar to or different from a typical adult system. Bernthal and Bankson illustrate this notion with final consonant deletion:

> One explanation for that process might be that the child misperceives the adult word, e.g., perceives [dɔg] as [dɔ]. A second explanation might be that the child's underlying lexical representation for dog is [dɔ], so the closest match in his store of lexical items is [dɔ]; thus, [dɔg] becomes [dɔ]. A third possible explanation is that the child's perceptual system functions appropriately and the lexical match between what the child perceives and what he or she has stored is consistent with the adult standard, but he or she has a phonological production rule that calls for the deletion of word-final stops. A fourth possibility is that the child has a motor production problem; in this case the child may have the appropriate perception but does not possess the necessary motor skill to make the physiological gesture to produce the sound. (1988, p. 279)

One might wonder how the clinician is to gain insight into a child's phonological knowledge. Although we are just beginning to understand this area, some procedures have been used by researchers. Due to difficulties inherent in assessing and interpreting a child's perceptual abilities (Locke, 1980) and the recent suggestion of independence between the perception and production systems (Dinnsen, 1985; Straight, 1980), most research has concentrated on data generated from a child's productive system. One example is provided by Maxwell and Rockman:

> [E]vidence can be adduced that shows that Jamie does know or does represent these words underlyingly with the appropriate postvocalic obstruents, that is, that he represents them the same way we do, but that his pronunciation of these words is governed by a phonological rule of final obstruent deletion . . . This evidence is available in his pronunciations of these words or morphemes in their inflected forms, that is, in morphophonemically related words. . . . These data reveal that for each morpheme the omitted consonant in question is not omitted when that consonant is in word-medial position. . . . For example, the morpheme meaning "duck" is pronounced [dʌ] without the final k in its uninflected form but as [dʌk] when the k is inflected with the diminutive morpheme [−i] as in [dʌki]. Morphophonemic evidence of this sort (e.g., k alternating with null) provides clear evidence that Jamie knows that the morpheme meaning "duck" must be represented underlyingly with a postvocalic k. (1984, pp. 11–12)

Elbert and Gierut (1986) have suggested a procedure for determining a child's productive phonological knowledge on a six-level continuum from least to most knowledge. Gierut et al. (1987) summarize the six types of knowledge. It is recommended by Elbert and Gierut (1986) that the clinician gather an extensive sample that includes all phonemes of English in all word positions with a variety of canonical shapes that provide multiple opportunities for phonemic contrast. After examining the child's phonetic and phonemic inventories, phonotactic rules, phonological rules, allophonic and neutralization rules, the clinician can categorize the types of phonological knowledge a child exhibits for individual sounds, sound classes, or the overall sound system. Gierut, Elbert, and Dinnsen (1987) found that the phonological knowledge continuum may relate to the amount of generalization to be expected in treatment. Basically, training of sounds with least phonological knowledge resulted in generalization across the entire phonological system, whereas training of sounds with most knowledge resulted in generalization to only the specific class of phoneme trained. Thus, the implication is that greater effects may be obtained by training phonemes for which the child has least knowledge. More research needs to be done in this area.

OTHER TESTING

Four additional areas of examination relate significantly to a competent evaluation of an articulation-disordered client depending on the type of case and the severity. The clinician should be prepared to assess these areas as appropriate.

1. *Language Assessment:*   The clinician examining a child's articulatory system should expect the bulk of these cases to exhibit some language deviations as well. Many authorities report the high co-occurrence of articulation and language disorders. Paul and Shriberg (1982) report that 86 percent of articulation-disordered children are also likely to exhibit syntactic delays. Shriberg et al. (1986) reported that only 20 to 25 percent of 114 phonologically disordered children studied did not have associated language problems. The clinician should routinely gather a spontaneous language sample and administer standardized language tests for each articulation-disordered client.

2. *Audiometric Screening:*   A second diagnostic procedure that should be routinely administered is an audiometric screening. It is critical that the possibility of hearing impairment be eliminated or confirmed prior to the administration of any standardized tests or measures of communicative competence. This becomes especially important if the parents report suspected auditory problems or if the child has a history of ear infections.

3. *The Oral-Peripheral Examination:*   This is an integral part of the articulation examination (see Chapter 9 for guidelines in conducting this procedure). Oral-peripheral examination results may be important in distinguishing a sensorimotor from a linguistic disorder of articulation. Fletcher (1972) provides some normative data on diadochokinetic (syllable repetition) rates for children, and this should also be included as part of the examination for sensorimotor difficulties.

4. *Auditory Discrimination:* This area has been classically explored in articulation evaluation. Historically, many investigations have shown that articulation-disordered children do not perform as well as normal speakers on auditory discrimination tasks (Bernthal & Bankson, 1988; Powers, 1971; Winitz, 1969). Early treatment programs incorporated an obligatory module of auditory discrimination training (Van Riper & Irwin, 1958) and many authorities continue to believe that the assessment of auditory discrimination is an important part of an evaluation (Winitz, 1975). Within the past 10 years, however, criticisms have emerged regarding our methods of auditory discrimination testing (Beving & Eblen, 1973; Schwartz & Goldman, 1974) and the efficacy of auditory discrimination training in treatment (Shelton et al., 1978; Williams & McReynolds, 1975). The most defensible position appears to be assessing the auditory discrimination of misarticulated sounds only (Bernthal & Bankson, 1988; Locke, 1980), rather than all phonemes, and to evaluate it in a way that avoids the use of paired comparisons (mass–math). It is presently not clear if auditory discrimination testing needs to be a part of routine articulatory evaluations or if it should be embarked upon only when some suspicion of a discrimination problem is evidenced in trial therapy. The present authors would favor the latter option.

SEVERITY AND INTELLIGIBILITY

Several investigators have considered the problem of assigning a severity rating to children's misarticulation problems. We often hear clinicians rate a child's difficulty as mild or moderate and when asked how this was determined, they often have no empirical basis. Shriberg and Kwiatkowski (1982) suggest the use of the percent of consonants correct (PCC) in a spontaneous sample as being a most reliable predicter of severity ratings. They had judges rank order variables that were thought to contribute to severity, and intelligibility was ranked first as the most influencing factor. They also had clinicians rate tape recordings of spontaneous speech on severity (mild, mild-moderate, moderate-severe, severe). Statistical analyses showed that the measure most predictive of severity rating was the percent of consonants correct (PCC). Basically, the PCC is a calculation of the number of correct consonants divided by the number of correct plus incorrect consonants. The resulting number is multiplied by 100 to arrive at the PCC. Shriberg and Kwiatkowski (1982b) outline specific procedures and a worksheet for use in the computation of the PCC. The point here is that the percentage of consonants correctly articulated relates to severity and severity relates to intelligibility. The number of errors a child has will obviously affect the PCC. Hodson and Paden (1983) offer the Composite Phonological Deviancy Score (CPDS) as a measure of severity. This system considers age in the calculation as well as a number of phonological processes occurring on the *Analysis of Phonological Processes (APP)*. Although both of these methods may be criticized by some, they are at least attempts to objectify severity in cases of articulation disorders and are available for use by practicing clinicians.

Another gauge of severity might be to have independent judges rate the severity of speech samples based on their perceptual judgments. Even though this is not a quantitative measure, it certainly is an indication of society's reaction to a person's phonological disorder. Garrett and Moran (1991) compared the ratings of experienced (speech-language pathology majors) and inexperienced (elementary education majors) listeners to more objective measures such as the PCC and CPDS. They found all measures to be highly intercorrelated. The two objective measures appeared to be useful as clinical indicators of severity. This is especially interesting since one of the measures (CPDS) is derived from a single-word sample and the other (PCC) from connected speech. Of course, the determination of the overall severity of a child's problem will also have to consider other variables in addition to phonology. For instance, if a child has a concomitant language disorder or hearing impairment, the overall severity level increases.

No matter how a child performs on an articulation test, a major concern of both the clinician and the parent is intelligibility in spontaneous speech. How understandable is the child in daily interactions? Intelligibility is difficult to measure since it is affected by many variables. For instance, a child will be more intelligible to family members because they have unconsciously decoded the "system" of substitutions and omissions. Another variable affecting intelligibility is the sound that the child misarticulates. Some sounds occur more frequently in the language than others, and if the child's error is on a sound that occurs frequently, intelligibility will be affected to a greater degree than when errors are on infrequently occurring phonemes. An obvious factor that could logically impact on intelligibility is the number of phonemes a child misarticulates, although Shriberg and Kwiatkowski (1982b) did not find high correlations between total number of errors and intelligibility.

Another variable affecting intelligibility may be the consistency of the error in the child's speech. This would also affect the PCC calculation. A final factor that could affect intelligibility is the type of error (omission, substitution, distortion) the child exhibits (Shriberg & Kwiatkowski, 1982).

Fudala (1970) recommends using a continuum for rating intelligibility similar to the following (however, we must remember that responses to these ratings would vary significantly from family members to strangers):

1. Speech not intelligible
2. Speech usually not intelligible
3. Speech difficult to understand
4. Speech intelligible with careful listening
5. Speech intelligible although noticeably in error
6. Speech intelligible with occasional error
7. Speech totally intelligible.

There are few data relating intelligibility to age although we know that children become more intelligible as they get older. Generally, a child of age three should be mostly intelligible to strangers, and the inability to understand a child of this age is reason for clinical intervention (Bernthal & Bankson, 1988).

Every assessment of articulatory ability should contain some judgment regarding intelligibility. This is a factor that can be an important deciding variable in making treatment recommendations.

COMPUTER-ASSISTED ANALYSIS OF PHONOLOGY

Much of the work in phonological analysis is detailed, laborious, and repetitive. Some of the major difficulties involve keeping track of the data on a host of different worksheets, tallying up percentages and frequency counts, and repeatedly cross-checking a variety of relationships found in different portions of the client's transcript. The nature of these tasks is ideally suited to computer analysis. The computer can take a corpus of language and the gloss of each utterance and produce more information than even the most zealous clinician would like to know about a child's phonological system. In some cases, computer analyses of human behavior are rather superficial and the programs available are just in the early stages of development. In the case of phonological analysis, however, the computer programs are detailed, user friendly, and here to stay! An analysis that might take a clinician several hours to accomplish can actually be completed in less than a few minutes by most programs. The software is compatible with the most popular types of microcomputers available in the majority of school systems, universities, and even households of prospective users. The cost of the programs varies from under $100 to just over $1,000. The programs differ in their scope, ranging from those designed to analyze the responses from a particular test of phonology to those focusing on the assessment of spontaneous samples of connected speech. Some of the available programs will be mentioned later; however, some words of caution are in order.

It would be ideal if the client simply talked into a microphone that was plugged into a computer, and in a few seconds a miraculous printout appeared that revealed the secrets of the phonological system. Unfortunately, this is not the case at the present time. The clinician must still obtain the sample, transcribe the sample, input the sample into the computer through the keyboard, and in many cases do some other work responding to menus and prompts produced on the screen. The tasks just described constitute a lot of painstaking work on the part of the clinician. Just transcribing a sample of connected speech can take hours of careful listening. The beauty of computer-assisted analysis is that the clinician does not have to spend several *more* hours organizing data, scanning the transcript over and over again, and performing mathematical operations. The computer also provides elegant summaries of the data, such as phonetic inventories, canonical shape analyses, positional inventories, phonological process analysis, measures of severity (e.g., PCC, CPDS), and even suggested treatment targets on some programs. Thus, one misconception some people might have is that computer analysis takes away all tedious work on the part of the clinician. The truth is, it takes away much of this work, but not all. A second misconception some people may have is that the computer will always come up with the "right answer" with regard to a client's

Table 6.4 Computer-Assisted Analysis of Misarticulations: Selected Programs

Computer Analysis of Phonological Processes. Hodson, B. (1985). Phonocomp, Box 46, Stonington, IL 62567.

Computerized Profiling. Long, S., & Fey, M. (1988). P.O. Box 740, Arcata, CA 95521.

Computer Managed Articulation Diagnosis. Fitch, J. (1985). Communication Skill Builders, P.O. Box 42050, Tucson, AZ 85733.

Diagnostic Articulation Analyzer. Parrot Software, P.O. Box 1139, State College, PA 16804.

LINGQUEST 2. Palin, M., & Mordecai, D., Charles E. Merrill Test Division, 1300 Alum Creek Dr., Box 508, Columbus, OH 43216.

Process Analysis. Weiner, F., Parrot Software, P.O. Box 1139, State College, PA 16804.

Programs to Examine Phonetic and Phonologic Evaluation Records (PEPPER). Shriberg, L. (1986). SDCD, University of Wisconsin, 1025 West Johnson St., Madison, WI 53706.

phonology. Even though the algorithms in most phonology programs are quite sophisticated, they have difficulty dealing with idiosyncratic processes and certain types of analyses. The one thing the clinician can expect, however, is output; it may not always be correct, but it *is* output. Thus, a clinician should be aware of the limitations of phonological analysis programs and practice by running phonological samples that they have done by hand to see if there is general agreement between the two methods. Table 6.4 includes a listing of some popular programs available for phonological analysis.

EVALUATION TASKS FOR REASSESSMENT DURING TREATMENT

Not all of the data we gather in the area of phonological disorders has to do with diagnosis. As we stated in Chapter 1, evaluation tasks are procedures that can be used in the diagnostic process, but they are also important in gauging the client's progress in treatment and determining the extent of a variety of types of generalization. The type of data used by the clinician in evaluation tasks for phonological disorders depends on a variety of factors.

1. *Type of Treatment Target Selected:* We mentioned earlier that misarticulations could have either a phonologic (linguistic) or a sensorimotor basis. If the clinician is working on an articulation error involving one or two single phoneme errors (e.g., /s/ or /r/), the probes may be specifically focused on these two sounds. If, on the other hand, the clinician has targeted a phonological process such as final consonant deletion, the treatment may involve some sounds included in the rule, and the probes would ideally focus on evaluating final consonant production in untrained elements. Interestingly, in the case of final consonant deletion, a correct response might be production of a final consonant, even if the phoneme is not the correct one (e.g., "dɔd" for "dɔg"). Thus, the notion of correct response changes from phoneme to process depending on what is being trained.

2. *Type of Generalization Probed:* There are several types of generalization reported in the literature on phonology (Bernthal & Bankson, 1988). One obvious type was discussed when probing of untrained phonemes was mentioned. Another type of generalization may have to do with different levels in a hierarchial treatment program. For example, many clinicians work on syllables, words, phrases, sentences, and conversation in certain types of phonological/articulatory treatment. Some research indicates generalization among these treatment levels that suggests that training on lower levels may transfer to higher levels of the program. So, if one works on the word level, does generalization occur to the sentence or conversational level? If one works in imitation, does some generalization to spontaneous productions occur? If one works with singletons, does generalization to consonant clusters occur? All of these questions could be answered effectively with a different type of evaluation probe.

The types of data that are typically found in research and clinical work are percentage correct scores or, in the case of phonological processes, percentage of occurrence scores. These are used primarily because simple frequency counts of number correct might vary due to different sample sizes. The percentage scores lend themselves to graphing at various probing intervals to determine if a client is improving, or if another more difficult level of treatment should be considered. A lot depends on the clinician's interest in either molar or molecular client behaviors. For example, a clinician might use the percent consonants correct (PCC) as one indication of overall treatment progress. It certainly would suggest that a client is more intelligible if, over time, the PCC went from 50 to 80. Another molar measure might be the whole word accuracy score (WWA) suggested by Schmitt, Howard, and Schmitt (1983). Even intelligibility ratings such as those suggested earlier by Fudala (1970) may be a general indication of treatment progress if done in a reliable manner. Another more general measure might be to descriptively compare phonetic and phonemic inventories at different points in time, or the number of phonological processes currently active in a child's system. On the more molecular side, a clinician may want to know the fate of a particular sound in a child's repertoire in terms of percent correct in conversation or a subconversational level such as words. A more molecular way to examine phonological processes is to determine their percent of occurrence and then track these over time to determine if obligatory processes have become optional and optional processes have reduced in their occurrence. For instance, if the final consonant deletion process at the beginning of treatment occurred 80 to 100 percent of the time and was found to be present in a later sample only 20–40 percent of the time, this documents change. Some clinicians may be interested in the number of phonetic elements involved in a process. The final consonant deletion process may have involved a total of 14 phones when treatment started and now may only involve three voiceless stops and two nasal consonants. The clinician could also take the concept of phonological knowledge and use it to document treatment progress by showing that a client began with many sounds on level 6 and at a later probe had no sounds below level 4.

There are many ways that a clinician can document treatment progress or change in a maturing child's phonological system. Many authorities are currently recommending techniques from single case experimental design to demonstrate that treatment has actually produced desired effects (Bernthal & Bankson, 1988; McReynolds & Kearns, 1983; Weiner, 1981). One of the most popular approaches is the multiple baseline design in which treatment of a given phoneme or process is conducted systematically, such that baseline data is taken on all behaviors of interest and then treatment is applied to one at a time while continuing to gather baseline information on untrained phonemes or processes. In this way, one can easily see that targets receiving training are changing while untrained behaviors are remaining stable. If the untrained items begin to change when training is applied only to one element, then one can assume these behaviors are either maturing spontaneously or generalizing from the trained element.

INTEGRATING DATA FROM THE ASSESSMENT

There are a variety of ways to assess articulatory ability and the broader the view taken by the clinician, the more realistic the picture obtained of the client. For instance, if only the results of a traditional articulation test are considered, the clinician may be able to summarize a phonetic inventory and make some preliminary judgments about distinctive feature acquisition, but perhaps an inventory of phonological processes may not be possible due to limited sampling. Further, the norms that might be used in comparing the child's phonetic inventory to other children (Sander, 1972; Templin, 1957) are not applicable to phonological processes. The areas of assessment discussed in this chapter are simply different ways of looking at the child's phonological/articulatory system. Many of the assessment tasks (traditional testing, oral-peripheral examination, audiological screening, detailed case history, language ability, construction of a phonetic/phonemic inventory) should at least be considered in every case presenting misarticulations. Then, further exploration might be undertaken in areas of concern, such as writing a phonology from a spontaneous speech sample if problems are indicated on measures such as a *PPA* or *APP*. If a child is noted to be missing entire classes of phonemes, then a more intensive distinctive feature analysis might be indicated. The point is that results from a variety of areas need to be considered and used as indicators for further analyses.

Figure 6.3 depicts some *hypothetical* decisions that a clinician could make in using some of the assessment procedures discussed in this chapter. One of the most difficult tasks for beginning clinicians is to decide which measures might be appropriate for a given case. It is equally confusing to decide where to go if the initial measure does not give you the type of information required to understand the client's problem. Figure 6.3 is meant to be an example of possible decision-making that could occur when dealing with cases on two extreme ends of the severity continuum. Clients in the middle of the continuum may require combinations of the decisions displayed in Figure 6.3. The figure

Figure 6.3 A Severity Continuum and Some Hypothetical Decision Points Demonstrating Differential Use of Assessment Techniques for Different Types of Cases. Decisions Do Not Have to Be Either/or; Many Clients Present Errors Requiring Assessment of Multiple Aspects of the System.

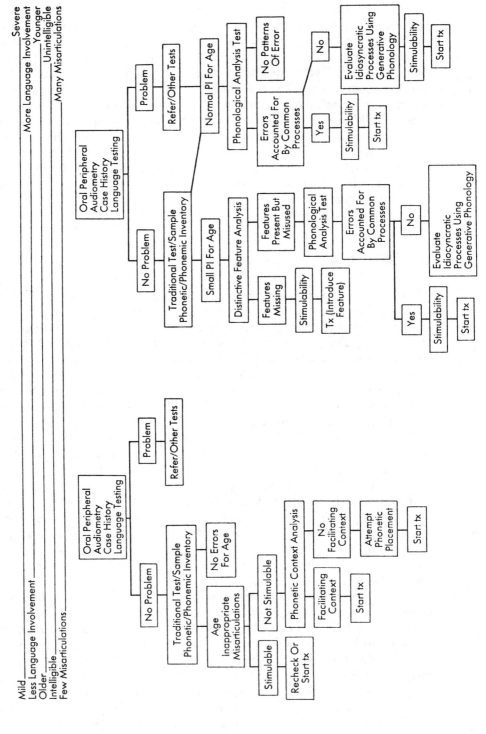

presents five continuua at the top that deal with severity, language involvement, age, intelligibility, and number of misarticulations. Generally, clients with only two or three error sounds are not particularly problematic for the speech-language pathologist. It is important for the beginning student to realize, however, that we do not necessarily have to perform every analysis technique in our armamentarium in such cases. On the other hand, cases with many errors and low intelligibility require greater skill and application of more assessment procedures. Students can follow the logic of the decisions made in the figure as an example of possible options to be considered in differing types of cases.

Shriberg and Kwiatkowski (1982a) have suggested that clinicians should consider possible causal correlates of articulation disorders. They recommended gathering data on each client in the areas of cognition/language, speech mechanism integrity, and psychological/social parameters. Consideration of these areas helps to keep the clinician from becoming too narrowly focused in the conception of articulation assessment and treatment. It also forces the clinician to at least consider the possibility of a variety of single or interactive maintaining factors in the articulation disorder. If a clinician is enamored with phonology and a linguistic interpretation of most articulation problems, such an approach forces the clinician to at least gather some information on psychosocial and speech mechanism variables. Conversely, if a clinician has a sensorimotor orientation, the approach forces the evaluation of more linguistic aspects. The findings of such a broad-based analysis may provide the clinician with important information on prognosis and treatment goals that would otherwise have not been considered.

BIBLIOGRAPHY

ALLEN, D., BLISS, L., & TIMMONS, J. (1981). Language evaluation: Science or art? *Journal of Speech and Hearing Disorders, 46,* 66–68.

AMERMAN, J., DANILOFF, R., & MOLL, K. (1970). Lip and jaw coarticulation for the phoneme /ae/. *Journal of Speech and Hearing Research, 13,* 148–161.

ANDERSON, V., & NEWBY, H. (1973). *Improving the child's speech* (2nd ed.). New York: Oxford University Press.

ANDREWS, N., & FEY, M. (1986). Analysis of the speech of phonologically impaired children in two sampling conditions. *Language, Speech and Hearing Services in Schools, 17,* 187–198.

AVANT, V., & HUTTON, C. (1962). Passage for speech screening in upper elementary grades. *Journal of Speech and Hearing Disorders, 27,* 40–46.

BATTLE, D., ALDES, M., GRANTHAM, R., HALFOND, M., HARRIS, G., MORGENSTERN-LOPEZ, N., SMITH, G., TERRELL, S., & COLE, L. (1983). Position paper—Social dialects. *Journal of the American Speech-Language-Hearing Association, 25,* 23–24.

BERNTHAL, J., & BANKSON, N. (1988). *Articulation disorders.* Englewood Cliffs, NJ: Prentice Hall.

BEVING, B., & EBLEN, R. (1973). Same and different concepts and children's performance on speech sound discrimination. *Journal of Speech and Hearing Research, 16,* 513–517.

BLACHE, S. (1978). *The acquisition of distinctive features.* Baltimore: University Park Press.

BRYANT, B., & BRYANT, D. (1983). *Test of articulation performance: Diagnostic.* Austin, TX: PRO-ED.

CAMARATA, S., & SCHWARTZ, L. (1985). Production of object words and action words: Evidence for a relationship between phonology and semantics. *Journal of Speech and Hearing Research, 28,* 323–330.

CAMPBELL, J., & SHRIBERG, L. (1982). Associations among pragmatic functions, linguistic stress and natural phonological processes in speech delayed children. *Journal of Speech and Hearing Research, 25,* 547–553.

CARNEY, E. (1979). Inappropriate abstraction in speech assessment procedures. *British Journal of Disorders of Communication, 14,* 123–135.

CARRELL, J., & TIFFANY., W. (1960). *Phonetics: Theory and application to speech improvement.* New York: McGraw-Hill.

CHOMSKY, N. (1957). *Syntactic structures.* The Hague: Mouton.

CHOMSKY, N., & HALLE, M. (1968). *The sound pattern of English.* New York: Harper & Row.

COMPTON, A. (1970). Generative studies of children's phonological disorders. *Journal of Speech and Hearing Disorders, 35,* 315–339.

COMPTON, A. (1976). Generative studies of children's phonological disorders. In D. Morehead & A. Morehead (Eds.), *Normal and deficient child language.* Baltimore: University Park Press.

COMPTON, A., & HUTTON, S. (1978). *Compton-Hutton Phonological Assessment.* San Francisco: Carousel House.

COSTELLO, J., & ONSTINE, J. (1976). The modification of multiple articulation errors based on distinctive feature theory. *Journal of Speech and Hearing Disorders, 41,* 199–215.

CYPREANSEN, L., WILEY, J., & LAASE, L. (1959). *Speech development, improvement and correction.* New York: Ronald Press.

DANILOFF, R., & MOLL, K. (1968). Coarticulation of lip rounding. *Journal of Speech and Hearing Research, 11,* 707–721.

DANILOFF, R., SCHUCKERS, G., & FETH, L. (1980). *The physiology of speech and hearing: An introduction.* Englewood Cliffs, NJ: Prentice Hall.

DARLEY, F. (1964). *Diagnosis and appraisal of communication disorders.* Englewood Cliffs, NJ: Prentice Hall.

DAVIS, B., & MACNEILAGE, P. (1990). Acquisition of correct vowel production: A quantitative case study. *Journal of Speech and Hearing Research, 33*(1), 16–27.

DICKSON, D., & MAUE-DICKSON, W. (1982). *Anatomical and physiological bases of speech.* Boston: Little, Brown.

DIEDRICH, W. (1983). Stimulability and articulation disorders. In J. Locke (Ed.), *Assessing and treating phonological disorders: Current approaches. Seminars in Speech and Language,* 4. New York: Thieme-Stratton.

DILLARD, J. (1972). *Black English: Its history and usage in the United States.* New York: Random House.

DINNSEN, D. (1984). Methods of empirical issues in analyzing functional misarticulation. *Phonological Theory and the Misarticulating Child, ASHA Monographs, 22,* 5–17.

DINNSEN, D. (1985). A re-examination of phonological neutralization. *Journal of Linguistics, 21,* 265–279.

DYSON, A. (1988). Phonetic inventories of 2 and 3 year old children. *Journal of Speech and Hearing Disorders, 53*(1), 89–93.

EDMONSON, W. (1969). *The Laradon Articulation Scale.* Denver, CO: Laradon Hall.

EISENSON, J., & OGILVIE, M. (1977). *Speech correction in the schools* (4th ed.). New York: Macmillan.

ELBERT, M., & GIERUT, J. (1986). *Handbook of clinical phonology: Approaches to assessment and treatment.* San Diego, CA: College-Hill.

EVELEIGH, K., & WARR-LEEPER, G. (1983). Improving efficiency in articulation screening.

Language, Speech and Hearing Services in Schools, 14, 223–232.

FAIRBANKS, G. (1960). *Voice and articulation drillbook* (2nd ed.). New York: Harper & Row.

FAIRCLOTH, M., & FAIRCLOTH, S. (1970). An analysis of the articulatory behavior of a speech defective child in connected speech and isolated word responses. *Journal of Speech and Hearing Disorders, 35,* 51–61.

FARQUHAR, M. (1961). Prognostic value of imitative and auditory discrimination tests. *Journal of Speech and Hearing Disorders, 26,* 342–347.

FISHER, H., & LOGEMANN, J. (1971). *The Fisher-Logemann Test of Articulation Competence.* Boston: Houghton Mifflin.

FLETCHER, S. (1972). Time-by-count measurement of diadochokinetic syllable rate. *Journal of Speech and Hearing Research, 15,* 763–770.

FLUHARTY, N. (1974). The design and standardization of a speech and language screening test for use with preschool children. *Journal of Speech and Hearing Disorders, 39,* 75–88.

FRISTOE, M., & GOLDMAN, R. (1968). Comparisons of traditional and condensed articulation tests examining the same number of sounds. *Journal of Speech and Hearing Research, 11,* 583–589.

FUDALA, J. (1970). *The Arizona Articulation Proficiency Scale.* Beverly Hills, CA: Western Psychological Services.

GALLAGHER, T., & SHRINER, T. (1975). Articulatory inconsistencies in the speech of normal children. *Journal of Speech and Hearing Research, 18,* 168–175.

GARBER, N. (1986). A phonological analysis classification for use with traditional articulation tests. *Language, Speech and Hearing Services in Schools, 17*(4), 253–261.

GARN-NUNN, P. (1986). Phonological processes and conventional articulation tests: Considerations for analysis. *Language, Speech and Hearing Services in Schools, 17*(4), 244–252.

GARRETT, K., & MORAN, M. (1991). A comparison of phonological severity measures. *Language, Speech and Hearing Services in Schools,* in press.

GIERUT, J., ELBERT, M., & DINNSEN, D. (1987). A functional analysis of phonological knowledge and generalization learning in misarticulating children. *Journal of Speech and Hearing Research, 30*(4), 462–479.

GODA, S. (1970). *Articulation therapy and consonant drillbook.* New York: Grune & Stratton.

GOLDMAN, R., & FRISTOE, M. (1986). *Goldman-Fristoe Test of Articulation.* Circle Pines, MN: American Guidance Service.

GRUNWELL, P. (1985). *Phonological assessment of child speech (PACS).* Windsor, UK: NFER-Nelson/San Diego, CA: College-Hill Press.

GRUNWELL, P. (1988). *Clinical phonology.* Baltimore: Williams and Wilkins.

HAYNES, W., HAYNES, M., & JACKSON, J. (1982). The effects of phonetic context and linguistic complexity on /s/ misarticulation in children. *Journal of Communication Disorders, 15,* 287–297.

HEJNA, R. (1963). *Development Articulation Test.* Ann Arbor, MI: Speech Materials.

HODSON, B. (1980). *The assessment of phonological processes.* Danville, IL: Interstate.

HODSON, B., & PADEN, E. (1983). *Targeting intelligible speech: A phonological approach to remediation.* San Diego: College-Hill Press.

HOFFMAN, P., SCHUCKERS, G., & RATUSNIK, D. (1977). Contextual-coarticulatory inconsistencies of /r/ misarticulation. *Journal of Speech and Hearing Research, 20,* 631–643.

INGRAM, D. (1971). *Edinburgh Articulation Test.* London: Edward Arnold Company.

INGRAM, D. (1976). *Phonological disability in children.* New York: Elsevier.

INGRAM, D. (1981). *Procedures for the phonological analysis of children's language.* Baltimore: University Park Press.

IRWIN, J. (1972). *Disorders of articulation.* Indianapolis: Bobbs-Merrill.

IRWIN, J., & WONG, P. (1983). *Phonological development in children 18 to 72 months.* Carbondale, IL: Southern Illinois University Press.

IRWIN, R. (1965). *Speech and hearing therapy.* Pittsburgh: Stanwix House.

JOHNSON, W., DARLEY, F., & SPRIESTERSBACH, D. (1963). *Diagnostic methods in speech pathology.* New York: Harper & Row.

KAHANE, J., & FOLKINS, J. (1984). *Atlas of speech and hearing anatomy.* Columbus: Charles E. Merrill.

KAHN, L., & LEWIS, N. (1986). *Kahn-Lewis Phonological Analysis.* Circle Pines, MN: American Guidance Service.

KENNEY, K., & PRATHER, E. (1984). *Coarticulation assessment in meaningful language.* Tucson, AZ: Communication Skill Builders.

KENT, R. (1982). Contextual facilitation of correct sound production. *Language, Speech and Hearing Services in Schools, 13,* 66–76.

KENT, R., & MINIFIE, F. (1977). Coarticulation in recent speech production models. *Journal of Phonetics, 5,* 115–133.

KLEIN, H. (1984). Procedure for maximizing phonological information from single word responses. *Language, Speech and Hearing Services in Schools, 15,* 267–274.

LARIVIERE, C., WINITZ, H., REEDS, J., & HERRIMAN, E. (1974). The conceptual reality of selected distinctive features. *Journal of Speech and Hearing Research, 17,* 122–133.

LEONARD, L. (1971). Preliminary view of information theory and articulatory omissions. *Journal of Speech and Hearing Disorders, 36,* 511–517.

LEONARD, L. (1973). Some limitations in the clinical application of distinctive features. *Journal of Speech and Hearing Disorders, 38,* 141–143.

LOCKE, J. (1980). The inference of speech perception in the phonologically disordered child. Part I: A rationale, some criteria, the conventional tests. *Journal of Speech and Hearing Disorders, 45,* 431–444.

LOCKE, J. (1983). Clinical phonology: The explanation and treatment of speech sound disorders. *Journal of Speech and Hearing Disorders, 48,* 339–341.

LOWE, R. (1986). *Assessment link between phonology and articulation.* Moline, IL: Linguisystems.

MCCAULEY, R., & SKENES, L. (1987). Contrastive stress, phonetic context and misarticulation of /r/ in young speakers. *Journal of Speech and Hearing Research, 30*(1), 114–121.

MCCLEAN, J. (1976). Articulation. In L. Lloyd (Ed.), *Communication assessment and intervention strategies.* Baltimore: University Park Press.

MCCLEAN, M. (1973). Forward coarticulation of velar movement at marked junctural boundaries. *Journal of Speech and Hearing Research, 16,* 236–246.

MCDONALD, E. (1964). *Articulation testing and treatment.* Pittsburgh: Stanwix House.

MCDONALD, E. (1968). *A Screening Deep Test of Articulation.* Pittsburgh: Stanwix House.

MCREYNOLDS, L., & ENGMANN, D. (1975). *Distinctive feature analysis of misarticulations.* Baltimore: University Park Press.

MCREYNOLDS, L., & HUSTON, K. (1971). A distinctive feature analysis of children's misarticulation. *Journal of Speech and Hearing Disorders, 36,* 155–166.

MCREYNOLDS, L., & KEARNS, K. (1983). *Single-subject experimental designs in communicative disorders.* Baltimore: University Park Press.

MADISON, C. (1979). Articulation stimulability reviewed. *Language, Speech and Hearing Services in Schools, 10,* 185–190.

MATHENY, N., & PANAGOS, J. (1978). Comparing the effects of articulation and syntax programs on syntax and articulation improvement. *Language, Speech and Hearing Services in Schools, 9,* 57–61.

MAXWELL, E., & ROCKMAN, B. (1984). Procedures for linguistic analysis of misarticulated speech. *Phonological Theory and the Misarticulating Child, ASHA Monographs, 22,* 69–84.

MAZZA, P., SCHUCKERS, G., & DANILOFF, R. (1979). Contextual-coarticulatory inconsistency of /s/ misarticulation. *Journal of Phonetics, 7,* 57–69.

MILISEN, R., ET AL. (1954). The disorder of articulation: A systematic clinical and experimental approach. *Journal of Speech and Hearing Disorders, Monograph Supplement 4.*

MOLL, K., & DANILOFF, R. (1971). Investigation of the timing of velar movements during speech. *Journal of the Acoustical Society of America, 50,* 678–684.

MONSEES, E., & BERMAN, C. (1968). Speech and language screening in a summer Headstart program. *Journal of Speech and Hearing Disorders, 33,* 121–126.

OLLER, K. D., ET AL. (1972). *Five studies in abnormal phonology.* Unpublished paper, University of Washington.

PADEN, E., & MOSS, S. (1985). Comparison of three phonological analysis procedures. *Language, Speech and Hearing Services in Schools, 16*(2), 103–109.

PALMER, J. (1984). *Anatomy for speech and hearing.* New York: Harper & Row.

PANAGOS, J., QUINE, H., & KLICH, P. (1979). Syntactic and phonological influences in children's articulations. *Journal of Speech and Hearing Research, 22,* 841–848.

PARKER, F. (1976). Distinctive features in speech pathology: Phonology or phonemics. *Journal of Speech and Hearing Disorders, 41,* 23–39.

PAUL, R., & SHRIBERG, L. (1982). Association between phonology and syntax in speech delayed children. *Journal of Speech and Hearing Research, 25,* 536–546.

PENDERGAST, K., DICKEY, S., SELMAR., T., & SODER, A. (1984). *Photo Articulation Test.* Danville, IL: Interstate.

POLLACK, E., & REES, N. (1972). Disorders of articulation: Some clinical applications of distinctive feature theory. *Journal of Speech and Hearing Disorders, 37,* 451–461.

POOLE, E. (1934). Genetic development of articulation of consonant sounds in speech. *Elementary English Review, 11,* 159–161.

POWERS, M. (1971). Functional disorders of articulation: symptomatology and etiology. In L. Travis (Ed.), *Handbook of speech pathology and audiology.* Englewood Cliffs, NJ: Prentice Hall.

PRATHER, E., HEDRICK, D., & KERN, C. (1975). Articulation development in children aged 2 to 4 years. *Journal of Speech and Hearing Disorders, 40,* 179–191.

PRATHER, E., & KENNEY, K. (1986). Coarticulation testing of kindergarten children. *Language, Speech and Hearing Services in Schools, 17,* 285–291.

RILEY, G. (1971). *Riley Articulation and Language Test.* Los Angeles: Western Psychological Service.

RITTERMAN, R., & FREEMAN, N. (1974). Distinctive phonetic features as relevant and irrelevant stimulus dimensions in speech sound discrimination learning. *Journal of Speech and Hearing Research, 17,* 417–425.

RITTERMAN, S., ZOOK-HERMAN, S., CARLSON, R., & KINDE, S. (1982). The pass/fail disparity among three commonly employed articulatory screening tests. *Journal of Speech and Hearing Disorders, 47,* 429–432.

ROGERS, W. (1972). *Picture Articulation and Screening Test.* Salt Lake City: Word Making Production.

RUDER, K., & BUNCE, B. (1981). Articulation therapy using distinctive feature analysis to structure the training program: Two case studies. *Journal of Speech and Hearing Disorders, 46,* 59–65.

SANDER, E. (1972). When are speech sounds learned? *Journal of Speech and Hearing Disorders, 37,* 55–63.

SCHISSEL, R., & JAMES, L. (1979). A comparison of children's performance on two tests of articulation. *Journal of Speech and Hearing Disorders, 44,* 363–372.

SCHMAUCH, V., PANAGOS, J., & KLICH, P. (1978). Syntax influences and accuracy of consonant production in language disordered children. *Journal of Communication Disorders, 11,* 315–323.

SCHMITT, L., HOWARD, B., & SCHMITT, J. (1983). Conversation speech sampling in the assessment of articulatory proficiency. *Language, Speech and Hearing Services in Schools, 14,* 210–214.

SCHWARTZ, A., & GOLDMAN, R. (1974). Variables influencing performance on speech sound discrimination tests. *Journal of Speech and Hearing Research, 17,* 25–32.

SCHWARTZ, R. (1983). Diagnosis of speech sound disorders in children. In B. Weinberg & I. Meitus (Eds.), *Diagnosis in speech-language pathology.* Baltimore: University Park Press.

SCRIPTURE, M., & JACKSON, E. (1927). *A manual of exercises for the correction of speech disorders.* Philadelphia: F. A. Davis.

SHELTON, R., JOHSON, A., RUSCELLO, D., & ARNDT, W. (1978). Assessment of parent-administered listening training for preschool children with articulation deficits. *Journal of Speech and Hearing Disorders, 43,* 242–254.

SHELTON, R., & MCREYNOLDS, L. (1979). Functional articulation disorders: Preliminaries to treatment. In N. Lass (Ed.), *Speech and language: Advances in basic research and practice* (Vol. 2). New York: Academic Press.

SHRIBERG, L., & KENT, R. (1982). *Clinical phonetics.* New York: Wiley.

SHRIBERG, L., & KWIATKOWSKI, J. (1977). *Phonological programming for unintelligible children in early childhood projects.* Paper presented to the convention of the American Speech and Hearing Association, Chicago.

SHRIBERG, L., & KWIATKOWSKI, J. (1980). *Natural process analysis.* New York: Wiley.

SHRIBERG, L., & KWIATKOWSKI, J. (1982a). Phonological disorders I: A diagnostic classification system. *Journal of Speech and Hearing Disorders, 47,* 226–241.

SHRIBERG, L., & KWIATKOWSKI, J. (1982b). Phonological disorders III: A procedure for assessing severity of involvement. *Journal of Speech and Hearing Disorders, 47,* 256–270.

SHRIBERG, L., & KWIATKOWSKI, J. (1988). A follow-up study of children with phonologic disorders of unknown origin. *Journal of Speech and Hearing Disorders, 53*(2), 144–155.

SHRIBERG, L., KWIATKOWSKI, J., BEST, S., HENGST, J., & TERSELIC-WEBER, B. (1986). Characteristics of children with phonologic disorders of unknown origin. *Journal of Speech and Hearing Disorders, 51,* 140–161.

SINGH, S. (1976). *Distinctive features theory and validation.* Baltimore: University Park Press.

SMIT, A. (1986). Ages of speech sound acquisition: Comparisons and critiques of several normative studies. *Language, Speech and Hearing Services in Schools, 17*(3), 175–186.

SMITH, N. (1973). *The acquisition of phonology.* Cambridge, England: Cambridge University Press.

SOMMERS, R. (1983). *Articulation disorders.* Englewood Cliffs, NJ: Prentice Hall.

STAMPE, D. (1969). *A dissertation on natural phonology.* Unpublished Ph.D. dissertation, University of Chicago.

STEED, S., & HAYNES, W. (1988). *Elicited articulatory system evaluation.* Austin, TX: PRO-ED.

STOEL-GAMMON, C. (1987). Phonological skills in 2 year olds. *Language, Speech and Hearing Services in Schools, 18*(4), 323–329.

STOLLER, P. (1975). *Black American English.* New York: Delta.

STRAIGHT, H. (1980). Auditory versus articulatory phonological processes and their development in children. In G. Yeni-Komshian, C. Kavanagh, & C. Ferguson (Eds.), *Child phonology: Perception* (Vol. 2). New York: Academic Press.

TAYLOR, O. (1986). Language differences. In G. Shames & E. Wiig (Eds.), *Human communication disorders: An introduction.* Columbus, OH: Merrill.

TEMPLIN, M. (1957). Certain language skills in children: Their development and interrelationships. *Institute of Child Welfare, Monograph 26.* Minneapolis: The University of Minnesota Press.

TEMPLIN, M., & DARLEY, F. (1969). *The Templin-Darley Tests of Articulation* (2nd ed.). Iowa City: University of Iowa Bureau of Educational Research and Service.

VAN RIPER, C. (1963). *Speech correction: Principles and methods* (4th ed.). Englewood Cliffs, NJ: Prentice Hall.

VAN RIPER, C., & ERICKSON, R. (1969). A predictive screening test of articulation. *Journal of Speech and Hearing Disorders, 34,* 214–219.

VAN RIPER, C., & IRWIN, J. (1958). *Voice and articulation.* Englewood Cliffs, NJ: Prentice Hall.

VAN RIPER, C., & SMITH, D. (1979). An introduction to general american phonetics (3rd ed.). New York: Harper & Row.

WALSH, H. (1974). On certain practical inadequacies of distinctive feature systems. *Journal of Speech and Hearing Disorders, 39,* 32–43.

WEINER, F. (1979). *Phonological process analysis.* Baltimore: University Park Press.

WEINER, F. (1981). Treatment of phonological disability using the method of meaningful minimal contrast: Two case studies. *Journal of Speech and Hearing Disorders, 46,* 97–103.

WEINER, F., & OSTROWSKI, A. (1979). Effects of listener uncertainty on articulatory inconsistency. *Journal of Speech and Hearing Disorders, 44,* 487–493.

WELLMAN, B., CASE, M., MENGERT, E., & BRADBURY, D. (1931). Speech sounds of young children. *University of Iowa Studies in Child Welfare. 5.*

WESTMAN, M., & BROEN, P. (1989). Preschool screening for predictive language errors. *Language, Speech and Hearing Services in Schools, 20,* 139–148.

WILLIAMS, G., & MCREYNOLDS, L. (1975). The relationship between discrimination and articulation training in children with misarticulations. *Journal of Speech and Hearing Research, 18,* 401–412.

WINITZ, H. (1969). *Articulatory acquisition and behavior.* Englewood Cliffs, NJ: Prentice Hall.

WINITZ, H. (1975). *From syllable to conversation.* Baltimore: University Park Press.

ZEMLIN, W. (1988). *Speech and hearing science.* Englewood Cliffs, NJ: Prentice Hall.

chapter

7

DISORDERS
OF FLUENCY

Stuttering is a curious, sometimes astonishing, and certainly a difficult way to talk. Why is the flow of speech, seemingly so easy and automatic for others, marred by tense interruptions? Unfortunately, the answer to that question still eludes clinicians and researchers—stuttering remains an enigma.

The puzzling nature of stuttering creates a dilemma for students. Confronted with a voluminous literature and a large number of treatment possibilities—each with its advocates—it is easy to give up in despair. Perhaps the negative attitude toward stutterers held by so many clinicians stems, in part, from overwhelming confusion about the disorder (Ragsdale & Ashby, 1982; St. Louis & Lass, 1981; Turnbaugh, Guitar, & Hoffman, 1979, 1981). Yet, for some beginning clinicians, the dramatic nature of the disorder and even the confusion among experts have a fascinating appeal; they present a challenge.

We will assume in this chapter that the reader has a good foundation concerning the nature of stuttering. Books by Bloodstein (1981) and Van Riper (1982) provide excellent discussions of the many aspects of stuttering. We present the following list of "facts" about stuttering that have diagnostic implications and have been gleaned from the literature. For purposes of exposition, we have eschewed lengthy lists of references. Each item can be documented, however, even though some might disagree with our particular selection or interpretation.

1. The basic speech characteristics of stuttering consist of relatively brief part-word (phonemic, syllabic) repetitions and prolongations. These oscillations and fixations may be audible or silent and tend to occur more frequently at the

beginning of an utterance and on words and phrases more complex motorically (such as long words and less frequently used words).

2. Stuttering is a disorder of childhood, generally having its onset before the age of six; rarely does it begin in older persons, and when it does it may be a distinct subtype of the disorder (such as neurotic stuttering).
3. Stuttering is found more frequently among males.
4. Stuttering tends to run in families.
5. Stuttering may be precipitated (and perpetuated) by certain environmental events, particularly the critical, demanding behaviors of significant others, usually parents.
6. Stuttering tends to appear more frequently in children described as "sensitive," who may be vulnerable or susceptible to stress. Stutterers may have a low threshold for autonomic arousal.
7. Stuttering tends to appear more frequently in children who were slow in acquiring speech or who manifest certain inadequacies of oral communication (articulation errors, language disturbances) other than fluency breakdowns.
8. Stuttering tends to exhibit cycles of frequency and severity in a given individual.
9. Stuttering is apparently "outgrown" by a significant number of individuals.
10. Stuttering tends to change in form and severity as the individual matures.
11. Stuttering is eliminated or markedly reduced in a variety of conditions: speaking while alone, choral speaking, singing, prolonged or slow speaking, talking in time to rhythm, or under masking conditions.
12. Stuttering, in its developed form, consists largely of escape and avoidance behavior; that is, much of the overt abnormality results from the individual's attempt to cope with the emission of the basic speech disfluency.
13. Stuttering is also characterized by speech and voice abnormalities other than disfluency (such as narrow pitch range, vocal tension, lack of vocal expression, muscular lags, and asynchronies) that can be detected in nonstuttered speech. These anomalies *may* reflect a basic impairment of phonation (difficulty in initiating phonation, making consonant-vowel transitions), respiration (abnormal reflex activity), neuromotor coordination, or cortical integration; they *may*, however, simply be effects of stuttering.
14. Stuttering, in its developed form, is often associated with an expectancy or anticipation of its occurrence.
15. Stuttering is a personal problem; individuals who stutter report fear, frustration, social penalties, dissatisfaction with themselves, lower level of aspiration, and felt loss of social esteem. There is a tendency for problems common to all human beings to become associated with the speech disturbance. However, there is no particular "stuttering personality," nor is the disorder a manifestation of psychoneurosis.

Even though the fluency disorder of stuttering remains a tantalizing mystery, there is much that we can do to help persons who seek our services.

DIFFERENTIAL DIAGNOSIS

Speech is fluent when words are produced easily, effortlessly, smoothly, quickly, and in a forward flow. Speech is disfluent when one word does not flow smoothly and quickly into the next. Obviously, then, all speakers are, at times, disfluent and these so-called normal disfluencies should be of no consequence. The speech-language pathologist needs to be able to differentiate normal from abnormal disfluencies; often this proves to be no easy feat with young children. If the clinician does identify a speaker's disfluencies as abnormal or clinically significant, the next decision is to distinguish the problem of stuttering from other conditions in which speech fluency is disrupted. A final aspect of the differential diagnosis process may be to identify subtypes within the stuttering population, so as to select the most appropriate form of treatment. Let us discuss these three aspects of differential diagnosis, but we will do so in a different order.

Sorting Out the Types of Fluency Disorders

Assuming that the clinician has already identified a speaker as having abnormal amounts and/or types of disfluencies, the diagnostic task is one of deciding *which* disorder of fluency is exhibited. Along with a behavioral analysis of the disfluencies, the case history information will go far in suggesting the disorder type. We will provide an overview of some of the fluency breakdowns that can be confused with the common variety of stuttering, called developmental stuttering (or simply stuttering).

Episodic Stress Reaction.   It is well known that most speakers exhibit some degree of disfluency—revisions, interjections, word and phrase repetitions, and occasionally even part-word repetitions and prolongations (Leeper et al., 1990; Pindzola, 1991; Yairi, 1981; Yairi & Clifton, 1972). Speech fluency is often considered a sensitive barometer of a person's psychological state. Stress, particularly communicative stress, tends to increase a speaker's disfluency. If minor stress can affect fluency, then more intense forms of psychological stress can certainly have a detrimental effect. Examples of conditions that can precipitate a fluency breakdown include battle conditions, intense excitement, emotional upheaval, and stage fright (Gavis, 1946; Grinker & Spiegal, 1945).

Fluency breakdowns due to episodic stress show a number of consistent identifying features: an acknowledged source of intense or prolonged stimulation; tension overflow throughout the body (including the oral area), which may also produce a tremulous voice; an exacerbation of "normal" disfluency, including broken words, incomplete phrases, interjections, and repetitions of whole and part-words; and no avoidance but feelings of fear. Finally, the most crucial characteristic is that the disfluency decreases markedly or stops when (or shortly after) the stress terminates. These acute, or episodic, periods of disfluency are usually not clinically significant.

Neurotic or Hysterical Stuttering.   Most stutterers, particularly confirmed adult cases, acquire a negative feeling about their problem. One of our clients summarized it succinctly when he said, "Stutterers are bugged because they are plugged." A few stutterers, however, show symptoms of a primary neurosis—they are "plugged because they are bugged." For these individuals, stuttering is a maladaptive solution to an acute psychological problem.

Case Example. Colleen, an eighth-grade parochial school pupil, began to stutter suddenly following the death of her parents in an automobile accident. She collapsed upon hearing the tragic news and remained mute, almost transfixed and catatonic, for several hours. During the planning for the funeral and the extended period of the wake, she started to stutter—a monotonous repetition of the initial syllable of words. She showed no struggle, no avoidance behavior. She looked directly at the listener when she spoke and smiled bravely. We followed this case closely until the remission of stuttering two months later, and her disfluency was always the same; it never varied in form or severity from situation to situation. When she read a passage several times, she did not show the typical reduction (adaptation) in stuttering. School documents, as well as interviews with several relatives, indicated that Colleen had no prior speech difficulty. One maternal aunt whom we interviewed did recall, however, that the girl had several "spells" of uncontrolled weeping and laughing during her first menses the year before. The child had received an incredible amount of attention and solace after her parents' death, perhaps even more so because of her "stuttering," from sympathetic adults.

Neurotic stuttering is a rare fluency disorder that is characterized by a sudden onset of rather severe stuttering. The onset may occur at any age, including adulthood, yet usually happens in an older child. Some severe (and lasting rather than episodic) psychological trauma, emotional upheaval, or stress seems to precipitate the occurrence of stuttering (Deal, 1982; Van Riper, 1982; Weiner, 1981). In contrast to the exacerbation of "normal" disfluencies seen in episodic stress, the neurotic stuttering pattern is severe from the beginning, with unvoiced prolongations, laryngeal blocks, tension, and/or lengthy repetitions typical. Although highly aware of these sudden and severe disfluencies, the person may or may not be frustrated by them. The level of concern and motivation to change are important elements for the speech-language pathologist to assess as they may shape the prognosis for change and the direction of intervention.

Neurogenic Stuttering. Stuttering, or a stutteringlike problem may occur following nervous system damage, such as from stroke, trauma, infection, or tumor. The designation establishes this as a fluency disorder that results from neurological damage. We have observed disfluency in clients suffering from Parkinson's disease, some types of cerebral palsy, apraxia, and other neurological impairments (Helms, Butler, & Canter, 1980; Koller, 1983; LeBrun, Retif, & Kaiser, 1983). There are also reports of fluency disruptions in alcoholics, drug addicts, and patients afflicted with AIDS (Fantry, 1990) and with dialysis dementia (Madison et al., 1977). Palilalia, perhaps a subtype of neurogenic stuttering, may be caused by bilateral subcortical brain damage. Individuals with palilalia repeat words and entire phrases, typically not sounds or syllables, and they do so with increasing speed and diminishing loudness (Kent & LaPointe, 1982; LaPointe & Horner, 1981). Canter (1971) classified neurogenic stuttering into subtypes, such as dysnomic stuttering, dysarthric stuttering, apraxic stuttering, and so forth.

Several aphasics with whom we have worked, particularly those clients who show good progress in word finding but have residual syntactic difficulty, exhibited fluency breakdowns superficially similar to stuttering.

Case Example. Mrs. Horn had suffered an aneurysm in the Circle of Willis, leaving her hemiplegic, apraxic, and with mild expressive aphasia. When we examined her, almost a year after the cerebral vascular episode, her speech pattern resembled clonic stuttering. She would begin a word, repeat a phoneme or syllable several times, back up, and try again; if blocked once more, a repetition might reverberate almost endlessly. She frequently pounded on the table as if to time her utterances. We could discern no evidence of fear or avoidance, just severe frustration. Interestingly, when she spoke or read swiftly her fluency increased dramatically; she also talked freely when distracted from closely monitoring the acts of speaking. Here is a sample of her speech taken from a tape recording during a group session: "I can't-I can't (sigh) . . . I-I-I-I have tr-trouble with my, ah, with my speech . . . and, ah, my leg is, is, you know is, stiff. . . . "

The disfluencies noted are rather typical: whole-word repetitions, revisions, interjections, broken words, and gaps in the flow of speech. This client had difficulty formulating messages and then programming the proper motor sequences to utter the thought. Unlike stutterers who have difficulty getting started, Mrs. Horn's fluency breakdowns occurred at any point in a sentence (Brown & Cullinan, 1981; Donnan, 1979; Rosenbek et al., 1978).

Cluttering. Cluttering is sometimes confused with stuttering, but it encompasses more than just a disorder of fluency. Cluttering has varied symptomatology and co-occurs with other speech, language, and behavioral disorders. According to Weiss (1964, 1968), cluttering symptoms may include: part- and whole-word repetitions, lack of awareness of the disorder, short attention span, perceptual weakness, poorly organized thinking, excessive speech rate (tachylalia), interjections, articulatory and motor disabilities, and grammatical difficulties. Other academic difficulties, noted by clinicians, teachers, and researchers, include reading and writing disorders, difficulty with many language-dependent skills (due to subtle language disorders), lack of rhythm and musical ability, and restlessness and hyperactivity (DeFusco & Menken, 1979; Irvine & Reis, 1980; Weiss, 1968).

Case Example. Ralph was referred to us as a stutterer by his industrial education supervisor during his semester of student teaching. When we examined him, he revealed no fears or avoidances, exhibited only a few short part-word repetitions, and had no fixations; he said that he enjoyed talking, did a lot of it, and that he was asked frequently to repeat himself, "especially when I talk fast." Ralph's difficulty seemed to take place on the phrase or sentence level; his interruptions broke the integrity of a *thought* rather than a *word*. In addition, he frequently omitted syllables and transposed words and phrases; he said "plobably," "posed," and "pacific" for "probably," "supposed," and "specific." Ralph's speech was sprinkled with spoonerisms (he said "beta dase" for "data base") and malapropisms (he described getting lost while hunting because the road he was following "dissipated" and told us he had a good "dialect" going with his roommate). His speech was swift and jumbled; it emerged in rapid torrents until he jammed up, and then he surged on again in another staccato outburst. In spontaneous talking, his message was characterized by disorganized sentences and poor phrasing. He gave the overall impression of being in great haste. When we asked him to slow down and speak carefully, there was a drastic improvement, but he soon forgot our admonishment and reverted to his hurried, disorganized style.

By and large, Ralph was unaware and indifferent to his fluency problem. He was an impatient, impulsive young man, always on the go. His coursework was characteristically done in a great, almost compulsive rush; he had difficulty reading, and his handwriting was a scrawl.

Distinguishing among Subtypes of Stuttering

Are there different kinds of (developmental) stuttering? Although there is no conclusive answer to that question, clinical opinion is that there must be—if only to explain the wide variety of clients, symptomatologies, and responses to intervention programs. Possibilities that come to mind include interiorized and exteriorized stutterers (Douglass & Quarrington, 1952); predominantly clonic (repetitive disfluencies) and predominantly tonic stutterers (with tension, prolongations, and blockages); clients who feature escape techniques; those who are addicted to avoidance; and those who can predict an occurrence of stuttering and those who cannot (Silverman & Williams, 1972). Perhaps there are even variations in stuttering that stem from cultural influences (Leith & Mims, 1975; Satcher, 1986; Shames, 1989). These distinctions may be useful in planning treatment. Researchers, too, are beginning to classify subgroups of stutterers, but as yet no one system has been accorded widespread acceptance.

Differentiating Normal Disfluencies from Stuttering

We saved this aspect of the differential diagnosis for last, although the clinician must determine it first. It is a vast topic. The literature shows good agreement regarding the general principles for distinguishing between normal and abnormal but often differs on the specifics. Where to draw the line segmenting normal types and amounts of disfluency from the abnormal is still a matter of clinical judgment; our data is not that precise. Van Riper (1982), however, comprised a useful list of distinguishing characteristics. Others have adapted this information for use on various clinical scales (Cooper, 1973; Pindzola, 1988).

Adams (1977) provides a clinical strategy for differentiating the normal child from one beginning to stutter. Also useful is the *Protocol for Differentiating the Incipient Stutterer* (Pindzola, 1988; Pindzola & White, 1986).

In making decisions about normal versus abnormal fluency (stuttering), the clinician should be guided by information available in the literature. The clinician then pulls together a vast array of information collected on and about the client to arrive at a diagnosis. We admit this is a judgment call on the part of the clinician, but if the evaluation is done thoroughly, it is an "informed" judgment call. Here are some guidelines.

The type of disfluency that predominates in a client's speech and the size of the speech unit affected by the breakdown influence society's judgment of normalcy. For example, repetitions of whole phrases are quite normal; whole-word repetitions are disfluencies typical of both stutterers and nonstutterers. Yet the predominance of part-word repetitions distinguishes stuttering from nonstuttering speakers of all ages, including preschoolers (Yairi & Lewis, 1984). Hesitations or pauses before phrases or before words may, likewise, be less innocuous than such gaps within words (i.e., preceding syllables or sounds). The rule of thumb suggested by Perkins (1971) is that the smaller the speech unit affected, the more abnormal the disfluency.

The frequency with which disfluent behaviors occur has long been recognized as important in the diagnosis of stuttering. Some authorities advocate the use of rate of stuttering (calculated as total stuttered words per minute of talking, SW/M) as a frequency measure of choice (Ryan, 1974; Shine, 1980); others use percentage of stuttered syllables or percentage of stuttered words. There are various norms in the literature; for example, frequencies in excess of 2 percent, 5 percent, or 10 percent may suggest a true stuttering disorder, depending on the strictness of the criterion selected by the clinician (Adams, 1977; Metraux, 1950; Van Riper, 1982; Yairi & Lewis, 1984). Being disfluent less than the cutoff percentage presumably indicates normalcy. Ryan (1974) suggests that disfluencies occurring an average of less than one word per two minutes of talking (0.5 SW/M) is within normal limits. Intervention is warranted, he says, if the rate of stuttering is 3 SW/M or more.

As part of the assessment, the clinician will gauge the duration of the client's disfluency. This is often expressed as an average number of reiterations of the repetition or as an average amount of time stuck in an audible or silent prolongation. If the typical duration of prolongations exceeds one second, or if repetitions involve numerous reiterations—say three to five or more, then these behaviors may be interpreted as signs of stuttering (Adams, 1977; Van Riper, 1982).

Audible signs of effort while speaking are generally not noted among normal speakers and therefore are indicative of abnormality (Pindzola, 1988; Pindzola & White, 1986). There are many signs of audible effort; some examples that are typically heard in stutterers include disrupted airflow, hard contacts (explosive, crisp articulation), effort or tension heard in the voice, and a pitch rise during a moment of stuttering.

Van Riper (1982) provides clinical reports that normal disfluencies and perhaps very early stutterings are characterized by repetitions that preserve the normal rhythm and rate of speech. Not until the tempo of the reiterations speeds up or their rhythm becomes irregular and choppy is there substantial reason for concern. The speech-language pathologist, then, should subjectively judge the client's rhythm, tempo, and speed of disfluencies when trying to make a differential diagnosis.

The presence of learned behaviors, or secondary behaviors, is strongly suggestive of stuttering, rather than normal fluency. The clinician therefore should determine whether the client uses concealment devices (such as word substitutions or circumlocutions), postponement devices, starting tricks, and so forth. Visually, the clinician may note physical involvement of the facial, head, and body regions. Frequently observed contortions are eye blinks, wrinkling of the forehead, distortions of the mouth, overt mandibular tension, head jerks, and the more subtle head turnings to divert eye contact.

Once the speech-language pathologist has made a differential diagnosis and determined that the client is stuttering, the next issue to be resolved is the developmental progression or severity of the disorder. In actuality, the information gathered to differentiate normal from abnormal speech is part of the same kind of information needed to determine the level of severity. On a continuum between normal and abnormal, the decision is now how far down the abnormal end of the continuum the client is placed. Just as data (e.g., percentage of stuttering, duration of the disfluencies) were used to segment normal from abnormal, so can they be used to categorize the problem as mild, moderate, and severe. Following that, the next decision that confronts the clinician is the recommended course of action. Is treatment warranted? If so, along what lines shall it be devised?

THE APPRAISAL OF STUTTERING

In our discussion of making a differential diagnosis, we glossed over the details of how to obtain the information necessary to make such a decision. What information is necessary? What published appraisal instruments are available to help collect and make sense of this information? (An annotated listing of some instruments can be found in Pindzola, 1986.) What less tangible factors need to be judged, albeit subjectively, by the clinician? We will now try to answer these questions. Bear in mind, however, that the "answers" may differ for different clients, depending on their age, intelligence, reading abilities, and so forth.

Case History Information and Parent Materials

We will discuss two forms of the case history intake: one done with the parents of a child who stutters or is beginning to stutter and one done with a teenager or adult who stutters.

Initial Interview with the Parents. The initial interview with the parents of a child beginning to stutter is of critical importance. We must establish our professional competence, demonstrate our genuine interest, and convince the parents that we can be trusted. In short, our primary task in this initial contact is to build a relationship for subsequent counseling sessions. We also listen carefully to the parents' presenting story: How do they see the child's problem? In their view, what might have caused it? What do they identify as their role in the onset of the child's stuttering? What expectations and apprehensions do they have regarding the nature and the outcome of treatment?

We like to regard the initial interaction between parents and clinician as a time for information-gathering and information-sharing. As we said, we first want to hear the presenting complaint—and encourage the telling of their child's speech story. We may opt to be more or less directive in our style with the parents, it does not matter, so long as the information we need unfolds. A parent's careful review of the many factors involved in the child's problem tends to foster objectivity. It also shifts the focus away from a general impression of "trouble" to the observation of specific behaviors. Here are some questions we use as guides in assembling information from parents:

1. When did the child begin exhibiting disfluencies?
2. What were the circumstances under which the disfluencies were noted?
3. How long has the child been exhibiting the disfluencies?
4. What changes have been noted in the frequency or form of the disfluencies?
5. What factors seem to increase or decrease the child's disfluency?
6. In what ways has the family tried to help the child?
7. What is the child's reaction to the family's efforts to help?

Additional items to assess in obtaining a case history include (1) a specific review of the familial incidence of stuttering; (2) the impact, if any, of siblings, relatives, teachers, or babysitters upon the child; (3) a description of how the child spends a typical day; and (4) a description of any prior professional treatment.

Case history collection forms, complete with specific questions and answer blanks for recording information, can be found in a number of books and intervention programs (Cooper, 1976; Goldberg, 1981; Luper & Mulder, 1966; Peins, McGough, & Lee, 1984; Peters & Guitar, 1991; Pindzola, 1988; Shine, 1980; Weiner, 1984; Wells, 1987; Wingate, 1976). The clinician may wish to adopt one or more of these styles.

The case history interview can be done either before or after the child has been seen and evaluated by the clinician. Consequently, this initial meeting may, in fact, involve several points of interaction or separate sessions. We try to refrain from being influenced by the parents' push for us to provide too much information prematurely; naturally, they want to know what caused their child's problem and what can be done (quickly) about it. We, however, do enlist the parents' help in collecting observations of the child's behavior in the home environment.

What things at home seem to promote fluency and what seems to promote disfluency? Is it all right for the parents to remind the child to "slow down" (as advocated by Shine, 1980 and Cooper, 1985) or is that counterproductive and something to be considered taboo (owing to the Wendell Johnson philosophy)? We do not know the answers to these questions for a *particular* child; the parents must find out. Parents' recordings of home behaviors have been advocated by many (Emerick, 1983; Pindzola, 1988; Shine, 1980; Zwitman, 1978).

We often find that simply asking parents to monitor the antecedents and consequences of their child's speech disfluencies is sufficiently motivating to engender change. Environmental events that disrupt a child's flow of speech typically become obvious when parents begin to chart.

Even though there is much information we simply cannot give the parents early on (often because we do not yet know the information), clinicians have a responsibility to help educate the parents. That is to say, we need to provide a good understanding of stuttering and its many ramifications. In addition to what we say, we like to provide the parents with reading materials; some are of our own preparation, while others are brochures and booklets from published sources. The interested reader might consider the materials by Johnson (1961), Robinson (1966), Cooper (1979), and Emerick (1983). The Speech Foundation of American (P.O. Box 11749, Memphis, TN 38111), the Stuttering Resource Foundation (123 Oxford Road, New Rochelle, NY 10804), the National Stuttering Project (4601 Irving Street, San Francisco, CA 94122), and the American Speech-Language-Hearing Association (10801 Rockville Pike, Rockville, MD 20852) have pamphlets or booklets available for parents. We find these more useful and up-to-date than the sources previously mentioned. Other tools that we use in helping parents are two excellent films: *Family Counseling* (Walle, 1975) and *Is It Me? Is It You?* (Walle, 1977). Both films are invaluable in helping parents understand how they can help children overcome the broken and hesitant speech often displayed between two and six years of age.

The clinician may wish to have one or both parents complete the *Parental Diagnostic Questionnaire* (Tanner, 1987). This paper and pencil questionnaire may prove useful in identifying parental perceptions and topics in need of exploration at subsequent counseling sessions. Checklists are also available to assess parental attitudes, which may be useful in determining the counseling needs of parents. Table 7.1 lists some of the available instruments for a clinician to consider in working with parents.

It is important that parents obtain some closure from these initial interviews. Let us demonstrate a typical conversation, showing how we relate our diagnostic findings to the parents of a client named Stephen.

> Stephen does indeed have some breaks in speech, more than normal for a child of his age. He is doing some stuttering, but it is still the "good kind": He is not struggling or avoiding and, most importantly, he doesn't seem to be very aware that talking is tough (we drew a rough sketch of the stuttering gauge depicted in Figure 7.1 and showed them that Stephen exhibited only the first three early danger signs of stuttering, based on the 1974 film by Walle). We want to prevent the disorder from developing further and cannot do anything without your help. We need to find out why he is having speech breaks; we need to know when he does it, under what circumstances. In short, we have to start looking at behaviors, at what he *does,* not a condition he *has.* In many cases like this, if we identify and alter certain environmental situations, the child stops stuttering. You were very wise to bring him in now, before the fear and frustration have a chance to develop. Let's plan on meeting again tomorrow, and together we can begin to review Stephen's background and then decide how to gather information on what is happening now.

Table 7.1 Some Assessment Instruments for Use with Parents of Young Stutterers

Parent Attitudes Toward Stuttering Checklist
(Cooper, 1976, 1985)

The Child Fluency Assessment Instrument
(Goldberg, 1981, contains parental questionnaire)

Parental Diagnostic Questionnaire
(Tanner, 1987)

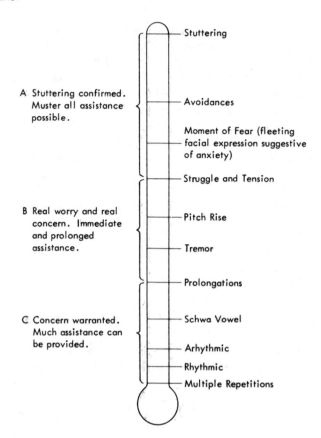

- Stuttering

A Stuttering confirmed. Muster all assistance possible.
- Avoidances
- Moment of Fear (fleeting facial expression suggestive of anxiety)
- Struggle and Tension

B Real worry and real concern. Immediate and prolonged assistance.
- Pitch Rise
- Tremor

C Concern warranted. Much assistance can be provided.
- Prolongations
- Schwa Vowel
- Arhythmic
- Rhythmic
- Multiple Repetitions

Figure 7.1 The Danger Signs of Developing Stuttering

Case History Interview with Older Clients. The case history and initial interview with an older client who stutters are obviously different from those we just described. Prior to undertaking formal observation and testing, we like to perform an intake interview. This brief preliminary discussion is designed to accomplish four objectives: (1) to inform the client what to expect in the diagnostic session; (2) to determine why the client is coming for treatment at this particular time; (3) to assemble historical information; and (4) to establish a working relationship.

Because we want the client to be a partner in the exploration of the problem, we feel it is important for the client to know *what* we intend to do and *why* we propose to do it. By structuring the clinical transaction so the stutterers know what role they are to play in their own recovery, we are establishing a therapeutic contract. The reader may also wish to consult Silverman (1980) who discusses the role of the client in defining treatment goals through the use of the *Stuttering Problem Profile.*

Case history questionnaires are readily available in many books and intervention programs. Examples include those by Wingate (1976), Goldberg (1981), Wells (1987), and Peters and Guitar (1991). Naturally, we ask about the duration of the problem, what professional help has been sought, recent changes in the speech, and a description of the current speaking difficulties.

We also like to determine why the client is coming (or being sent) to a speech-language pathologist at this particular point in time. Has the individual undergone a "bottoming-out" experience, a severe crisis in his/her social, occupational, or educational life? What does he/she expect from treatment? What do others expect? Answers to these questions are useful in determining the client's motivation and in making a prognosis. All in all, the initial contact with a client is of inestimable importance in establishing a working relationship.

Differentiating and Predictive Scales

As we discussed earlier in this chapter, one of the clinician's major responsibilities is differentiating normal speakers having usual disfluencies from persons who are stuttering. This may be obvious in the evaluation of some clients, but it may be quite difficult with others—particularly young children.

Complicating the issue further with young children is the notion of spontaneous recovery. Estimates are that as many as 80 percent of the children who begin to stutter spontaneously recover or "outgrow" the problem (Andrews & Harris, 1964). We should also report that Young (1975) and Martin and Lindamood (1986) concluded, after a critical review of the literature, that the 80 percent recovery figure is too high; spontaneous recovery rates may be as low as 30 percent. Still, the clinician needs to know which disfluent children will likely outgrow the problem and which seem destined for chronic difficulties and therefore need clinical intervention. Although we are far from being able to precisely differentiate these two types of children, we do have assessment instruments that help us in our predictions. We cite *A Stuttering Chronicity Prediction Checklist* (Cooper, 1973, 1976, 1985) and the *Stuttering Prediction Instrument for Young Children* (Riley, 1981) as examples. In the hands of an experienced clinician, all assessment indices provide information useful in "guessing" who will and who will not outgrow stuttering without help. Table 7.2 lists many of the available assessments instruments, useful for a variety of purposes.

Severity Scales

The clinician's primary mission in the evaluation of a stutterer is to perform a careful analysis of the individual's speech disfluency behavior. Not only is this necessary for differential diagnosis, but also for the appraisal of the severity of the disorder. With regard to treatment, the disfluency assessment also accomplishes two basic purposes: It delineates the behaviors to be altered, and it provides a base measure to which the clinician can refer when monitoring the impact of treatment. The majority of published assessment instruments help the clinician determine the extent of the speech problem. We will call these *severity scales*, whether or not the "score" from the test yields a severity modifier, such as mild to very severe.

Table 7.2 listed some of the available instruments that assess the overt features of stuttering. Many aspects of the stuttering problem can be tapped by

Table 7.2   Some Available Instruments for the Assessment of Overt Features of
Stuttering, including Diagnostic, Severity, and Predictive Scales

Southern Illinois Behavior Checklist
    (Brutten & Shoemaker, 1974)

Syracuse University Fluency Diagnostic Summary Sheet
    (Conture, 1990)

A Stuttering Chronicity Prediction Checklist
    (Cooper, 1973, 1976, 1985)

Concomitant Stuttering Behavior Checklist
    (Cooper, 1976, 1985)

Stuttering Frequency and Duration Estimate Record
    (Cooper, 1976, 1985)

Client and Clinician Perceptions of Stuttering Severity Ratings
    (Cooper, 1976, 1985)

The Preschool Fluency Baseline Record
    (Culp, 1984)

Severity Scale (S-Scale)
    (Erickson, 1969)

The Child, Adolescent, Adult Fluency Assessment Instrument
    (Goldberg, 1981, three multifaceted assessment systems)

Scale for Rating the Severity of Stuttering
    (Johnson, Darley, & Spriestersbach, 1963)

The Stuttering Severity Scale (SS Scale)
    (Lanyon, 1967)

Stuttering Diagnostic and Evaluative Checklist
    (Luper & Mulder, 1966)

Checklist of Physical Behaviors Accompanying Stuttering
    (Peins, McGough, & Lee, 1984)

A Protocol for Differentiating the Incipient Stutterer
    (Pindzola & White, 1986; Pindzola, 1988)

Stuttering Severity Instrument for Children and Adults
    (Riley, 1972, 1980)

Stuttering Prediction Instrument for Young Children
    (Riley, 1981)

Stuttering Interview (Forms A and B)
    (Ryan, 1974)

Assessment Form: Systematic Fluency Training for Young Children
    (Shine, 1980)

The Stocker Probe Technique for Diagnosis and Treatment of Stuttering in Young Children
    (Stocker, 1980)

Profile of Stuttering Severity: A Revised Scale
    (Van Riper, 1982)

Stutterers' Physiological Assessment
    (Wells, 1987)

Severity Rating Guide
    (Wingate, 1976)

using a variety of these instruments, including the frequency of disfluency, the duration of the disfluency, the physical behaviors that accompany speech attempts, and so forth. Judging from the length of this (nonexhaustive) list, there are many severity scales from which to choose. We will highlight one.

In wide use is the *Stuttering Severity Instrument* (Riley, 1972, 1980). This SSI, as it is often known, is useful with both children and adults and has provisions for testing those who can and cannot read. The number of words stuttered and the number of total words spoken are computed by the speech-language pathologist as the client reads and/or is engaged in conversation. Frequency, expressed as a percentage of stuttering, is then computed (number of stuttered words divided by total words spoken times 100 = percentage) and converted to a corresponding task score. The clinician also monitors the amount of time the client blocks and averages the three longest. This measure is converted into a task score. Lastly, the clinician watches and carefully listens to the client during reading and/or conversation samples and rates the presence and conspicuousness of physical behaviors concomitant to the speech attempts. A separate rating (on a 0 to 5 scale) is made for each anatomical area (facial, head, and extremity) and for distracting sounds; their sum constitutes this task score. Frequency, duration, and physical concomitant task scores are then combined for a total score. The severity of the client's stuttering can be ascertained by comparing the total score to the normative data provided in the test manual. Stuttering severity may be described as very mild, mild, moderate, severe, or very severe in this manner.

At this point, we would like to mention that the Individualized Education Program (IEP) format adopted by most school districts requires a statement regarding the educational and psychological severity of a student's handicapping condition. The speech-language pathologist who works in the public schools, then, must categorize the severity of the student's stuttering along the continuum of very mild to very severe. The ease of administration and the usefulness of the results may account for the popularity of the SSI among clinicians, especially those employed by the schools (e.g., Howard County, MD, 1985). (Treatment approaches with built-in IEP formats include those by Cooper, 1985 and Pindzola, 1988.)

The appraisal of the overt symptoms of stuttering need not require administration of a published test. The clinician's analysis, whether using a formal published test or an informal look at a speech sample, should include a thorough description of the stuttering pattern (topography) and measures of the relative frequency with which various features of the pattern occur. Descriptions of the process can be found in the writings of Conture (1990), Starkweather, Gottwald, and Halfond (1990), and Peters and Guitar (1991).

The Assessment Process

We will now walk the reader through our assessment process. The first step in the disfluency analysis is to obtain a representative sample of the client's speech. The operative word here is *representative;* stuttering is an intermittent disorder, and the amount of difficulty an individual has is contingent on the speaking task, the situation, and other variables. If it is possible, there are obvious advantages to collecting samples of the client's "real" communication in naturalistic settings—the playground, informal group situations, the family dinner table. Generally, however, clinicians rely on data obtained from speaking tasks, such as reading aloud a standard passage, giving a monologue, or conversing. Be sure to tape-record, or, even better, videotape, the session and note the time elapsed for each segment of the total sample: It will then be easier to specify rather precise frequency and severity values. We always ask the stutterer to discuss both neutral topics (hobbies, sports, vacations) and threatening topics (family, school, dating) to ensure that we obtain a range of speaking difficulty. It is important to know what produces stress and how the individual responds to it; we experiment in the session with things like hurrying the client, feigning listener loss, and asking the client to repeat.

An Overall Description. We begin the analysis with a global description of the individual's speech behavior. What is his/her normal speech like in terms of rate, rhythm, degree of tension, articulation, and voice? What are the salient features of the stuttering pattern?

Core Behaviors. The lowest common denominators of the problem of stuttering seem to be repetitions (oscillative phenomena) and prolongations (fixative phenomena). Although most individuals have either predominately repetitive or predominately tense disfluency patterns, all stutterers exhibit a variety of forms of the speech interruption. A key feature of the disfluency analysis, therefore, is a precise description of these core behaviors.

With respect to *repetitions,* we want to identify the size of the unit (phrase, whole word, syllable), the number of oscillations per unit (e.g., b-boy versus b-b-b-b-boy), their tempo and degree of tension involved, and how they are terminated. Are there silent oscillations of articulatory postures? Does the client have difficulty finding the proper vowel during the course of the repetitions?

In terms of *prolongations,* we are interested in the anatomical site of the fixations, whether they are silent or audible, how long they last, the degree of tension involved, and how they are terminated.

Struggle-Tension Features. Very rarely does a client exhibit *only* repetitions and prolongations. Anyone who has observed stutterers knows that they appear tense and often make irrelevant sounds and movements while attempting to speak. Stutterers display a wide variety of these mannerisms, and they may vary in frequency of occurrence and degree of involvement in particular clients; some individuals manifest an astounding array of eye blinking, head jerking, postponement rituals, and other behaviors, whereas others appear relatively quiescent, at least overtly. The clinician should take note of these "accessory features." Several scales listed in Table 7.2 can be used as well. For example, the *Southern Illinois Behavior Checklist* (Brutten & Shoemaker, 1974) lists 97 different behaviors and is designed so that both the client and the clinician can record the presence of various mannerisms.

Covert Measures.   In developed stuttering, the overt symptoms may be only the tip of the problem. After years of difficulty speaking, especially since the amount of difficulty varies with the speaking situation, it is only natural that the person would develop hidden feelings and attitudes about speech. The negative feelings may be generalized but are often directed toward particular speaking situations, conversational partners, and even particular word and phoneme combinations. Following on the heels of apprehension, dislike, and fear of these events comes the avoidance of them. Therefore, measuring the covert side of a client's stuttering problem is often part of the diagnostic process. Early on, perhaps in the initial session, we attempt to discuss with the client his/her feelings, attitudes, fears, and experiences. This helps us "get to know" the client and better understand the depth of the problem. Counseling may need to be part of the treatment program for some clients. In addition to discussions of feelings, the clinician can utilize published instruments. Sentence completion tasks and adjective checklists help to identify attitudes and personality traits. Several are listed in Table 7.3.

Table 7.3   Some Available Instruments for the Assessment of Covert Features of Stuttering, including Perception/Attitude Scales and Situation/Avoidance Checklists

Iowa Scale of Attitude Toward Stuttering
   (Ammons & Johnson, 1944)

Modified Erickson Scale of Communication Attitudes
   (Andrews & Cutler, 1974)

Communication Attitude Test
   (Brutten & Dunham, 1989)

Fear Survey Schedule
   (Brutten & Shoemaker, 1974)

Speech Situation Checklist
   (Brutten & Shoemaker, 1974)

Stuttering Attitudes Checklist
   (Cooper, 1976, 1985)

Situation Avoidance Behavior Checklist
   (Cooper, 1976, 1985)

Adjective Checklist
   (Erickson, 1969)

Role Construct Repertory Test
   (Fransella, 1972)

A-19 Scale for Children Who Stutter
   (Guitar & Grims, 1977)

Stutterer's Self-Ratings of Reactions to Speech Situations (ARSF Scale)
   (Shumak, 1955)

Perceptions of Stuttering Inventory (PSI)
   (Woolf, 1967)

Hierarchy Ranking
   (Wells, 1987, several versions)

We would be remiss if we did not acknowledge that some behavioral clinicians opt not to measure, or clinically deal with, covert feelings and attitudes. The focus of intervention may, indeed, be to train fluency and let the covert aspects drop out of the client's repertoire on their own, in due time. Likewise, the clinician may use an attitude scale as a baseline measure, proceed with a behavioral approach that focuses only on the overt side of stuttering, and then probe for attitudinal change as a consequence of successful fluency.

We *are* interested in avoidance behaviors that the client exhibits. We feel that, clinically, avoidance behavior is an important feature to deal with because it tends to reinforce and compound the stutterer's difficulty. Rather than diminishing, fears tend to incubate and grow when a person recoils from them; avoidances keep the apprehension high and the problem expanding.

Avoidance is characterized by reduction or cessation of communication: The stutterer retreats from the act of talking. The clinician can discern the types of speaking situations and listeners that increase or decrease the client's stuttering. This can be accomplished by interview or by having the client fill out a checklist. The clinician can devise a form for recording data (simply list different speaking situations, topics of conversation, and so forth) or use a published inventory. Table 7.3 listed assessment instruments useful with the covert side of stuttering. We will highlight a few.

The *Speech Situation Checklist* (Brutten & Shoemaker, 1974) has the client rate his/her degree of emotional response and severity of speech disruption in 51 life situations. Although no formal instrument is supplied, Shames and Egolf (1976) list various circumstances (audience size, specific people, different talking situations) and suggest tactics for sampling actual speech behavior under those conditions. In addition to listing the conditions under which stuttering is increased or reduced, the clinician may ask the client to rank-order the items in terms of speech difficulty and emotional impact, as done by Wells (1987).

In addition to situation fears, many stutterers report that they have particular difficulty with certain words and speech sounds. We make a list of these items and then examine the speech sample to determine if in fact there is more stuttering on some sounds or words. During attempts at trial treatment, we like to show the client ways of ameliorating the stuttering and often use his/her most feared words as stimuli.

Any assessment of stuttering should also include the client's own perceptions of the magnitude of the problem. The clinician can obtain the stutterer's self-rating of severity in many of the instruments listed in Tables 7.2 and 7.3. In particular, we like to administer the *Perceptions of Stuttering Inventory* (Woolf, 1967). The PSI, as it can be called, is an instrument devised to assess three dimensions of stuttering behavior: struggle, avoidance, and expectancy, as perceived by the person who stutters. It yields a profile that the clinician can then compare to scores obtained by a reference group of stutterers.

Having now discussed the predictive instruments, severity scales, and covert measures typically used in the evaluation of stuttering, let us turn our attention to some general evaluation principles and special considerations for clients of various ages.

EVALUATION AT THE ONSET OF STUTTERING

Experienced clinicians agree that the problem of stuttering is much easier to prevent or manage in children than to treat in chronic adult clients. Indeed, the early detection and management of children beginning to stutter is one of the most significant contributions a speech clinician can make. The speech-language pathologist must seek answers for a great many questions: Is the child stuttering? If so, how far has the disturbance progressed? When did it begin? What factors were associated with the onset of the problem? How aware is the child of the speech disturbance? How do listeners attempt to help, and how does this affect the child's efforts? How can we alter the child's environment to prevent the problem from getting worse?

Throughout this book, we have repeatedly suggested that diagnosis and treatment are not separate undertakings. The careful assessment of a client's problem is often therapeutic; only by working with an individual (and his/her parents) for a period of time do we truly come to know the dimensions of the problem. This is particularly true in the management of children beginning to stutter.

In many cases, a physician is the first professional to be consulted by parents. The clinician is wise to enlist the support of local pediatricians in the early identification of children beginning to stutter.

We agree with Wyatt (1969) that the onset of stuttering is a crisis situation in which swift intervention is absolutely essential. In planning for the evaluation, we delineate several objectives that will guide our efforts:

1. Determine if the child is stuttering (problem–no problem determination).
2. If so, identify to what stage or level of development the disorder has progressed (severity determination).
3. Obtain the parent's perception of the onset and current status of the problem.
4. Sample the child's general level of functioning in regard to auditory, motor, social, articulatory, and cognitive-linguistic abilities.
5. Commence the development of a counseling relationship with the parents.

We have already discussed much of this. Various assessment instruments are available to help the clinician make a differential diagnosis, determine the severity of the speech difficulties, appraise the home situation and parental attitudes, and begin a healthy dialogue with the parents of the child beginning to stutter. What remains to be discussed are the ancillary areas that need to be assessed in the young child.

Several authorities recommend assessing the child's rate of speech, as well as the parents' rates (Peters & Guitar, 1991; Starkweather, Gottwald, & Halfond, 1990). Normative data for children can be found in Pindzola, Jenkins, and Lokken (1989). Speech rate is a basic element of fluency and therefore warrants assessment. The rate at which parents talk may be demanding of fluency in the child.

Speed and coordination of repetitive oral movements may be tested using Fletcher's (1972) norms for diadochokinesis. Also, Riley and Riley (1986) have published the *Oral Motor Assessment Scale.*

Phonological disorders seem to co-occur frequently with stuttering, as do language delays or disorders (Conture, 1990). Various articulation and language tests should be used as part of a thorough fluency evaluation. Information contained in Chapters 4, 5, and 6 certainly pertains. The presence of speech and language disorders concomitant with stuttering will impact on the planning of an appropriate treatment program.

Along with these areas of assessment, we routinely screen the oral mechanism, voice, and hearing. We advocate referral for additional testing of cognitive, motoric, and psychological status, as needed, with particular clients.

A Direction for Treatment

Even though it is beyond the scope of this chapter to discuss the myriad of treatment programs available, we do wish to point out to the reader that different philosophies exist regarding the treatment of young stutterers, such as those between the ages of two and nine years. Also, although many preschoolers will continue to receive intervention services in clinics and through private practitioners, with the implementation of PL 94-457, more and more will be treated by the public school speech-language pathologist. School systems are currently servicing children ages three to five and will soon be responsible for the birth through age two population. Four treatment options may be considered.

In the first option, environmental treatment, the speech-language pathologist determines that the most prudent course of action is to work through the significant others in the child's life—parents and teachers—to modify the daily environment. The goal is to structure the child's environment to make it more conducive to fluency. The child is not seen for treatment; typically, parents and teachers meet regularly with the clinician to discuss environmental modifications and results. Opting for only environmental treatment is commonly done for the child "at risk" for developing stuttering, or for the beginning stutterer who displays early developed symptoms. Modifying parental and teacher reactions to disfluencies; altering the pace and organization of home and school; and generally educating significant others about fluency, disfluency, and the modeling of good speech habits are beneficial. Reduction in communicative pressures that the child is vulnerable to are a necessary and important aspect of treatment.

A second treatment option is to combine the environmental treatment with direct, but modified, therapy for the child. Sessions may be individual but are often in groups. The treatment is considered modified as it does not focus on specific symptoms of stuttering. Rather, treatment may emphasize the concept of rhythm by having children sing, speak to a rhythm, practice rhymes, use choral speaking, and just generally experience much success in easy, fluent speech. Modified treatment often involves language treatment. The language skills of a young stutterer may be somewhat delayed. The length and complexity of utterances affect the likelihood of even normal speakers having a disfluency.

By shoring up weak language skills, and by systematically controlling the linguistic output of young clients (e.g., sentence length and syntactic complexity), speech-language pathologists are able to reduce or eliminate stuttering. Additionally, some speech-language pathologists may include in the modified program mention of "smooth" and "bumpy" speech and train the children to identify samples of each. Altering the "bumpy" speech, however, is not done in this form of treatment.

A third option of treatment for the young stutterer is to combine the environmental approach with direct intervention. The child attends individual or group treatment sessions (depending upon the severity of the problem) with the purpose of modifying specific stuttering symptoms. A variety of therapeutic emphases are possible. The student may be taught a new, fluent way of talking by learning patterns such as "slow speech," "breathy speech," "stretchy speech," the "easy speaking voice," "slow, easy speech," and other similar strategies for fluency. Discussions of feelings and attitudes are often a component of the treatment program for children ready to address personal issues surrounding their speech difficulties.

The fourth option of direct stuttering modification alone expands the details involved in mastering strategies, techniques, or targets for fluency. The absence of co-occurring environmental treatment may be a function of (1) the setting in which services are provided (parents may not be available to participate fully in the intervention program); or (2) the child's stuttering symptoms may have progressed beyond the level where environmental manipulations would be expected to have much effect. In such cases, efforts need to be focused on direct treatments using greater specificity.

Prognosis with Young Children

We are very impressed with the efficacy of treatment for young children beginning to stutter. When the clinician can intervene before the child develops fear and avoidance reactions, and if the parents are amenable to counseling, the prognosis for recovery is excellent. There are several factors that the clinician must consider when estimating a client's prospects for recovery:

1. How long has the child been stuttering? The older the child is and the longer his/her exposure to adverse environmental reactions, the poorer the prognosis.
2. What type and intensity of environmental reactions has the child been exposed to? In our experience, children who have been slapped or have suffered other forms of physical abuse had the worst problems.
3. Is the child aware of speaking difficulties? The more heedful the child is of speech interruptions, the less positive the prognosis. (This may be argued as evidence of the progression of the disorder, hence the less favorable prognosis.)
4. What type of speech disfluency characteristics are present? The more danger signs present—in particular, cessation of phonation, stoppage of airflow, dysrhythmia, tension, and fear—the poorer the prognosis.
5. How amenable are the parents to counseling? An all-out concerted effort at the home front is ideal, perhaps essential, for amelioration.

6. What is the child's level of intelligence? We have had more limited success with "slow" children.

7. Are there organic or neurotic factors that figure in the onset of stuttering? Chances for recovery are more limited if either is present.

Our clinical success or failure with children beginning to stutter is also related to the characteristic pattern of factors present at the onset of stuttering. Apparently, there are several ways of becoming a stutterer (Van Riper, 1982; Yairi, 1983). We find the model developed by Myers and Wall (1982) useful for synthesizing diagnostic information and making a prognosis about a young disfluent child. The many variables that may be involved in the onset of stuttering are organized into three major categories: physiological, psycholinguistic, and psychosocial (Figure 7.2). Note how the three categories overlap. For example, a child delayed in language development and deficient in motor skills could be particularly susceptible to high parental standards or communication competition with siblings. These same thoughts are amplified by Wells (1987) and by Starkweather, Gottwald, and Halfond (1990).

One question continues to nag clinicians who work with young children. Would they have gotten better without our help, due simply to the passage of time and some internal recovery potential in the child? Although we cannot answer that question with any authority, we do see that in most instances, the child's recovery from stuttering occurred too swiftly after the initiation of treatment (two weeks to several months) to be attributed to spontaneous recovery.

Figure 7.2 Factors Influencing Early Childhood Stuttering

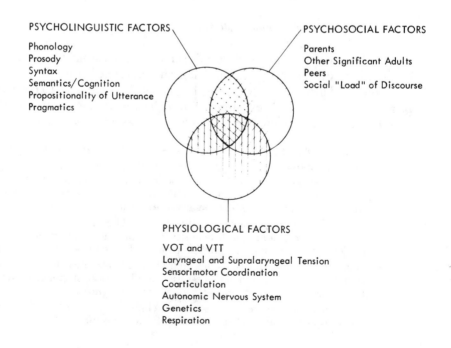

PSYCHOLINGUISTIC FACTORS

Phonology
Prosody
Syntax
Semantics/Cognition
Propositionality of Utterance
Pragmatics

PSYCHOSOCIAL FACTORS

Parents
Other Significant Adults
Peers
Social "Load" of Discourse

PHYSIOLOGICAL FACTORS

VOT and VTT
Laryngeal and Supralaryngeal Tension
Sensorimotor Coordination
Coarticulation
Autonomic Nervous System
Genetics
Respiration

The interested reader may consult the work of Wyatt (1969) for a list of variables contributing to and inhibiting progress.

EVALUATION OF THE SCHOOL-AGED STUDENT

Elementary Students

Appraising and treating elementary school stutterers is particularly challenging. This group of children, approximately seven- to 12-years-old, is no longer beginning to stutter; they are not simply repeating and hesitating. They struggle noticeably when speaking and attempt to avoid or disguise their difficulty; they are frustrated and it is now necessary to deal directly with the stuttering.

The clinician is faced with several thorny problems when planning an examination of a young stutterer: (1) Young children frequently lack the insight and cooperation necessary to analyze their problem objectively and rationally. (2) Children are reluctant or unable to verbalize their internal feelings freely. (3) The speech clinician is associated in the child's mind with the teaching personnel, who may in some cases be penalizing or disturbing listeners. In addition, the clinician may be identified with authority figures; this tends to undermine a trusting relationship. (4) Last, and perhaps most significantly, the child usually has no choice about entering treatment; most likely the student is brought for evaluation by the parents, referred by a teacher, or identified in a screening by a speech clinician.

The clinician may find that these students respond to an honest, straightforward clinical approach. With early elementary school children, we use descriptive language, such as "tensing" or "getting stuck," to inquire about their speaking difficulty, not out of any fear of the word stuttering, but simply because the term either doesn't mean much to the child or, in some cases, is too negatively charged. With older elementary school children, we use a frank, direct style. Establish trust and confidence by showing the client that the clinician is competent and *knows* about the problem of stuttering.

The evaluation of a student does not differ greatly in substance from an assessment of an older individual except that with young children, environmental, parental, and school factors are more important. In order to reveal the range of information generally sought, Figure 7.3 outlines an assessment plan prepared by a diagnostic team composed of a faculty member and graduate students. The plan was compiled for the evaluation of a 10-year-old child referred to a university speech clinic by a public school clinician.

Junior and Senior High School Students

The assessment and treatment of stuttering in older students is even more challenging than with the youngsters. Denial of the problem, lack of cooperation, and lack of motivation seem typical in the teenagers we have seen.

Figure 7.3 *Assessment Plan for Alan Schlicher*

I. *Identifying Information*

Obtain all the usual information regarding address, grade level, and so on. This can be obtained from Mrs. Hronkin, the referral source, or in the parent interview. Be sure to inquire about living arrangements: Ms. Hronkin mentioned that a parental grandfather may reside with the family and apparently he is a dominant force in the family (reportedly, he is against Alan's receiving speech therapy and insists he overcame stuttering by eating mashed potatoes!).

II. *Description of Stuttering*

A. Global description: What are the salient descriptive features of Alan's stuttering behavior? Is it basically fixative or oscillative? Are there long silent periods of internal struggle, or does he exhibit a more overt pattern?

B. Core behaviors: Make an analysis of the repetitions and prolongations observed—the number of oscillations per unit, tempo, duration, and so forth.

C. Tension-struggle features: Note the occurrence and location of any ancillary behaviors.

D. Frequency: This analysis will serve as our baseline for reevaluation of Alan, so we need to be especially precise. Collect data (count repetitions, prolongations, other salient features of his moments of stuttering) on at least three types of speech samples—reading, paraphrasing, and spontaneous speech. We can compute the relative frequency of stutterings per minute, or per total words uttered, by analyzing the videotape later.

E. Severity: We will use the *Stuttering Severity Instrument* (Riley, 1980); this instrument employs the three dimensions of frequency, duration, and physical concomitants and yields a score that can be converted to a percentile. A severity measure like this (particularly when it allows the examiner to score a client on a common scale of 0 to 100) is useful when communicating the results of the evaluation to the parents, teacher, even the child himself.

F. Variations in frequency/severity: Explore with the child and his parents whether his stuttering comes and goes in cycles, which situations or listeners provoke variations in his problem, and whether there are any words or sounds that are particularly difficult. Determine what impact delayed auditory feedback and masking noise have on his speech.

G. How does the child try to control his stuttering? What techniques has he devised for coping with speech interruptions? How effective are they? Additionally, we need to identify which speech-altering strategies—slowing, easy onset, and so forth—induce fluency. Use Cooper's (1982) *Disfluency Descriptor Digest* as a checklist to record observations.

H. Can the child predict when he is about to stutter? Ask him if he can; but also have him underline words he thinks he might stutter on as he reads silently a simple passage. Have him read it aloud and determine the degree to which he can accurately predict his stuttering.

I. What is the client's poststuttering behavior? Does he continue talking, give up, become angry, or cry? Does he appear indifferent?

III. *Attitude Dimension*

This is the most difficult and least reliable aspect of the evaluation. Some information can be obtained through observation of Alan and his parents and by what they say about the problem. We can also administer several self-inventory scales such as the A-19 Scale developed by Guitar, 1977. What is the child's attitude toward treatment? How much does he know about stuttering? Has he been teased at school or home because of his problem?

IV. *Case History*

We will want to obtain background information with respect to four basic areas: history of general development (motor, language, social), onset and development of stuttering, medical history, and family history. These areas can be explored in the parent interview.

V. *Present Functioning*

A. Personality: Describe the child's personality in general terms (shy, aggressive, and so on) and identify any special features (fears, tics, nail biting, and the like) that may apply to him. Ascertain his special interests or hobbies.

B. School: Obtain information relevant to his academic and social adjustment in school.
C. Related testing: Is a psychological or medical referral indicated? Perform screening evaluations on the child's motor behavior, hearing, and language ability. The latter is particularly important, as there is some evidence that children who stutter may have a language disability. Plan to use the testing format suggested by Riley and Riley (1982). They advocate evaluating the following skills:
  1. *Attending behavior.* Is the child distractible? Does he perseverate?
  2. *Auditory processing.* Does he delay in responding to tasks? Does he request repetitions of instructions?
  3. *Sentence formulation.* Is there any evidence of a breakdown in word order?
  4. *Oral motor.* What is the child's diadochokinetic rates for /p/, /k/, and /t/? Is there any evidence of articulatory imprecision?
D. Diagnostic session: How did the child behave during the diagnostic session? What could be discerned about his level of motivation? How did he respond when put under communicative stress? How did he respond to trial therapy?

Figure 7.3 *(Continued)*

The assessment outline does not differ much from the example shown for Alan Schlicher. The process, however, is very adultlike; environmental and parental factors are downplayed.

Direction for Treatment

The treatment of stuttering among some older children, adolescents, and adults is of the direct type. Obviously, programs differ in complexities and emphases for these disparate age groups. As negative feelings and attitudes develop late in the evolution of stuttering, treatment for the older student often involves explorations into these psychological topics. The emotional crisis of stuttering escalates during the teenage years when social interactions become so critical. (Students may benefit from reading *Do You Stutter: A Guide for Teens,* published by the Speech Foundation of America.) Physiological modifications of speech are often components in adolescent and adult fluency programs. Physiological targets may include breath, voice onset, and rate, as well as a host of others. Computerized instrumentation may help in the training of these speech targets. Much practice is necessary to habituate new speaking patterns, and support from family, friends, and school personnel can be critical to success.

Prognosis

What factors are crucial for improvement with students? What variables should the clinician consider when making a prognosis? We believe that the most significant improvement in treatment is noted in cases with the following operative factors:

1. No prior record of unsuccessful treatment; an absence of treatment seems more conducive to success than a history of therapeutic failure.
2. Cooperative parents, willing to participate meaningfully in a program of counseling.

3. More severe stuttering pattern; mild stutterers typically show little improvement.

4. A predominantly clonic stuttering pattern featuring struggle and escape (students adept at avoidance generally have more difficulty).

5. Cooperative teachers and other school personnel.

6. No other significant problems (reading difficulty, a scholastic problem independent of stuttering, and so on).

7. Other available resources (expertise in scouting, athletics, music).

8. A schedule of intensive therapy (at least three, preferably four, contacts a week).

ASSESSMENT OF THE ADULT STUTTERER

The disorder is fully developed in the adult client: Speech interruptions are more complex and characteristically compulsive; fears and apprehensions become chronic; avoidance, disguise, and negative attitudes hamper and distort the individual's relationships with others. At this stage, a speech breakdown is not simply a response, it is also a stimulus—the problem has become cyclic and self-reinforcing. Clinicians agree that the treatment of stuttering at this advanced stage is complicated—but far from impossible. There is a bewildering array of treatment approaches (and indices of their successes); we, however, will not attempt to summarize them here.

Prognosis

Making a prognosis about success and failure in stuttering is an inexact science. Recent research efforts have tried to delineate some factors that may be involved in determining successful outcomes. The reader is referred to the works of Guitar (1976), Boberg, Howie, and Woods (1979), and Perkins (1983). We present an incomplete and heuristic list of factors that help in making prognoses. The items are presented in random order, for at present we have no data that would allow us to assign weight to them.

1. *Severity:* Paradoxically, the more severe stutterers, other factors being equal, seem to make better progress than do milder stutterers.

2. *Motivation and Attitude:* Motivation to change is, of course, a most significant variable in all intervention programs. The better the client's pretreatment attitude, the more successful the outcome of treatment is likely to be.

3. *Timing:* A client's motivation for treatment is often related to crucial life experiences. Stutterers who have reached a critical stage and feel blocked by their disordered speech; barred from job advancement, education, or marriage; and voluntarily seek treatment have a more favorable prognosis.

4. *Age:* Adolescents, particularly between the ages of 13 and 16, are especially resistant to treatment. Similarly, clients over 40 tend to do poorly in treatment.

5. *Sex:* Women seem to be more difficult to treat than men.

6. *Nonstuttered Speech:* The more well integrated the client's nonstuttered speech is, in terms of prosody, the better the prognosis.

7. *Type of Stuttering:* Predominantly repetitive stutterers make more rapid progress than do predominantly fixative stutterers; clients who feature escape reactions are easier to work with than chronic avoiders. Interiorized stutterers—especially those manifesting laryngeal blocking—are very resistant to treatment.

8. *Concomitant Problems:* Clients presenting with organic complications (e.g., sensory, intellectual, or motor impairments) or psychological symptoms require more prolonged treatment and do less well than clients without concomitant problems.

9. *Prior Treatment and Intensive Treatment:* Clients with a history of therapeutic failure have a poor prognosis. Token treatment may be worse than no treatment at all. When intensive treatment (minimum daily contact of at least one hour) is available and the client can participate in a comprehensive program, the prospects for recovery are more favorable.

BIBLIOGRAPHY

ADAMS, M. (1977). A clinical strategy for differentiating the normally nonfluent child and the incipient stutterer. *Journal of Fluency Disorders, 2,* 141–148.

AMMONS, R., & JOHNSON, W. (1944). Studies in the psychology of stuttering. *Journal of Speech Disorders, 9,* 39–49.

ANDREWS, G., & CUTLER, J. (1974). Stuttering therapy: The relation between changes in symptom level and attitudes. *Journal of Speech and Hearing Disorders, 39,* 312–319.

ANDREWS, G., & HARRIS, M. (1964). *The syndrome of stuttering.* Clinics in Developmental Medicine No. 17. London: William Heinemann.

BLOODSTEIN, O. (1981). *A handbook on stuttering.* Chicago: National Easter Seal Society.

BOBERG, E., HOWIE, P., & WOODS, L. (1979). Maintenance of fluency: A review. *Journal of Fluency Disorders, 4,* 93–116.

BROWN, C., & CULLINAN, W. (1981). Word-retrieval difficulty and disfluent speech in adult anomic speakers. *Journal of Speech and Hearing Research, 24,* 358–365.

BRUTTEN, E., & DUNHAM, S. (1989). The Communication Attitude Test: A normative study of grade school children. *Journal of Fluency Disorders, 14,* 371–377.

BRUTTEN, E., & SHOEMAKER, D. (1974). *The Southern Illinois Behavior Check List.* Carbondale, IL: Southern Illinois University.

CANTER, G. J. (1971). Observations on neurogenic stuttering: A contribution to differential diagnosis. *British Journal of Disorders of Communication, 6,* 139–143.

CONTURE, E. G. (1990). *Stuttering* (2nd ed.). Englewood Cliffs, NJ: Prentice Hall.

COOPER, E. B. (1973). The development of a Stuttering Chronicity Prediction Checklist: A preliminary report. *Journal of Speech and Hearing Disorders, 38,* 215–223.

COOPER, E. B. (1976). *Personalized fluency control therapy.* Allen, TX: DLM/Teaching Resources.

COOPER, E. B. (1979). *Understanding stuttering: Information for parents.* Chicago: National Easter Seal Society.

COOPER, E. B. (1982). A disfluency descriptor for clinical use. *Journal of Fluency Disorders, 7,* 355–358.

COOPER, E. B. (1985). *Personalized fluency control therapy—Revised.* Allen, TX: DLM/Teaching Resources.

CULP, D. M. (1984). The preschool fluency development program: Assessment and treatment. In M. Peins (Ed.), *Contemporary approaches in stuttering therapy.* Boston: Little, Brown.

DEAL, J. (1982). Sudden onset of stuttering: A case report. *Journal of Speech and Hearing Disorders, 47,* 301–304.

DEFUSCO, E., & MENKEN, M. (1979). Symptomatic cluttering in adults. *Brain and Language, 8,* 25–33.

DONNAN, G. A. (1979). Stuttering as a manifestation of stroke. *Medical Journal of Australia, 1,* 44–45.

DOUGLASS, E., & QUARRINGTON, B. (1952). The differentiation of interiorized and exteriorized secondary stuttering. *Journal of Speech and Hearing Disorders, 17,* 377–385.

EMERICK, L. (1983). *With slow and halting tongue.* Danville, IL: Interstate Printers and Publishers.

ERICKSON, R. (1969). Assessing communication attitudes among stutterers. *Journal of Speech and Hearing Research, 12,* 711–724.

FANTRY, L. (1990). AIDS-related acquired stuttering. *Quo Vadis, 2*(2), 6.

FLETCHER, S. (1972). Time-by-count measurement of diadochokinetic syllable rate. *Journal of Speech and Hearing Research, 15,* 763–770.

FRANSELLA, F. (1972). *Personal change and reconstruction.* London: Academic Press.

GAVIS, L. (1946). Bombing mission no. 15. *Journal of Abnormal and Social Psychology, 41,* 189–198.

GOLDBERG, S. A. (1981). *Behavioral cognitive stuttering therapy.* Tigard, OR: C.C. Publications.

GRINKER, R., & SPIEGAL, J. (1945). *War neuroses.* Philadelphia, PA: Blakiston.

GUITAR, B. (1976). Pretreatment factors associated with the outcome of stuttering therapy. *Journal of Speech and Hearing Research, 19,* 590–600.

GUITAR, B., & GRIMS, S. (1977). *Developing a scale to assess communication attitudes in children who stutter.* Paper presented at the convention of the American Speech-Language-Hearing Association, Atlanta, GA.

HELMS, N. A., BUTLER, R. B., & CANTER, G. J. (1980). Neurogenic acquired stuttering. *Journal of Fluency Disorders, 5,* 269–279.

HOWARD COUNTY (MD) PUBLIC SCHOOL SYSTEM (1985). *Communication rating scales, service delivery model, and dismissal criteria for speech-language services.* Paper presented at the convention of the American Speech-Language-Hearing Association, Washington, DC.

IRVINE, T., & REIS, R. (1980). Cluttering as a complex of learning disabilities. *Language, Speech and Hearing Services in Schools, 11,* 3–14.

JOHNSON, W. (1961). *Stuttering and what you can do about it.* Minneapolis, MN: University of Minnesota Press.

JOHNSON, W., DARLEY, F., & SPRIESTERSBACH, D. (1963). *Diagnostic methods in speech pathology.* New York: Harper & Row.

KENT, R, & LAPOINTE, L. (1982). Acoustic properties of pathological reiterative utterances: A case study of palilalia. *Journal of Speech and Hearing Research, 25,* 95–99.

KOLLER, W. (1983). Disfluency (stuttering) in extrapyramidal disease. *Archives of Neurology, 40,* 175–177.

LANYON, R. I. (1967). The measurement of stuttering severity. *Journal of Speech and Hearing Research, 10,* 836–843.

LAPOINT, L., & HORNER, J. (1981). Palilalia: A descriptive study of pathological reiterative utterances. *Journal of Speech and Hearing Disorders, 46,* 34–38.

LeBRUN, Y., RETIF, J., & KAISER, G. (1983). Acquired stuttering as a forerunner of motor neuron disease. *Journal of Fluency Disorders, 8,* 161–167.

LEEPER, L., CULATTA, R., PINDZOLA, R., & DUCHIN-CESKA, S. (1990). *Elderly speakers' rate/fluency: What we know, what it means.* Paper presented at the convention of the American Speech-Language-Hearing Association, Seattle, WA.

LEITH, W., & MIMS, H. (1975). Cultural influences in the development and treatment of stuttering: A preliminary report. *Journal of Speech and Hearing Disorders, 40,* 459–466.

LUPER, H. L., & MULDER, R. L. (1966). *Stuttering therapy for children.* Englewood Cliffs, NJ: Prentice Hall.

MADISON, D., BAEHR, E. T., BAZELL, M., HARTMAN, R. W., MAHURKAS, S. D., & DUNEA, G. (1977). Communicative and cognitive deterioration in dialysis dementia: Two case studies. *Journal of Speech and Hearing Disorders, 42,* 238–243.

MARTIN, R. R., & LINDAMOOD, L. P. (1986). Stuttering and spontaneous recovery: Implications for the speech-language pathologist. *Language, Speech and Hearing Services in Schools, 17,* 207–218.

METRAUX, R. (1950). Speech profiles of the preschool child 18 to 54 months. *Journal of Speech Disorders, 15,* 37–53.

MYERS, F., & WALL, M. (1982). Toward an integrated approach to early childhood stuttering. *Journal of Fluency Disorders, 7,* 47–54.

PEINS, M., McGOUGH, W. E., & LEE, B. S. (1984). Double tape recorder therapy for stutterers. In M. Peins (Ed.), *Contemporary approaches in stuttering therapy.* Boston: Little, Brown.

PERKINS, W. H. (1971). *Speech pathology: An applied behavioral science.* St. Louis, MO: C. V. Mosby.

PERKINS, W. H. (1983). Learning from negative outcomes in stuttering therapy. II. An epiphany of failures. *Journal of Fluency Disorders, 8,* 155–160.

PETERS, T. J., & GUITAR, B. (1991). *Stuttering: An integrated approach to its nature and treatment.* Baltimore: Williams & Wilkins.

PINDZOLA, R. H. (1986). A description of some selected stuttering instruments. *Journal of Childhood Communication Disorders, 9,* 183–200.

PINDZOLA, R. H. (1988). *Stuttering Intervention Program: Age 3 to Grade 3.* Austin, TX: PRO-ED.

PINDZOLA, R. H. (1991). Disfluency characteristics of aged, normal-speaking black and white males. *Journal of Fluency Disorders,* in press.

PINDZOLA, R. H., JENKINS, M., & LOKKEN, K. (1989). Speaking rates of young children. *Language, Speech and Hearing Services in Schools, 20,* 133–138.

PINDZOLA, R. H., & WHITE, D. (1986). A protocol for differentiating the incipient stutters. *Language, Speech and Hearing Services in Schools, 17,* 2–15.

RAGSDALE, J., & ASHBY, J. (1982). Speech-language pathologists' connotation of stuttering. *Journal of Speech and Hearing Research, 25,* 78–80.

RILEY, G. (1972). A Stuttering Severity Instrument for Children and Adults. *Journal of Speech and Hearing Disorders, 37,* 314–322.

RILEY, G. (1980). *Stuttering Severity Instrument for Children and Adults.* Tigard, OR: C.C. Publications.

RILEY, G. (1981). *Stuttering Prediction Instrument for Young Children.* Tigard, OR: C.C. Publications.

RILEY, G., & RILEY, J. (1986). *Oral motor assessment and treatment.* Tigard, OR: C.C. Publications.

ROBINSON, F. B. (1966). *What parents and teachers should know about children who stutter.* Washington, DC: National Association of Hearing and Speech Agencies.

ROSENBEK, J., MESSERT, B., COLLINS, M., & WERTZ, R. (1978). Stuttering following brain damage. *Brain and Language, 6,* 82–96.

RYAN, B. (1974). *Programmed therapy for stuttering in children and adults.* Springfield, IL: Charles C Thomas.

SATCHER, D. (1986). Research needs for minority populations. In F. H. Bess, B. S. Clark, & H. R. Mitchell (Eds.), *Concerns for minority groups in communication disorders.* Rockville, MD: ASHA Reports 16.

SHAMES, G. H. (1989). Stuttering: An RFP for a cultural perspective. *Journal of Fluency Disorders, 14,* 67–77.

SHAMES, G. H., & EGOLF, D. (1976). *Operant conditioning and the management of stuttering.* Englewood Cliffs, NJ: Prentice Hall.

SHINE, R. E. (1980). *Systematic fluency training for children.* Austin, TX: PRO-ED.

SHUMAK, I. (1955). A speech situation rating sheet for stutterers. In W. Johnson (Ed.), *Stuttering in children and adults.* Minneapolis, MN: University of Minnesota Press.

SILVERMAN, F. (1980). Stuttering Problem Profile: A task that assists both client and clinician in defining therapy goals. *Journal of Speech and Hearing Disorders, 45,* 119–123.

SILVERMAN, F., & WILLIAMS, D. (1972). Prediction of stuttering by school age stutterers. *Journal of Speech and Hearing Research, 15,* 189–193.

STARKWEATHER, C. W., GOTTWALD, S. R., & HALFOND, M. M. (1990). *Stuttering prevention: A clinical method.* Englewood Cliffs, NJ: Prentice Hall.

ST. LOUIS, K., & LASS, N. (1981). A survey of communication disorder students' attitudes toward stuttering. *Journal of Fluency Disorders, 6,* 49–79.

STOCKER, B. (1980). *The Stocker probe technique.* Austin, TX: PRO-ED.

TANNER, D. (1987). *Parental Diagnostic Questionnaire* (rev.). Austin, TX: PRO-ED.

TURNBAUGH, K., GUITAR, B., & HOFFMAN, P. (1979). Speech clinicians' attribution of personality traits as a function of stuttering severity. *Journal of Speech and Hearing Research, 22,* 37–45.

TURNBAUGH, K., GUITAR., B., & HOFFMAN, P. (1981). The attribution of personality traits: The stutterer and nonstutterer. *Journal of Speech and Hearing Research, 24,* 288–291.

VAN RIPER, C. (1982). *The nature of stuttering* (2nd ed.). Englewood Cliffs, NJ: Prentice Hall.

WALLE, E. (1974). *The prevention of stuttering. I. Identifying danger signs* (a film). Memphis, TN: Speech Foundation of America.

WALLE, E. (1975). *The prevention of stuttering. II. Parent counseling and elimination of the problem* (a film). Memphis, TN: Speech Foundation of America.

WALLE, E. (1977). *The prevention of stuttering. III. SSStuttering and your child. Is it me? Is it you?* (a film). Memphis, TN: Speech Foundation of America.

WEINER, A. (1981). A case of adult onset of stuttering. *Journal of Fluency Disorders, 6,* 181–186.

WEINER, A. (1984). Vocal control therapy for stutterers. In M. Peins (Ed.), *Contemporary approaches in stuttering therapy.* Boston: Little, Brown.

WEISS, D. A. (1964). *Cluttering.* Englewood Cliffs, NJ: Prentice Hall.

WEISS, D. A. (1968). Cluttering: Central language imbalance. *Pediatric Clinics of North America, 15,* 705–720.

WELLS, G. B. (1987). *Stuttering treatment: A comprehensive clinical guide.* Englewood Cliffs, NJ: Prentice Hall.

WINGATE, M. E. (1976). *Stuttering theory and treatment.* New York: Irvington Publishers.

WOOLF, G. (1967). The assessment of stuttering as struggle, avoidance, and expectancy. *British Journal of Disorders of Communication, 2,* 158–171.

WYATT, E. (1969). *Language learning and disorders of communication in children.* New York: Free Press.

YAIRI, E. (1981). Disfluencies of normally speaking two-year-old children. *Journal of Speech and Hearing Research, 24,* 490–495.

YAIRI, E. (1983). The onset of stuttering in two- and three-year-old children: A preliminary report. *Journal of Speech and Hearing Disorders, 48,* 171–177.

YAIRI, E., & CLIFTON, N. F. (1972). Disfluent speech behavior of preschool children, high school seniors, and geriatric persons. *Journal of Speech and Hearing Research, 15,* 714–719.

YAIRI, E., & LEWIS, B. (1984). Disfluencies at the onset of stuttering. *Journal of Speech and Hearing Research, 27,* 155–159.

YOUNG, M. (1975). Onset, prevalence, and recovery from stuttering. *Journal of Speech and Hearing Disorders, 40*(1), 49–58.

ZWITMAN, D. (1978). *The disfluent child.* Baltimore: University Park Press.

chapter

8

ASSESSMENT OF APHASIA AND ADULT LANGUAGE DISORDERS

When an adult suddenly loses the easy use of language, it is a devastating experience for the individual and for the family. Aphasia, and other adult language disorders, affect that which makes us uniquely human—our ability to communicate with each other by a system of language symbols.

THE NATURE OF APHASIA

Aphasia is the most common disorder of communication resulting from brain injury. Damage occurs in the hemisphere of the brain that is dominant for language; for most of us, this is the left hemisphere. An adult with aphasia has a basic interference with *comprehension* and *use* of language in its many forms. More specifically, aphasia is a syndrome of language deficits resulting from destruction of cortical tissue and is characterized by one or more of the following symptoms:

1. Disturbance in receiving and decoding symbolic materials via auditory, visual, or tactile channels; although the individual can still hear and see, there is difficulty deciphering the learned associations of messages
2. Disturbance in central processes of meaning, word selection, and message formulation
3. Disturbance in expressing symbolic materials by means of speech, writing, or gesture.

Aphasia may result from trauma, brain tumors, certain inflammatory processes, and degenerative diseases. The vast majority of aphasias, however, are the consequence of a cerebrovascular accident (CVA) or stroke.

The cerebral vascular accident is a relatively common illness that affects approximately a half million persons each year. In the United States, CVA now stands as the third leading cause of death (outdistanced only by heart disease and cancer). No one knows precisely how many surviving stroke victims are left with language impairment; estimates suggest at least a quarter of the victims present some degree of aphasia that warrants treatment.

Etiology can influence the onset, progress, and type of aphasia symptoms. According to Rosenbek, LaPointe, and Wertz (1989), the onset of symptoms is likely to be insidious when caused by tumor, and abrupt when due to CVA. They go on to state that improvement is more likely if the aphasia is caused by a CVA than by a tumor, and patients with tumors may have wide differences in abilities across modalities (reading, writing, listening, speaking). Such large differences are less likely from a CVA. Aphasia resulting from trauma is often accompanied by a greater variety of cognitive deficits, but it shows a faster recovery than aphasia resulting from CVA.

There are a host of other disorders that may resemble aphasia and have brain damage as their basis. These include the language of confusion, language of intellectual deterioration (dementia), communication deficit subsequent to a nondominant lesion (usually right hemisphere damage), language associated with psychosis, and motor speech disorders. These disorders will be discussed later in this chapter as part of the differential diagnosis process.

The severity of aphasia can vary greatly, from minimal, temporary language dysfunction to almost total and permanent inability to use and comprehend language. It is important to remember that the impoverishment of language observed in aphasia is *not* due to loss of mental capacity, impairment of sensory organs, or paralysis of the speech apparatus. These problems, however, can co-occur with aphasia, making differential diagnosis important.

Classifying a patient as to the *type* of aphasia displayed can be an important feature of diagnosis and treatment planning. Many labels and classification systems have been put forth through the years for this purpose. Three methods are currently in wide use: (1) fluent-nonfluent dichotomy, which is based on the patient's length of utterance; (2) the "Boston" classification system by Goodglass and Kaplan (1983); and (3) the *Western Aphasia Battery* (WAB) taxonomy by Kertesz (1979, 1980). The Boston and WAB systems are quite similar and use fluency, auditory comprehension, repetition, and naming abilities for arriving at a diagnostic label. Table 8.1 lists characteristics of each of the major types of aphasia (Fitch-West, 1984; Goodglass & Kaplan, 1983).

Although there is some controversy as to our ability to localize language functions in the brain, there is fairly good agreement with site of lesion information and the language characteristics seen in individual patients. Primary language areas of the left hemisphere and associated aphasias are shown in Figure 8.1. As can be seen, anterior lesions generally produce nonfluent aphasia, such as Broca's and transcortical motor aphasias. Posterior lesions are associated with

Table 8.1   Neurolinguistic Features of the Major Types of Aphasia

Broca's Aphasia

  impaired fluency; limited verbal output

  relatively good auditory comprehension

  impaired articulatory agility

  stereotyped grammar

  telegraphic and agrammatic (especially reduced use of articles,
    prepositions, auxiliaries, copulas, and derivational endings)

  prosodic alterations

Transcortical Motor Aphasia

  preserved ability to repeat

  nonfluent

  some auditory comprehension impairment, similar to Broca's aphasia

  naming ability superior to spontaneous speech

Global Aphasia

  severe loss of all receptive modalities

  severe loss of all expressive modalities

  speech almost totally absent

  stereotypic utterances (perhaps with normal melody and intonation)

Wernicke's Aphasia

  fluent; copious verbal output

  impaired auditory comprehension (often severe)

  paraphasias frequent (especially semantic types)

  neologisms and jargon, if severe

  normal articulatory agility

  normal prosody

  normal or supranormal phrase length

  full range of grammatical forms

  syntax preserved

  impaired naming and repetition abilities

Transcortical Sensory Aphasia

  Preserved ability to repeat

  conversation resembles symptoms of Wernicke's aphasia

  extreme difficulty with nouns

  excessive paraphasias

  impaired auditory comprehension, resembles Wernicke's

Conduction Aphasia

  poor repetition ability

  fluent speech; good articulation and phrase length

  paraphasias frequent (especially literal types)

  some auditory comprehension impairment

  acute awareness of errors

Table 8.1   *(Continued)*

Anomic Aphasia

  severe word-finding deficits

  frequent circumlocutions

  paraphasic errors minimal

  fluent speech; good articulation and phrase length

  appropriate grammatical forms

  good auditory comprehension

the fluent aphasias, such as Wernicke's, conduction, and transcortical sensory aphasias.

Site of lesion (anatomical areas affected) and type of lesion (tumor, CVA, and so forth) can usually be determined by modern methods of brain imaging such as computerized tomography (CT), positron emission tomography (PET), and magnetic resonance imaging (MRI). An example of a CT scan is shown in Figure 8.2. These methods have contributed greatly to aphasiology and are reviewed by Metter and Hanson (1985). Although such anatomical evidence supplied by the neuroradiologist is diagnostically valuable, the speech-language pathologist may be wise to focus on carefully describing what the individual can and cannot do with respect to language. The clinician must first and foremost delineate the patient's ability to talk, listen, read, and write.

In our zeal to identify the neurolinguistic dimensions of aphasia, it is possible to forget that brain injury is a grave health problem. The individual has suffered a major life crisis that has profound medical, psychological, and social consequences. In addition to the language impairment, the patient may present paralysis or paresis of the extremities (generally the right side, sometimes including the face), sensory abnormalities, and behavioral disturbances. There seems to be little, if any, relationship between these difficulties and the

Figure 8.1   Areas of the Left Hemisphere Associated with Some of the Types of Aphasia

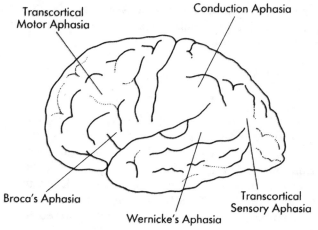

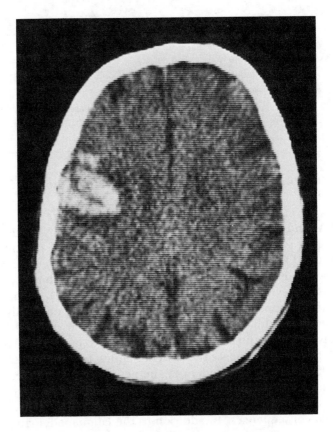

Figure 8.2 Computed Tomographic (CT) Scan (x-ray pictures taken from many angles and computerized) Showing a Lesion in the Left Hemisphere. The Patient Had a Broca's Aphasia. (Photograph courtesy of D. Shah, M.D., Hines V.A. Hospital)

extent of the language impairment. Above all, the clinician must remember that aphasia is both a personal catastrophe and a family crisis, as Buck (1968) so eloquently points out.

CASE HISTORY

As speech-language pathologists, it is wise for us to remember that we work with *persons* who have aphasia, not aphasia. Language treatment for an adult aphasic has to be very personalized. Therefore, we need to know as much as possible about our clients when planning a rehabilitation program. What sort of people were they before the stroke? How did they meet their problems? What educational level was achieved? What was their occupation? Their avocations? What changes in behavior, if any, have occurred following the brain injury?

The style, pace, and content of treatment will be based on the answers to these and many other questions.

Unfortunately, the aphasic patient is often in no position to provide the kind of detailed information we seek. In some instances, official records (educational tests, military records) and personal documents (diaries, letters) are helpful. Usually, however, we must rely on the accuracy and veracity of informants who are familiar with the patient. The most common method of assembling information about the language-impaired individual is a case history form that is filled out by a spouse or other close relative. Sample questions from a typical case history form are listed in Table 8.2. Ideally, the clinician also interviews the respondent to clarify any ambiguities in the written information and to permit additional questioning. Keep in mind, however, that a long-term marriage partner typically sees the patient as less impaired than objective language testing may show (Helmick, Watamori, & Palmer, 1976). On the contrary, Holland (1977) points out that acontextual tests of language do not measure communication and the client may, in fact, perform better in a "real" setting.

The interview of a family member also allows us to learn something of the family dynamics that may impact on treatment outcome. There are many difficulties with which the family of an aphasic must cope—often, unfortunately, without professional guidance (Derman & Manaster, 1967; Porter & Dabul, 1977). We may want to consider the following: In terms of life cycle, at what stage is the family? Are there young or adolescent children? Is it a middle-aged couple, now alone and with leisure and peak earning power? What premorbid marital problems existed? Will they be exacerbated or will the family unit draw more closely together to meet the threat? Does the spouse have health problems? How does the family handle the fear of recurring stokes? Are there financial difficulties? Is there any guilt? How are they coping with the communication impairment? What are their impressions of the physical changes?

It is wise to remember as we conduct the interview that relatives of aphasics need information, reassurance, and an outlet for frustration (Derman & Manaster, 1967). Thus, there is only an imaginary line between case history interviewing and the start of family counseling.

In addition to the case history, the speech-language pathologist may wish to prepare an index that reflects the severity of the patient's total disability. The SLP can choose from several published scales, among them the *Maryland Disability Index, Communication Status Chart* (Wisconsin Division of Health, 1966), the *Pulses Profile and Barthel Index* (Granger & Albrecht, 1979), the *Functional Performance Assessment* (Harvey & Jellinek, 1983), and the *Functional Life Scale* (Sarno & Sarno, 1973). We prefer the latter device because it provides a quantitative measure of the individual's ability to participate in all phases of daily activity—in the home, outside the home, and in social interaction. It should also be mentioned that other ways to assess the psychosocial impact of adult language impairment have been put forth by Evans and Northwood (1983) and by Muller, Code, and Mugford (1983).

Health history of the patient is ascertained, in part, during the case history interview (recall Table 8.2), but medical records provide greater specificity.

Table 8.2 Sample Questionnaire Topics for a Case History

Personal

Marital status

Name and occupation of spouse

Names and locations of children

Information about grandchildren

Amount of education

Occupation

Current employment status (retired?)

Hobbies and special interests

Preferences in reading material, television entertainment, and use of writing

Which hand was preferred?

What was native language? Knowledge of others?

Description of personality

Describe involvement in group activities (e.g., bowling leagues, church fellowships)

Since the injury, describe any changes in mood, personality, ability to care for self, and the like

Medical

Date of injury

Cause of injury (accident, stroke, disease)

Length of unconsciousness, if any

Describe paralysis, if any

Any complaints of dizziness, faintness, headaches?

Describe any visual or hearing problems

Describe any other problems, illnesses, or injuries

Communicative

What was the patient's speech like at the onset of the problem?

How has it changed?

Check the appropriate column as it applies to the patient *now:*

CAN	CANNOT	
___	___	Indicate meaning by gesture
___	___	Repeat words spoken by others
___	___	Use one or a few words over and over
___	___	Use swear words (often)
___	___	Use some words spontaneously
___	___	Say short phrases
___	___	Say short sentences
___	___	Follow requests and understand directions
___	___	Follow radio or television speech
___	___	Read signs with understanding
___	___	Read newspapers, magazines
___	___	Tell time
___	___	Write name without assistance
___	___	Write sentences, letters
___	___	Do simple arithmetic
___	___	Handle money, make change

Information concerning the current medical episode is particularly useful in differential diagnosis and treatment planning. Rosenbek, LaPointe, and Wertz (1989) suggest that the following medical data be collected:

1. Major and secondary medical diagnoses (e.g., thrombosis of left middle cerebral artery, organic brain syndrome, diabetes, CVA with right hemiparesis, and the like)
2. Date of onset as regards etiology of communication disorder
3. Localization of brain damage (hemisphere and lobes affected) and source of data (e.g., CT, MRI, and other techniques)
4. Previous CNS involvement (type and date of onset)
5. Brain stem signs (e.g., facial weakness, extraocular movement, dysphagia, other bulbar signs)
6. Limb involvement
7. Vision (acuity, corrective lens, visual field deficits, etc.)
8. Hearing (acuity, discrimination, amplification, etc.).

Access to the patient's medical chart is therefore essential to the SLP. In addition to the physician/neurologist report, entries by the neuroradiologist, social worker, nurse, and other health care professionals are enlightening. Note the information gained from this telegraphic chart note entered by a neurologist:

> This alert, oriented adult male suffered a CVA on 3-19-90. Expressive-receptive aphasia. Right hemiplegia. Babinski sign on the right. Gross motor functioning of involved leg is returning; arm and hand are doubtful. Electroencephalography revealed a focal lesion in the left parietal-temporal region. Site of lesion confirmed by CT scan. Right side astereognosis. Right homonomous hemianopsia.

This brief report told us several important things about the patient: The brain damage was apparently localized and was not widespread; the aphasia was probably not transitory, as lesions in the region cited generally result in more persistent language impairment; he could not identify objects by touch when they were placed in his right hand; and he could not see in the right field of vision. This last anomaly would require that we present testing materials from the patient's left side. Information assembled by the neurologist is, of course, very useful to the SLP. In addition to the size and locale of the lesion, the nature of the injury may be pertinent diagnostically. (For example, patients incurring traumatic brain injury often experience a different course of recovery from persons' suffering vascular episodes.) The chart note also underscores the importance of being familiar with pertinent medical terminology.

After garnering case history information, the SLP should have a rather detailed description of the salient aspects of the patient's premorbid personality, health history and current status, and social orientation. But what impact would this sudden illness have? How much change could be expected, and in what areas? Would the patient's responses to the language impairment and physical disabilities merely be an exaggeration of earlier behavior patterns?

There are only limited answers to these questions. We suspect, however, that the nature of the illness, the treatment the patient receives, and premorbid factors are all crucial in determining the impact of the problem upon the individual. In summary, any and all information about the individual that can be pulled together is important and may shape our course of assessment and treatment.

DIAGNOSIS AND FORMAL TESTING

A comprehensive evaluation of an adult aphasic includes several clinical tasks: (1) a review of pertinent medical information and the sequence of events leading up to the referral; (2) a preliminary interview with the patient's spouse or other close relatives; (3) a case history, including information about the impact of brain injury on the patient and how much natural or spontaneous recovery has taken place; (4) an inventory of the client's language/communication performance; (5) observation and related testing (including informal assessments, oral peripheral examination, hearing test, and the like); and (6) a diagnostic determination with recommendations as to the nature of treatment and a judgment about the individual's prospects for recovery. In arriving at a diagnosis, the clinician first determines whether or not a communication problem exists and, if it does, what kind of problem. This involves sorting out among various possible conditions and among subtypes within specific conditions. This decision-making process is shown schematically in Figure 8.3.

Having already discussed the first three tasks in the list, let us now turn our attention to the fourth and see how the evaluation process leads to a diagnosis. The speech-language pathologist may need a quick idea of the client's language abilities and disabilities in order to determine the need for further

Figure 8.3 Diagnosis Decision Matrix

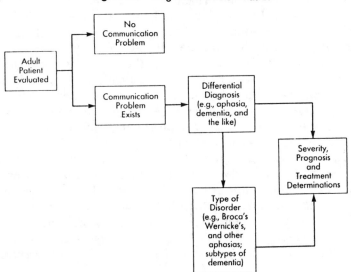

testing and to better choose the most appropriate standardized tests to employ. A screening test, therefore, may be administered.

Screening for Aphasia

A screening instrument is designed to swiftly evaluate a patient's language abilities before the administration of a more thorough (and lengthy) examination. One reason for using a screening instrument is that it allows the SLP to quickly advise relatives and health care professionals about the best means of communicating with the patient. Additionally, patients' symptoms change rapidly during the first days and months following brain injury; screenings allow for frequent reassessments to document the patient's progress (or lack of progress) and to modify suggestions as to how best to communicate with the patient. Frequent readministrations of formal, standardized tests—many lasting one to six hours—would not be practical.

Some screening tests were designed as screening devices per se; others are merely shortened versions of published language examinations for aphasia. Table 8.3 lists some of the available screening tests for aphasia.

Many experienced clinicians design their own screening device—usually one that is more cursory than published tests. In some work settings, for example, the SLP must quickly (in five minutes or so) interview and screen all newly admitted patients to determine if a communication problem exists and to decide

Table 8.3 Some Screening Tests for Aphasia

Halstead-Wepman Aphasia Screening Test
(Halstead & Wepman, 1949)

Short Examination for Aphasia
(Schuell, 1957)

Sklar Aphasia Scale (SAS)
(Sklar, 1966)

A Short Form of the Token Test
(Spellacy & Spreen, 1969)

Screening Test of Aphasia
(Emerick & Coyne, 1972)

Aphasia Language Performance Scales (ALPS)
(Keenan & Brassell, 1975)

Shortened Version of the PICA (4 subtests)
(DiSimoni et al., 1975)

Shortened Version of the PICA (2 of the objects in 17 subtests)
(DiSimoni, Keith, & Darley, 1980)

Very Short Form of the Minnesota Aphasia Test
(Powell, Bailey, & Clark, 1980)

Whurr Aphasia Screening Test
(Whurr, 1983)

Bedside Evaluation and Screening Test of Aphasia (BEST)
(Fitch-West & Sands, 1987)

Acute Aphasia Screening Protocol
(Crary & Haak, in press)

whether to suggest that the physician order a speech-language consult. This is done because third-party reimbursement agencies require that evaluations be medically necessary and physician-ordered. Typically, the SLP will elicit spontaneous conversation and judge it for contextual accuracy, topic maintenance, length of utterance, syntactic variety, facility with word selection, and fluency. Limited or absent conversation may lead the SLP to quickly assess more basic skills, such as naming and pointing to objects in the room, repeating, following commands (nonverbally), and responding to yes/no questions (verbally or gesturally). Such a quick, albeit incomplete screening permits the clinician to judge (1) whether or not a communication problem exists on a gross level, (2) the need for further testing (and hence the need for a physician-ordered consult), and (3) which formal tests would be best suited to the patient's level of functioning.

No matter which form of screening is done, before the patient leaves the hospital or rehabilitation center, the speech-language pathologist should enter a summary note in the patient's medial chart. An example follows:

> The results of the screening test are encouraging. Mr. Tenhave has good auditory recognition (pointing to objects and pictures when named) and his comprehension for auditory materials is good within his limited auditory memory span. His listening is accurate for simple, short messages. He seems to understand more than he really does because he is alert and well oriented, and he picks out a crucial word in a sentence. He has a good supply of automatic (counting, emotional language) and reactive speech. He frequently gives associations when asked to name objects or pictures; for example, he said "pedal" for "brake." His gestures are not more complex than his verbal output. I did not ask him to write at this time, but it is my impression that his language deficit cuts across all modalities. No dysarthria was observed, although he did simplify complex words such as "Methodist." He is making a great many attempts at self-correction. On balance, then, I would say that he has a good prognosis for functional use of language.

We offer a final word of caution: Screening tests were not designed to replace longer, more comprehensive evaluations. As Schuell (1966) points out, screening tests fail to sample behaviors in all communicative modalities, and they do not provide a sufficient sample in the modalities that are tested to make a confident differential diagnosis or to plan treatment.

Standardized Testing

In order to devise a plan of treatment, as well as to predict the probable course and outcome of treatment, the speech-language pathologist needs a comprehensive appraisal of the patient's present language abilities. Where is the patient having difficulty? Which modalities are working best? How are errors made and are there discernible patterns to the errors? To answer these and other questions, we inventory the patient's language.

The SLP has many published tests from which to choose; Table 8.4 lists some of the more commonly used tests of aphasia. Many of these instruments have been reviewed in detail elsewhere (Buros, 1978; Darley, 1979; Davis, 1983; Kertesz, 1979; Rosenbek, LaPointe, & Wertz, 1989; Tikofsky, 1984).

Table 8.4   Commonly Used Tests for Aphasia

Aphasia Language Performance Scales (ALPS)
   (Keenan & Brassell, 1975)

Appraisal of Language Disturbance (ALD)
   (Emerick, 1971)

Boston Diagnostic Aphasia Examination (BDAE)
   (Goodglass & Kaplan, 1983)

Communicative Abilities in Daily Living
   (Holland, 1980)

Functional Communication Profile
   (Sarno, 1969)

Minnesota Test for Differential Diagnosis of Aphasia (MTDDA)
   (Schuell, 1973)

Neurosensory Center Comprehensive Examination for Aphasia
   (Spreen & Benton, 1977)

Porch Index of Communicative Ability (PICA)
   (Porch, 1971)

Sklar Aphasia Scale
   (Sklar, 1966)

Western Aphasia Battery
   (Kertesz, 1980)

Only a cursory discussion of the more popular—and different—tests will be presented here.

Beginning clinicians often ask which aphasia test they should select for examining patients. We prefer not to advocate any particular instrument but instead ask the clinicians to specify their purposes in testing. What do they want the test to show? If prediction of the course of the patient's recovery is important, the *PICA* (Porch, 1971) is the instrument of choice; if the clinician is more interested in the site of the lesion, the *Boston Diagnostic Aphasia Examination* (Goodglass & Kaplan, 1983) or the Western Aphasia Battery (Kertesz, 1980) are indicated; if the clinician wants to know how the patient performs on basic-to-complicated language functions, then the *Minnesota Test for Differential Diagnosis of Aphasia* (Schuell, 1973) is a good choice. To sample a patient's communication ability in natural settings, the checklist called the *Functional Communication Profile* (Taylor, 1963) or the more extensive *Communicative Abilities in Daily Living* (Holland, 1980) would be the instruments of choice.

In the hands of a skilled and perceptive clinician who is thoroughly familiar with the materials, *any* of the published tests will provide a detailed description of an aphasic patient's language disturbance. As we pointed out earlier in this book, a test is only a tool, a way to help the clinician make relatively precise observations of a particular individual. Nation and Aram state the issue succinctly: "A good diagnostician relies on the feelings that have resulted as much as on the tools that were administered" (1977, p. 258). None of the published aphasia tests is pure, none is sacrosanct. With this in mind, let us discuss four popular tests that are very different in philosophy and content.

The Porch Index of Communicative Ability. Better known as the *PICA* (Porch, 1971), this is a psychometrically well-constructed test that assesses verbal, gestural, and graphic responses to common objects. The test features a multidimensional scoring system, using one to 16 categories, that allows the clinician to make precise observations of the patient's responses. Scores with percentile norms, performance plots, and recovery curves are generated through data manipulation. Speech-language pathologists have found the overall score (as a single index of communication ability) and the recovery predictions extremely useful information to share with physicians.

In mild criticism of the *PICA*, we dislike the rigidity of the test and feel that the standard procedure breaks down the patient-clinician relationship. As Keenan and Brassell state, "a badly presented item is a minor error, far less important than an impersonal or mechanical response to the patient" (1975, p. 36). Additionally, we find that starting the examination with the most difficult task often overwhelms the aphasic and disturbs his/her subsequent performance. The *PICA* offers only limited information about a patient's verbal ability: Only four of the 18 subtests elicit verbal behavior; only one of the four, "describing how objects are used," affords any insight into how the patient talks. Finally, we do not feel that a clinician should abrogate his/her personal clinical responsibility for judgment by deferring to a test or the numerical scores it generates. A combination of clinical intuition, patient observations, lesion information, *and* test scores/performances should shape our diagnoses and predictions.

The Boston Diagnostic Aphasia Examination. The *BDAE* (Goodglass & Kaplan, 1983, 2nd ed.) operates on the localization premise that test scores and profiles correspond to specific types of aphasia. We particularly recognize as a strength the conversational and expository speech section that rates six features: melodic line, phrase length, articulatory agility, grammatical form, paraphasia, and word finding. Subtests cover a wide variety of skills and modalities, making it a well-rounded examination. Supplementary tests are included for use with related disorders. We, however, do find that the *BDAE* is a lengthy test and one that may frustrate low-level patients.

Communicative Abilities in Daily Living. Holland (1980) designed the *CADL* to sample the patient's functional communication skills in naturalistic situations. It is to supplement traditional tests of aphasia, not replace them. As such, it does not lend itself to differential diagnosis. The content of the *CADL* is unique; it includes categories such as role-playing situations, utilizing nonverbal context, and analyzing speech acts. All in all, it is a test that measures what it purports—communication in daily activities.

Aphasia Language Performance Scales. The *ALPS*, by Keenan and Brassell (1975), is a quick-to-administer test that emphasizes an informal conversational approach. It contains four 10-item scales: listening, talking, reading, writing. Items are presented in an increasingly complex order and may be omitted if judged too difficult or too easy for a patient. We find the *ALPS* a useful test for low-level patients but also consider it rather cursory for differential diagnosing and treatment planning.

Regardless of the test used, the evaluation process permits the clinician to identify islands of communication ability the patient retains. In many instances, however, the speech-language pathologist will want to do additional, more extensive testing in particular areas. Some specialized tests follow:

1. *Auditory Comprehension:* Almost every comprehensive aphasia battery has at least one section that evaluates auditory comprehension. Since the integrity of the auditory modality is so crucial in predicting recovery, several specialized tests have been published. The most notable of them include the *Token Test* (DeRenzi & Vignolo, 1962) and its many versions, the most popular of which is the *Revised Token Test* (McNeil & Prescott, 1978); the *Auditory Comprehension Test for Sentences (ACTS)* (Shewan, 1980); and the *Functional Auditory Comprehension Task (FACT)* (LaPointe & Horner, 1978).

2. *Expressive Abilities:* Early aphasia batteries have been criticized for not evaluating the spontaneous speech of patients. The *Boston Diagnostic Aphasia Examination* (Goodglass & Kaplan, 1983), in contrast, does elicit conversational and expository speech. The test's "Cookie Theft" picture description task and ratings based on the patient's verbal output are well known. Recently, *discourse analysis* has become refined and the work of Ulatowska and colleagues shows clinical promise (Ulatowska, North, & Macaluso-Haynes, 1981; Ulatowska & Bond, 1983; Ulatowska et al., 1983). On a syntactic level, the *Sentence Completion Test* (Goodglass et al., 1972) is useful in assessing sentence construction abilities and the patient's use of derivations.

3. *Reading Ability:* The *Reading Comprehension Battery* (LaPointe & Horner, 1979) and the *Battery of Adult Reading Function* (Gonzales-Rothi, Costett, & Heilman, 1984) are useful in-depth measures of reading ability.

4. *Intelligence:* The *Coloured Progressive Matrices* (Raven, 1963) is useful in assessing nonverbal skills, while the *Wechsler Adult Intelligence Scale* (Wechsler, 1955) is a traditional battery with many useful subtests.

5. *Others:* Additional special testing almost surely includes an oral-peripheral and motor examination and a test of hearing acuity, as well as others deemed necessary for particular patients.

DIFFERENTIAL DIAGNOSIS

The speech-language pathologist must often distinguish between aphasia and a number of other conditions involving abnormality in language and/or speech. A variety of special tests may be needed to supplement standard aphasia batteries in order to facilitate differential diagnosing. Table 8.5 lists some tests useful in differentiating aphasia from other adult language disorders, as culled from

Table 8.5 Useful Tests for Cognitive-Communicative Assessments of "Nonaphasic" Disorders

Assessment of Cognitive Abilities
   (Adamovich & Henderson, 1985)

Hooper Visual Organization Test
   (Hooper, 1958)

F-A-S Word Fluency Measure
   (Borkowski, Benton, & Spreen, 1967)

Boston Naming Test
   (Kaplan, Goodglass, & Weintraub, 1976)

Selected subtests of the *Wechsler Adult Intelligence Scale* (WAIS)
   (Wechsler, 1955)

Wechsler Memory Scale
   (Wechsler & Stone, 1948)

Selected subtests of an aphasia battery, such as the *Boston Diagnostic Aphasia Examination*
   (Goodglass & Kaplan, 1983)

Peabody Picture Vocabulary Test —Revised
   (Dunn & Dunn, 1981)

Nonsense Syllable Learning Task
   (Alexander, 1973)

Geriatric Mental Status Interview (GMS)
   (Gurland et al., 1976)

Geriatric Rating Scale (GRS)
   (Plutchik et al., 1970)

Mental Status Questionnaire (MSQ)
   (Goldfarb & Antin, 1975)

Selected subtests of the *Illinois Tests of Psycholinguistic Abilities* (ITPA)
   (Kirk, McCarthy, & Kirk, 1968)

Selected subtests of the *Detroit Test of Learning Aptitude* (DTLA)
   (Baker & Leland, 1959)

Developmental Test of Visual Perception
   (Frostig, 1963)

Ross Test of Higher Cognitive Processes
   (Ross & Ross, 1976)

Nonverbal Test of Cognitive Skills
   (Johnson & Boyd, 1981)

Coloured Progressive Matrices
   (Raven, 1963)

Luria-Nebraska Neuropsychological Battery
   (consult Lezak, 1983 for description)

Halstead-Reitan Battery
   (revised frequently; consult Lezak, 1983 for description)

Blessed Orientation and Memory Examination
   (Blessed, Tomlinson, & Roth, 1968)

Mini-Mental State Examination (MMS)
   (Folstein, Folstein, & McHugh, 1975)

Mattis Dementia Rating Scale (MDRS)
   (Mattis, 1976)

Global Deterioration Scale of Primary Degenerative Dementia (GDS)
   (Reisberg, Ferris, & Crook, 1982)

Benton Revised Visual Retention Test (BVRT-R)
   (Benton, 1974)

the literature (Bayles, 1984; Hagen, 1984; Marquardt, 1982; Myers, 1984). Special tests delineate patient's strengths and weaknesses beyond the realm of language; areas such as intelligence, cognition, perception, mood, and behavior need to be tapped.

We present the following brief discussion of some disorders that might be confused with aphasia. Keep in mind, however, that impairment of symbolic functioning can coexist with any of these conditions.

Psychosis

Although it is rather easy for the professional to distinguish aphasia from *psychosis,* it is understandable why laypersons are often confused. The aphasic may say yes when he/she means no, use obscenities and other antisocial language or gestures freely, laugh or cry often, lapse into euphoria, deny his/her symptoms, or withdraw into severe depression and despair. The distinguishing features of psychosis are, however, rather obvious: severe personality decomposition—not just frustration or emotional overflow when trying to comprehend or speak—and distortion of, or loss of contact with, reality. The vast majority of aphasic patients do not show evidence of mental deterioration or gross disturbances in processing reality. Additionally, the aphasic will generally try hard to communicate with others; for the psychotic, interpersonal contact is irrelevant.

Considering all the frustrations aphasics encounter, we have often wondered why they do not behave in a more abnormal manner than they do. Indeed, their demeanor and social interaction, aside from the language impairment, are remarkably normal. Nevertheless, some individuals with aphasia do experience psychotic episodes and periods of severe depression.

Language of Confusion

The *language of confusion,* according to Darley (1982), describes patients with irrelevant and confabulatory language, unclear thinking, reduced recognition of the environment, faulty memory, and disorientation to time and place. Syntax, word retrieval, auditory comprehension, and ability to repeat are usually not impaired. The patient's relatively good language is, therefore, unlike aphasia.

In persons who exhibit the language of confusion, the injury to the brain is widespread—usually bilateral—and often due to trauma. The following case example illustrates the irrelevance and confusion:

Tom Snively, a 20-year-old college junior, suffered a closed head injury in a skiing accident. He was in a coma for two weeks. Now, two months post onset, he is an inpatient in the Marquette Rehabilitation Center. When evaluated with a standard test of aphasia, Tom showed no disturbance of vocabulary or syntax; he did have some limited word-finding difficulty. The examiner noted, however, that the young man had trouble attending and staying in touch with the test situation. The patient tended to give responses that, although syntactically correct, were often irrelevant. Additionally, Tom was disoriented and particularly in response to open-ended questions gave rambling, fabricated answers. Here is a portion of an interview conducted by a medical social worker that reveals the patient's disorientation and tendency to confabulate:

WORKER: Where are you?

TOM: Ah, in training camp. Colorado Springs. And tomorrow we do time trials for the giant slalom.

WORKER: But, what is this place?

TOM: A training center. I had a hamstring pull and need whirlpool treatments.

In addition to language confusion and other cognitive symptoms, patients may show changes in personality as well. Areas to be assessed include orientation, memory, reasoning, story retelling, and verbal explanations, to name but a few. The speech-language pathologist may wish to select from tests presented in Table 8.5. Regarding prognosis, the confusion may range from mild and temporary, such as in concussion or hypothermia, to profound and chronic, as in head injury or drug overdose.

Language of Generalized Intellectual Deterioration

Dementia refers to a group of disorders that feature generalized intellectual decline. The deterioration of emotional control, cognitive skills, and language use is caused by diffuse, bilateral subcortical and cortical brain injury or atrophy. Dementia is caused by, among other factors, infectious diseases, tumor, multiple strokes, and Parkinson's and Alzheimer's diseases. Unlike language confusion, dementia often has a gradual, insidious onset.

Before a clinical diagnosis of dementia can be confirmed, several key features must be present (Berg et al., 1982):

1. A sustained deterioration of *memory,* plus a disturbance in at least three of the following areas: (a) orientation in time and place; (b) judgment and problem solving (dealing with everyday situations); (c) community affairs (shopping, handling finances); (d) home and avocations; and (e) personal care
2. A gradual onset and progression
3. A duration of at least six months or longer.

Generalized intellectual decline and cognitive dysfunction are hallmarks of dementia that are evident in the patient's overt language. Table 8.6 highlights differences between dementia and aphasia (Bayles & Kaszniak, 1987; Rosenbek, LaPointe, & Wertz, 1989).

In order to illustrate the salient behavioral and communicative symptoms observed in dementia, we include a portion of a diagnostic report on a patient in the second phase of Alzheimer's disease (Powell & Courtice, 1983):

This 64-year-old patient manifested the following behaviors: lowered drive and energy level; memory loss; slow reaction time; and difficulty making decisions.

ASSESSMENT OF APHASIA AND ADULT LANGUAGE DISORDERS **243**

Table 8.6 Cognitive and Communicative Differences between Aphasia and Dementia

VARIABLE	APHASIA	DEMENTIA
Progression	Rapid onset; improvement typical	Slow onset; progressive deterioration
Cognition	Generally intact	Mildly to profoundly impaired; worsens with the condition; poor problem-solving
Memory	Generally intact	Mildly forgetful to profoundly impaired or amnesic; worsens with the condition
Emotionality	Mood typically appropriate with occasional periods of depression or frustration	Typically labile, apathetic and withdrawn; intermittently shows agitation; can exhibit depression or mania
Pragmatics	Socially appropriate skills are evident despite some comprehension failures; communication efforts typically show relevance	Mildly to severely affected; inappropriate behaviors and irrelevant comments typical; disorganized thought processes
Repetition Ability	Slightly to severely impaired	Generally intact unless the condition is severe
Semantics	Word retrieval difficulties can be mild to severe; semantic and literal paraphasias may be used	Ranges from mild word retrieval difficulties to visual misrecognitions to severe vocabulary reductions
Syntax	Affected to varying degrees; can be classified as fluent or nonfluent based on length of utterance	Intact when disorder is mild; reduction of syntactic complexity as the disorder progresses
Phonology	Impaired in nonfluent aphasia; may be present as literal paraphasia in fluent aphasia	Generally intact unless the condition is severe; dysarthria possible

Her personality has changed in the past year so that now she typically is dull, bland, and unresponsive socially.

Mrs. Davis's language abilities are only mildly impaired at this time. She can match objects; point to and name pictures; and repeat words, phrases, and short sentences. Phonologically and syntactically, her speech is within normal limits. She does have limited output, however, and restricted usage. The patient's speech performance is slow and often, after trying to respond to a task, she will say, "I don't know."

The patient's language disturbance was more evident on tasks requiring greater intellectual effort and abstraction. For example, Mrs. Davis was unable to find and correct semantic errors in sentences ("My sister is an only child") or discern the ambiguity in sentences ("Visiting relatives can be a nuisance").

Unfortunately, a battery of language tests for evaluating dementia (and the subtypes or levels of dementia) does not exist. As Bayles states, "Clinicians must plan evaluations based on literature reports about the nature of such patient's intellectual and linguistic deterioration" (1984, p. 231). Areas to be tested in a battery for assessing the cognitive and communicative deficits in dementia might include memory, orientation, associative thought, intelligence, reasoning (both verbal and nonverbal), story retelling, object descriptions, explanations, and vocabulary. Many of the tests listed in Table 8.5 would be appropriate to use.

Right Hemisphere Impairment

Most individuals are left hemisphere dominant for language; yet, injury to the right hemisphere can cause communication deficits. According to Myers (1984), problems are mostly perceptual and prosodic. Linguistic deficits become apparent only with higher order, complex tasks. The communicative inefficiencies resulting from right hemisphere damage do not resemble aphasic symptoms. Table 8.7 summarizes deficits typically seen in patients with right hemisphere damage (Myers, 1984).

There is, as yet, no single test of right hemisphere communication impairment. Typically, speech-language pathologists and/or neuropsychologists form a test battery using selected subtests from standard tests of aphasia, learning aptitude tests, perceptual tests, and others (recall Table 8.5). Informal test items are also often part of the assessment battery. Of particular importance are the patient's abilities/disabilities with visuospatial perception, prosody, judgment, and high-level communication.

Table 8.7   Sequelae of Right Hemisphere Damage

General Symptoms

1. Neglect of the left half of space
2. Denial of illness
3. Impaired judgment
4. Impaired self-monitoring
5. Poor motivation

Visuospatial Deficits

1. Visual memory and imagery problems
2. Facial recognition difficulties (disorientation to person)
3. Geographic and spatial disorientation (to place)
4. Visual field deficits (especially left)
5. Visual hallucinations
7. Visuoconstructive deficits (constructional apraxia)

Deficits in Affect and Prosody

1. Indifference reaction
2. Reduced sensitivity to emotional tone
3. Impaired prosodic production and comprehension

Linguistic Deficits

1. Problems with figurative language (interprets literally)
2. Impaired sense of humor
3. Linquistic deficits, including
    Comprehension of complex auditory material
    Word fluency
    Word recognition and word-picture matching
    Paragraph comprehension
4. Higher order communication deficits, including
    Difficulty organizing information
    Tendency to produce impulsive answers with unnecessary detail
    Insensitive to contextual cues and pragmatic aspects of communication

Motor Speech Disorders

Motor speech disorders often coexist with language disorders, particularly aphasia. The presence of a speech disorder certainly affects the language treatment goals and procedures. For example, facilitative articulation techniques must often be incorporated into the total management program. The evaluation of a patient with brain damage, therefore, should include tasks to determine the existence of either *apraxia of speech* or *dysarthria*. We will discuss these disorders, and the process of differential diagnosis, in Chapter 9.

Determining the Type of Aphasia

Once the speech-language pathologist has narrowed down the diagnostic options and determined that the patient has aphasia, the next step is to decide which *type* of aphasia is exhibited. The characteristics of the various types of aphasia were summarized in Table 8.1. Communicative abilities and disabilities are considered in "fitting" the patient into a diagnostic category. Many of the published tests facilitate this decision-making process by profiling patient scores from the various subtests. Clinical experience and expertise are often invaluable, as well.

Summary

What is aphasia and what is not aphasia remain controversial, even among the experts. Many definitions of aphasia exist—some broad and all-encompassing and others quite specific and limiting. Speech-language pathologists will be wise to keep this in mind as they seek to differentiate aphasia from other speech and language disorders. In the final analysis, labels we use reflect speech-language diagnoses, not medical diagnoses. The evaluation process is likened to taking an inventory of the patient's communicative strengths and weaknesses; this can be done informally as well.

THE ART OF INFORMAL ASSESSMENT

Regardless of which standardized test the clinician administers, for treatment planning it is important to examine *how* the patient made the errors. Did the patient seem to perseverate? At what level of complexity did responses break down? Did the patient give synonyms or associations for words when asked to name pictures or objects? For example, when asked to name a picture of a dollar bill, a patient who says, "Put it . . . pocket . . . wallet . . . " is making a "better error" than a response of "soup" or "don't know." Was the patient attempting to correct the errors? Are responses significantly delayed? How did the patient respond to various cueing techniques? What strategies, if any, were used to assist in word retrieval—using gestures, writing, semantic, or phonetic cues? Answers to these questions are based more on clinician observations during the testing process than on test scores. Informal assessment with activities that probe treatment levels and cueing needs may be most insightful.

In evaluating a patient, it is not *necessary* to use a "test" at all; some speech-language pathologists prefer to rely on observation of the patient in the natural environment. The *Functional Communication Profile* (Taylor, 1963) and the informal assessment tasks prepared by Ulatowska, Macaluso-Haynes, and Mendel-Richardson (1976) are useful in providing a structure for observing the patient's communication abilities in real situations. Ideas may also be borrowed from the *CADL* (Holland, 1980), without actually administering the test, for clinical insights of the patient's functional use of language in contrived situations. Functional communication skills exhibited by the patient are relevant to designing treatment. Questions that should come to the mind of the clinician include: Which of the patient's strategies should be capitalized on and reinforced? Which can be made more effective? Which strategies are counterproductive and interfering? Should alternative modes of communication be employed to develop functional responding? The evaluation provides an excellent time to observe *patient-generated facilitation strategies,* such as gesturing an action to aid in word retrieval, finger tapping to pace speech production, requesting repetitions or using a delay to gain extra processing time, and the like. Also, before designing a management program, the speech-language pathologist must consider *characteristics of the stimulus* and which *cues and prompts* may be presented to the patient to increase the likelihood of response accuracy. Treatment probes to determine these things may be initiated during the evaluation stage but should continue to be used throughout the management program to maintain efficiency. (Patient progress is often uneven and "steps" in the program may be skipped from time to time.)

Characteristics of the stimulus affect the patient's ability to respond. The prevailing clinical assumption is that parameters of the stimulus can be hierarchically arranged to produce a level of responding that is not only continual but also correct (appropriate) more than half of the time (Marquardt, 1982). The writings of Darley (1976), Duffy (1981), and Marquardt (1982) provide good reviews of stimulus attributes and their therapeutic applications. Some general guidelines can be summarized here; the clinician may want to probe the patient's needs regarding these stimulus characteristics:

1. Presentation of a stimulus through more than one modality increases the likehood of a correct response. This also provides more contextual information.
2. Salient and nonambiguous stimuli affect performance positively—for example, large pictures without distracting backgrounds, or intense auditory stimuli with a favorable signal-to-noise ratio.
3. Reduced length and complexity of presentation, such as using short words or short and grammatically simple sentences, improves comprehension and production accuracy.
4. Presentation of stimuli at reduced rates for longer periods of time and with an imposed response delay affects performance favorably.

Various cues and prompts may be presented to increase the likelihood of response accuracy. These may be provided by the clinician initially and later, through training, may be faded from use or become self-generated cues, thus

Table 8.8   A Hierarchy for Word Retrieval

Step 1.   "Say (word)." (Patient imitates.)
Step 2.   Sentence completion with first and second phonemes supplied (e.g., You sleep in a be ____.).
Step 3.   Sentence completion with first phoneme supplied (e.g., You sleep in a b____.).
Step 4.   Sentence completion with first phoneme silently articulated [e.g., You sleep in a . . . (form /b/ on lips)].
Step 5.   Sentence completion (e.g., You sleep in a ____.).
Step 6.   State function, demonstrate function, and supply a carrier phrase (e.g., You sleep on it . . . motion sleep . . . it's a ____.).
Step 7.   State function and supply a carrier phrase (e.g., You sleep on it; it's a ____.).
Step 8.   Direct the patient to demonstrate the function (e.g., Show me what you do with it.).
Step 9.   Direct the patient to state the function (e.g., What do you do with this?).
Step 10.   Request the name (e.g., What's this?).

helping the patient become a self-sufficient, functional communicator. McDearmon and Potter (1975) categorized types of cues and their work should be consulted by the interested reader. "Associational" cues include such things as the use of sentence completion, first sounds, function, or rhyme to trigger word retrieval. "Symbolic" prompts are written, printed, or spoken words, whereas "realistic" prompts show attributes of the stimulus. Examples of realistic prompts include a picture of an object, the object itself, or sensory properties of the stimulus, such as the ticking of a clock to evoke the response "clock" or the feel of water to evoke its name. Cueing characteristics and optimal hierarchies are an often researched area in aphasiology. Table 8.8 lists a 10-level cueing hierarchy, based on the work of Linebaugh and Lehner (1977), which is useful in assisting patients with word retrieval problems. Cue the patient at the highest step possible to initially aid in word recall and back down the steps, supplying more assistance, as needed. Table 8.9 explains strategies suggested by Whitney (1975) that might prove helpful during the informal assessment and that later can be integrated into treatment. We have often used such stop-and-go strategies to elicit optimal, elaborate, on-target responses from our patients in both assessment and treatment situations.

SUMMING UP THE FINDINGS

Patient abilities and disabilities are determined through the formal and informal evaluation process. Such information permits the SLP to diagnose the type of aphasia (or other communication disorder), if any. The diagnostic label is useful as a "summary statement." The information collected is used in determining the patient's prognosis for recovery. Furthermore, it shapes the direction that treatment will take. Of course, the ultimate goal of evaluation and diagnosis is to ensure that the patient's symptoms are managed appropriately.

Prognosis

Selecting patients for treatment who have the best chance of recovery from aphasia is an unsettling task. Rather than abandon anyone, the clinician's

Table 8.9 Compensatory Strategies for Aphasia

Comprehension Strategies

1. Repeat the utterance for the patient; later have the patient assume the responsibility of requesting repeats.
2. Augment verbal material with the same information in writing; patient eventually should ask for material to be written if this modality aids comprehension.

"Stop" Strategies

These strategies are useful with patients who have fluent aphasia. They assist in controlling fluency and monitoring empty speech or paraphasic errors.

1. Clinician can model a slow rate of speech and monitor the patient's pace, stopping to correct when needed.
2. Encourage the patient to listen to himself/herself. Frequent verbal reminder to "listen" may be employed.
3. Clinician may need to actively stop the patient's speech output. This can be done by touching the lips, saying "stop," using a gesture signal (such as hand up) or any combination of these that successfully terminate the jargon. Fading of the stop cue should be incorporated into the treatment plan.
4. Encourage self-correction in the patient. Direction to use another strategy, such as a word retrieval technique, may be helpful.

"Go" Strategies

These strategies are useful with patients who have nonfluent aphasia. Go strategies encourage the patient to keep communication going by using telegraphic speech, gestures, or graphics on which to expand.

1. Get the patient started; the clinician can suggest a gesture or "key word" to initiate a telegraphic response.
2. Keep the patient going; the clinician can replay or feed back to the patient what was initially said and encourage expansion or elaboration.

---

impulse is to attempt to work with every aphasic even though prospects for improvement in cases of severe language impairment are dim (Sarno, Silverman, & Sands, 1970). When there is little real progress, the patient's labors are like those of Sisyphus.

How, then, can the SLP identify aphasic patients with the best potential? A list of interrelated factors that we have found helpful for making a prognosis is presented here; however, we trust the reader's forecasting will be guided by three important maxims: (1) Do not make a final prognosis on the basis of a single evaluation session—a period of trial therapy is always highly informative; (2) do not make a prognosis solely on the basis of a single measure of behavior (such as one test); and (3) be sure you understand the value of predictors—they can be potent self-fulfilling prophecies.

1. *Initial Severity:* Initial severity of aphasia is the single best predictor of recovery, according to Kertesz (1979). The more severe the patient's language impairment is at the time of assessment, the poorer the prognosis. Three aspects of language functioning are particularly important in predicting recovery:

- *Auditory recognition.* Patients who make errors (even a few errors—two or three out of 10 items—are significant) when identifying pictures or common objects named by the examiner have an unfavorable prognosis; an impairment at this level is apparently irreversible (Schuell, 1973).

- *Comprehension.* Patients who have marked difficulty in comprehending verbal messages make poor candidates for treatment. In fact, a reliable index of the severity of language impairment in aphasia is the degree of disturbance in comprehension (Schuell, 1973).
- *Speech fluency.* Patients who speak more fluently seem to make better recoveries. But the presence of jargon, especially when it is coupled with lack of self-monitoring, euphoria, or denial, is a poor clinical sign.

2. *Time Elapsed since Onset:*   Many studies have concluded that patients who receive language treatment before six months have elapsed since the cerebral insult show the most significant gains in treatment. The longer the time elapsed since onset of aphasia and the beginning of treatment, the poorer the prognosis (Fitch-West, 1984). Habits of dependence, withdrawal, and possible secondary gains accruing from a nonverbal role tend to defeat therapeutic intervention.

3. *Type of Aphasia:*   Recovery of aphasia seems to follow a pattern of evolution (Kertesz, 1979). Progress in global aphasia is often poor, but when improvement occurs it is toward the symptoms of Broca's aphasia. Broca's aphasia typically shows fair-to-good recovery; when symptoms diminish, the patient usually retains word-retrieval difficulty and dysfluency. Wernicke's aphasia carries a split prognosis, with some patients doing fairly well and others poorly. Although the symptoms of Wernicke's aphasia often persist, recovery can occur with symptoms evolving toward conduction or anomic types of aphasia. Conduction aphasia improves toward symptoms of anomic aphasia or may recover completely. Anomic aphasia also shows complete recovery or recovery with only the persistence of mild word-retrieval difficulties.

4. *Etiology:*   Depending on the location and extent of the lesion, patients who have suffered traumatic brain injury tend to make better recoveries than do individuals who have had thrombotic or other vascular episodes and tumors (Rosenbek, LaPointe, & Wertz, 1989).

5. *Age:*   The importance of age as a prognostic variable is not clear, as it often overlaps with factors such as etiology. For example, trauma patients tend to be younger than CVA patients. However, it can generally be said that younger patients recover faster and more adequately than do older patients. Presumably this is because younger brains show more plasticity and older patients may have more widespread cerebral damage due to arteriosclerosis. In addition, aphasic patients in or near retirement may lack the energy and motivation to persist in a treatment program.

6. *Presence of Other Health Problems:*   In our clinical experience, aphasic patients presenting health problems in addition to the brain injury (such as diabetes, systemic vascular disease, or kidney disease) often do poorly in treatment.

7. *Family Response:*   Patients whose families provide supportive understanding and appropriate stimulation and permit the individual to regain his/her role within the family unit have a more favorable prognosis.

8. *Extent of the Lesion:* The more extensive the brain injury, the poorer the prospects for recovery.

9. *Location of the Lesion:* This variable overlaps with type of aphasia. In general, damage occurring posterior to the fissure of Rolando, especially at the junction of the parietal and temporal lobes, tends to result in more persistent aphasia (Fitch-West, 1984).

10. *Premorbid Personality:* The more outgoing, flexible individual generally responds better to treatment than does an inhibited, introverted person. Personality and temperament are often said to have altered as a result of brain damage. Behavior patterns seen in some aphasic patients have been labeled "egocentricity," "catastrophic response," "concretism," and the like. Despite the tremendous frustration and alteration in self-concept that aphasia produces, most of our clients have not exhibited much change in their basic personality traits.

11. *Intelligence and Education:* The more intelligent, better educated patients make better candidates for treatment. Although this is generally true, a few of our most highly educated patients were so vividly aware of the discrepancy between their premorbid abilities and their present condition, they simply withdrew in futility.

12. *Self-Monitoring:* Patients who are aware of their errors and attempt to correct them have a more favorable prognosis than those who do not.

13. *Handedness:* Left-handed patients have better prognoses than right-handed ones (Fitch-West, 1984). However, it may be that left-handed individuals are more likely to become aphasic regardless of which hemisphere of the brain is damaged, suggesting that left-handers show bilateral language representation.

The reader may want to consult the following references for further information regarding prognosis in aphasia: Keenan and Brassell (1974), Kertesz and McCabe (1977), Marshall and Phillips (1983), Fitch-West (1984), and Crary and Haak (1988).

Early Intervention

We cannot overemphasize the critical importance of early intervention in the clinical management of aphasic clients; this position becomes obvious when we consider that aphasia is a personal and family catastrophe (Buck, 1968). Early support and counseling for the patient and for the family are greatly needed. Early initiation of language stimulation is also wise. We offer the following five concluding points for consideration in early intervention with acute patients: (1) Nurses and others who work with the patient should receive inservice training on how to deal adequately with aphasic patients. Consult the work of Leutenegger (1975) and Haynes and Greenberg (1976) for useful material for inservice training. (2) There should be information-sharing and planning conferences with professional team members—the physician, physical therapist, occupational therapist, social worker, and others concerned with the rehabilitation of the patient. (3) Supportive interviews with the aphasic patient should be conducted to provide release of feelings and to offer reassurance that a professional clinician is concerned and attempting to do something about the language problem. (4) Family counseling is most important. Families are confronted with a crisis when an adult member is suddenly afflicted with a potentially deadly, often mysterious illness that results in such profound physical and psychological alterations. A serious illness disrupts communication patterns, dissolves or shifts roles, and forces family members to assume unfamiliar responsibilities. The resolution of the crisis situation and the manner in which members reorganize the family structure will have profound implications for the patient's rehabilitation (Kinsella & Duffy, 1978). The maintenance of a supportive, nonthreatening environment for the brain-injured patient is crucial to recovery. (5) Last, design a treatment program that is appropriate for the patient and modify it as the patient's abilities and disabilities change. With recovery from brain damage, the patient's symptoms will evolve, making dynamic treatment with frequent reassessments a necessity.

A discussion of treatment philosophies and treatment approaches is beyond the scope of this book. The reader is encouraged to consult many of the fine books on the clinical management of adult communication deficits. Among them are Schuell, Jenkins, and Jimenez-Pabon (1964); Jenkins et al. (1975); Johns (1978); Rosenbek, LaPointe, and Wertz (1989); Chapey (1981); Eisenson (1984); Davis and Wilcox (1985); and Shewan and Bandur (1986).

BIBLIOGRAPHY

ADAMOVICH, B. B., & HENDERSON, J. A. (1985). *Assessment of cognitive abilities.* In B. B. Adamovich, J. A. Henderson, and S. Auerbach (Eds.), *Cognitive rehabilitation of closed head injured patients.* San Diego, CA: College-Hill Press.

ALEXANDER, D. A. (1973). Some tests of intelligence and learning for elderly psychiatric patients: A validation study. *British Journal of Social and Clinical Psychology, 12,* 188–193.

BAKER, H. J., & LELAND, B. (1959). *Detroit Test of Learning Aptitude.* Indianapolis, IN: Bobbs-Merrill.

BAYLES, K. A. (1984). Language and dementia. In A. L. Holland (Ed.), *Language disorders in adults: Recent advances.* San Diego, CA: College-Hill Press.

BAYLES, K. A., & KASZNIAK, A. W. (1987). *Communication and cognition in normal aging and dementia.* San Diego, CA: College-Hill.

BENTON, A. L. (1974). *Revised Visual Retention Test: Clinical and experimental application* (4th ed.). New York: The Psychological Corp.

BERG, L., HUGHES, C. P., COBEN, L. A., DANZIGER, W. L., & MARTIN, R. L. (1982). Mild senile dementia of Alzheimer type: Research diagnostic criteria, recruitment, and description of a population study.

Journal of Neurology, Neurosurgery and Psychiatry, 45, 962–968.

BLESSED, G., TOMLINSON, B. E., & ROTH, M. (1968). The association between quantitative measures of dementia and of senile change in the cerebral grey matter of elderly subjects. *Journal of Psychiatry, 114,* 797–811.

BORKOWSKI, J. G., BENTON, A. L., & SPREEN, D. (1967). Word fluency and brain damage. *Neuropsychologia, 5,* 135–140.

BUCK, M. (1968). *Dysphasia.* Englewood Cliffs, NJ: Prentice Hall.

BUROS, O. (Ed.). (1978). *The Eighth Mental Measurements Yearbook* (Vol 2). Highland Park, NJ: Gryphon Press.

CHAPEY, R. (1981). *Language intervention strategies in adult aphasia.* Baltimore: Williams & Wilkins.

CRARY, M., & HAAK, N. J. (in press). *Acute Aphasia Screening Test.* New York, NY: The Psychological Corp.

CRARY, M. A., & HAAK, N. J. (1988). One perspective on recovery in aphasia. *NSSLHA Journal, 16* (1), 76–92.

DARLEY, F. L. (1976). Maximizing input to the aphasic patient: A review of research. In R.

Brookshire (Ed.), *Clinical aphasiology conference proceedings*. Minneapolis, MN: BRK Publishers.

DARLEY, F. L. (1979). *Evaluation of appraisal techniques in speech and language pathology*. Reading, MA: Addison-Wesley.

DARLEY, F. L. (1982). *Aphasia*. Philadelphia: W. B. Saunders.

DAVIS, G. A. (1983). *A survey of adult aphasia*. Englewood Cliffs: NJ: Prentice Hall.

DAVIS, G. A., & WILCOX, M. J. (1985). *Adult aphasia rehabilitation: Applied pragmatics*. San Diego, CA: College-Hill Press.

DeRENZI, E., & VIGNOLO, L. A. (1962). The Token Test: A sensitive test to detect receptive disturbances in aphasics. *Brain, 85*, 665–678.

DERMAN, S., & MANASTER, A. (1967). Family counseling with relatives of aphasic patients. *Journal of American Speech and Hearing Association, 8*, 175–177.

DiSIMONI, F. G., KEITH, R. L., & DARLEY, F. L. (1980). Prediction of PICA overall score by short versions of the test. *Journal of Speech and Hearing Research, 23*, 511–516.

DiSIMONI, F. G., KEITH, R. L., HOLT, D. L., & DARLEY, F. L. (1975). Practicality of shortening the Porch Index of Communicative Ability. *Journal of Speech and Hearing Research, 18*, 491–497.

DUFFY, J. (1981). Schuell's stimulation approach to rehabilitation. In R. Chapey (Ed.), *Language intervention strategies in adult aphasia*. Baltimore: Williams & Wilkins.

DUNN, L. M., & DUNN, L. M. (1981). *Peabody Picture Vocabulary Test — Revised*. Circle Pines, MN: American Guidance Service.

EISENSON, J. (1984). *Aphasia in adults*. Englewood Cliffs, NJ: Prentice Hall.

EMERICK, L. (1971). *Appraisal of language disturbance*. Marquette: Northern Michigan University Press.

EMERICK, L., & COYNE, J. (1972). *Screening Test of Aphasia*. Danville, IL: Interstate Printers and Publishers.

EVANS, R., & NORTHWOOD, L. (1983). Social support needs in adjustment to stroke. *Archives of Physical Medicine and Rehabilitation, 64*, 61–64.

FITCH-WEST, J. (1984). Aphasia rehabilitation. In S. Dickson (Ed.), *Communication disorders: Remedial principles and practices*. Glenview, IL: Scott Foresman and Co.

FITCH-WEST, J., & SANDS, E. S. (1987). *The Bedside Evaluation Screening Test (BEST)*. Frederick, MD: Aspen Publishers, Inc.

FOLSTEIN, M. F., FOLSTEIN, S. E., & McHUGH, P. R. (1975). Mini-mental state: A practical method for grading the cognitive state of patients for the clinician. *Journal of Psychiatric Research, 12*, 189–198.

FROSTIG, M. (1963). *Developmental Test of Visual Perception*. Chicago, IL: Follett.

GOLDFARB, A. I., & ANTIN, S. (1975). Unpublished data. In R. Goldman & M. Rockstein (Eds.), *The*

physiology and pathology of human aging. New York: Academic Press.

GONZALES-ROTHI, L. J., COSTETT, H. B., & HEILMAN, K. M. (1984). *Battery of adult reading function*. Unpublished, experimental test of the Veteran's Hospital, Gainesville, FL.

GOODGLASS, H., GLEASON, J. B., BERNHOLTZ, N. D., & HYDE, M. R. (1972). Some linguistic structures in the speech of a Broca's aphasic. *Cortex, 8*, 191–212.

GOODGLASS, H., & KAPLAN, E. (1983). *The Assessment of aphasia and related disorders*. Philadelphia, PA: Lea & Febiger.

GRANGER, C., & ALBRECHT, G. (1979). Outcome of comprehensive medical rehabilitation: Measurement by PULSES Profile and Barthel Index. *Archives of Physical Medicine and Rehabilitation, 60*, 145–154.

GURLAND, B. J., COPELAND, J., SHARPE, L., & KELLEHER, M. (1976). The Geriatric Mental Status Interview (GMS). *International Journal of Aging and Human Development, 7*, 303–311.

HAGEN, C. (1984). Language disorders in head trauma. In A. Holland (Ed.), *Language disorders in adults: Recent advances*. San Diego, CA: College-Hill Press.

HALSTEAD, W. C., & WEPMAN, J. M. (1949). The Halstead-Wepman aphasia screening test. *Journal of Speech and Hearing Disorders, 14*, 9–15.

HARVEY, R., & JELLINEK, H. (1983). Patient profiles: Utilization in functional performance assessment. *Archives of Physical Medicine and Rehabilitation, 64*, 268–271.

HAYNES, W., & GREENBERG, B. (1976). *Understanding aphasia*. Danville, IL: Interstate Printers and Publishers.

HELMICK, J., WATAMORI, T., & PALMER, J. (1976). Spouses' understanding of the communication disorders of aphasic patients. *Journal of Speech and Hearing Disorders, 41*, 238–243.

HOLLAND, A. (1977). Comment on "Spouses' understanding of the communication disorders of aphasic patients." *Journal of Speech and Hearing Disorders, 42*, 307–308.

HOLLAND, A. (1980). *Communicative abilities in daily living*. Baltimore: University Park Press.

HOOPER, E. (1958). *The Hooper Visual Organization Test*. Los Angeles, CA: Western Psychological Services.

JENKINS, J., JIMÉNEZ-PABÓN, E., SHAW, R., & SEFER, J. W. (1975). *Aphasia in adults* (2nd ed.). New York: Harper & Row.

JOHNS, D. (1978). *Clinical management of neurogenic communicative disorders*. Boston: Little, Brown.

JOHNSON, G. O., & BOYD, H. F. (1981). *Nonverbal Test of Cognitive Skills*. Columbus, OH: Charles E. Merrill.

KAPLAN, E., GOODGLASS, H., & WEINTRAUB, S. (1976). *Boston Naming Test*. Philadelphia, PA: Lea and Febiger.

KEENAN, J., & BRASSELL, E. (1974). A study of factors related to prognosis for individual aphasic patients. *Journal of Speech and Hearing Disorders, 39*, 257–269.

KEENAN, J., & BRASSELL, E. (1975). *Aphasia language performance scales.* Murfreesboro, TN: Pinnacle Press.

KERTESZ, A. (1979). *Aphasia and associated disorders: Taxonomy, localization and recovery.* New York: Grune & Stratton.

KERTESZ, A. (1980). *Western aphasia battery.* London, Ontario: University of Western Ontario.

KERTESZ, A., & MCCABE, P. (1977). Recovery patterns and prognosis in aphasia. *Brain, 100*, 1–18.

KINSELLA, G., & DUFFY, F. (1978). The spouse of the aphasic patient. In Y. LeBrun & R. Hoops (Eds.), *The management of aphasia.* Amsterdam: Swets and Zeitlinger.

KIRK, S. A., MCCARTHY, J., & KIRK, W. D. (1968). *Illinois Test of Psycholinguistic Abilities.* Champaign, IL: University of Illinois Press.

LAPOINTE, L., & HORNER, J. (1978). The functional auditory comprehension task (FACT): Protocol and test format. *FLASHA Journal,* Spring, 27–33.

LAPOINTE, L., & HORNER, J. (1979). *Reading comprehension battery for aphasia.* Tigard, OR: C.C. Publications.

LEUTENEGGER, R. (1975). *Patient care and rehabilitation of communication impaired adults.* Springfield, IL: Charles C Thomas.

LEZAK, M. D. (1983). *Neuropsychological assessment* (2nd ed.). New York: Oxford University Press.

LINEBAUGH, C., & LEHNER, L. (1977). Cueing hierarchies and word retrieval: A therapy program. In R. Brookshire (Ed.), *Clinical aphasiology: Conference proceedings.* Minneapolis, MN: BRK Publishers.

MCDEARMON, J., & POTTER, R. (1975). The use of representational prompts in aphasia therapy. *Journal of Communication Disorders, 8*, 199–206.

MCNEIL, M., & PRESCOTT, T. (1978). *Revised Token Test.* Baltimore: University Park Press.

MARQUARDT, T. P. (1982). *Acquired neurogenic disorders.* Englewood Cliffs, NJ: Prentice Hall.

MARSHALL, R., & PHILLIPS, D. (1983). Prognosis for improved verbal communication in aphasic stroke patients. *Archives of Physical Medicine and Rehabilitation, 64*, 597–600.

MATTIS, S. (1976). Mental status examination for organic mental syndrome in the elderly patient. In R. Bellack & B. Karasu (Eds.), *Geriatric psychiatry.* New York: Grune & Stratton.

METTER, E. J., & HANSON, W. R. (1985). Brain imaging as related to speech and language. In J. K. Darby (Ed.), *Speech and language evaluation in neurology: Adult disorders.* Orlando, FL: Grune & Stratton.

MULLER, D., CODE, C., & MUGFORD, J. (1983). Predicting psychosocial adjustment to aphasia. *British Journal of Disorders of Communication, 18*, 23–29.

MYERS, P. S. (1984). Right hemisphere impairment. In A. L. Holland (Ed.), *Language disorders in adults: Recent advances.* San Diego, CA: College-Hill Press.

NATION, J., & ARAM, D. (1977). *Diagnosis of speech and language disorders.* St. Louis, MO: C. V. Mosby.

PLUTCHIK, R., CONTE, H., LIEBERMAN, M., BAKUR, M., GROSSMAN, J., & LEHRMAN, N. (1970). Reliability and validity of a scale for assessing the function of geriatric patients. *Journal of the American Geriatrics Society, 18*, 491–500.

PORCH, B. (1971). *Porch Index of Communicative Ability.* Palo Alto, CA: Consulting Psychologists Press.

PORTER, J., & DABUL B. (1977). The application of transactional analysis to therapy with wives of adult aphasic patients. *Journal of the American Speech and Hearing Association, 19*, 244–248.

POWELL, G., BAILEY, S., & CLARK, E. (1980). A very short form of the Minnesota Aphasia Test. *British Journal of Social and Clinical Psychology, 19*, 189–194.

POWELL, L., & COURTICE, K. (1983). *Alzheimer's disease.* Reading, MA: Addison-Wesley.

RAVEN, J. (1963). *Guide to using the coloured progressive matrices, Sets A, B, Ab.* London: H. K. Lewis.

REISBERG, B., FERRIS, S. H., & CROOK, T. (1982). Signs, symptoms, and course of age-associated cognitive decline. In S. Corkin, K. L. Davis, J. H. Growdon, E. Usdin, & R. L. Wurtman (Eds.), *Aging* (Vol. 19): *Alzheimer's disease: A report of progress.* New York: Raven Press.

ROSENBEK, J. C., LAPOINTE, L., & WERTZ, R. T. (1989). *Aphasia: A clinical approach.* Boston: College-Hill Press.

ROSS, J. D., & ROSS, C. M. (1976). *Ross Test of Higher Cognitive Processes.* Novato, CA: Academic Therapy Publications.

SARNO, M. T. (1969). *Functional communication profile.* New York: Institute of Rehabilitation Medicine.

SARNO, J., & SARNO, M. (1973). The Functional Life Scale. *Archives of Physical Medicine and Rehabilitation, 54*, 214–220.

SARNO, M. T., SILVERMAN, M., & SANDS, E. (1970). Speech therapy and language recovery in severe aphasia. *Journal of Speech and Hearing Disorders, 13*, 607–623.

SCHUELL, H. (1957). A short examination for aphasia. *Neurology, 7*, 625–634.

SCHUELL, H. (1966). A re-evaluation of the short examination for aphasia. *Journal of Speech and Hearing Disorders, 31*, 137–147.

SCHUELL, H. (1973). *The Minnesota Test for Differential Diagnosis of Aphasia.* Minneapolis, MN: University of Minnesota Press.

SCHUELL, H., JENKINS, J., & JIMENEZ-PABON, E. (1964). *Aphasia in adults.* New York: Harper & Row.

SHEWAN, C. M. (1980). *Auditory Comprehension Test for Sentences.* Chicago, IL: Biolinguistics Clinical Institutes.

SHEWAN, C. M., & BANDUR, D. L. (1986). *Treatment of aphasia: A language-oriented approach.* San Diego, CA: College-Hill Press.

SKLAR, M. (1966). *Sklar Aphasia Scale.* Los Angeles, CA: Western Psychological Services.

SPELLACY, F., & SPREEN, O. (1969). A short form of the Token Test. *Cortex, 5,* 390–397.

SPREEN, O., & BENTON, A. (1977). *Neurosensory center comprehensive examination for aphasia.* Victoria, BC: University of Victoria.

TAYLOR, M. (1963). *Functional communication profile.* New York: New York University Medical Center.

TIFOSKY, R. (1984). Assessment of aphasic disorders. In J. Eisenson (Ed.), *Adult aphasia.* Englewood Cliffs, NJ: Prentice Hall.

ULATOWSKA, H. K., & BOND, S. (1983). Aphasia: Discourse considerations. *Topics in Language Disorders, 3,* 21–34.

ULATOWSKA, H. K., FREEDMAN-STERN, R. F., DOYLE, A. W., MACALUSO-HAYNES, S., & NORTH, A. J. (1983). Production of narrative discourse in aphasia. *Brain and Language, 19,* 317–334.

ULATOWSKA, H. K., MACALUSO-HAYNES, S., & MENDEL-RICHARDSON, S. (1976). The assessment of communicative competence in aphasia. In R. H. Brookshire (Ed.), *Clinical aphasiology conference proceedings.* Minneapolis, MN: BRK Publishers.

ULATOWSKA, H. K., NORTH, A. J., & MACALUSO-HAYNES, S. (1981). Production of discourse and communicative competence in aphasia. In R. H. Brookshire (Ed.), *Clinical aphasiology conference proceedings.* Minneapolis, MN: BRK Publishers.

WECHSLER, D. (1955). *Manual for the Wechsler Adult Intelligence Scale.* New York: The Psychological Corp.

WECHSLER, D., & STONE, C. (1948). *Wechsler Memory Scale.* New York: The Psychological Corp.

WHITNEY, J. L. (1975). *Developing aphasics' use of compensatory strategies.* Paper presented at the annual convention of the American Speech and Hearing Association, Washington, DC.

WHURR, R. (1983). *Whurr Aphasia Screening Test.* London: M. Phil.

Wisconsin Division of Health. (1966). *Communication status chart.* Madison, WI: Division of Health.

9

MOTOR SPEECH
DISORDERS AND
THE ORAL EXAM

Motor speech disorders is an umbrella term that includes many diverse, neurologically based problems. Those that may come to mind first are the many adult dysarthrias. The cerebral palsies originate in infancy, and the speech impairment that may coexist with the movement disorder is also considered dysarthria. Neuromuscular difficulties may result in swallowing disorders or dysphagia, which may or may not co-occur with speech disorders. Then, there are the apraxias that may affect various parts of the body, in particular the control of oral muscles, leading to oral (nonverbal) apraxia or apraxia of speech (verbal apraxia). All in all we have our work cut out for us in this chapter! In order to adequately cover evaluation and diagnosis of such a broad spectrum of motor disorders, we will discuss each in individual sections of the chapter; furthermore, we will limit our discussion to disorders affecting the processes underlying speech. (Consequently, dysphagia will not be covered in this text.) This chapter also provides the logical place for the discussion of "how to do an oral-motor examination" of a patient. Information important to the diagnosis of motor speech disorders will come, in part, from the oral exam. We will, however, attempt to be generic in our discussion of the oral examination to make it applicable for clients of any age (child to adult) or with any speech-language disorder (e.g., articulation, cleft palate, dysarthria). With our territory now laid before us, let us begin our journey.

APRAXIA OF SPEECH IN ADULTS

The Greek word *praxis* means action. The performance of action can go awry with damage to the central nervous system, and the resulting disruption of movement control can affect various body parts and abilities (Wertz, LaPointe, & Rosenbek, 1984). Limb apraxia, constructional apraxia, and a myriad of apraxic conditions have been reported; we will focus our discussion on apraxia of speech with brief mention of its close cousin, oral (nonverbal) apraxia.

Cortical damage to the inferior-posterior region of the frontal lobe in the left (dominant) hemisphere can impair oral movements and, in particular, articulate speech production. This condition has been called by many names but is generally known as *apraxia of speech*. Controversy continues as to whether the disturbance in articulatory programming is the *same* as Broca's aphasia, a condition that *coexists* with Broca's aphasia, or a condition that can occur in *isolation* of language impairment (Benson, 1979; Johns & LaPointe, 1976; Martin, 1974). Prevailing opinion, and the perspective of this chapter, is that apraxia is a nonlinguistic speech disorder (Darley, Aronson, & Brown, 1975; Wertz, LaPointe, & Rosenbek, 1984). It can coexist with other disorders and is frequently observed in concert with aphasia and/or dysarthria. Wertz, Rosenbek, and Deal (1970) found that 65 percent of patients with apraxia of speech also demonstrated aphasia, 14 percent had a combination of apraxia, aphasia, and dysarthria, 13 percent had apraxia only, and 8 percent showed apraxia combined with dysarthria. As we shall see, the differential diagnosis of a patient is important in shaping the appropriate management program. Treatment strategies need to be tailored to the specific type(s) of speech motor programming deficit.

The Characteristics of Adult Apraxia of Speech

According to Kent and Rosenbek (1983), apraxia of speech is the impaired volitional production of articulation and prosody. The articulation and prosodic disturbances, however, do not result from muscle weakness or slowness, but from inhibition or impairment of the central nervous system's programming of oral movements. Wertz, LaPointe, and Rosenbek (1984) traced the evolution of our clinical knowledge regarding the characteristics of apraxia of speech and have discarded much of "what we thought we knew." They state that the salient, clinical characteristics of apraxia of speech are

1. Effortful, trial and error, groping articulatory movements and attempts at self-correction
2. Dysprosody unrelieved by extended periods of normal rhythm, stress, and intonation
3. Articulatory inconsistency on repeated productions of the same utterance
4. Obvious difficulty initiating utterances.

Many investigators have analyzed articulation error patterns of persons with apraxia of speech. Clinicians hold that substitution errors occur more frequently than do errors of distortion, omission, or addition. Perceptual studies support this observation but recent acoustical investigations suggest that articulatory distortions are more commonplace. This revelation challenges our traditional differential diagnostic guideline where we once said apraxics make substitution errors while dysarthrics make errors of distortion. Wertz, LaPointe, and Rosenbek (1984) conclude that, in general, apraxic errors are "in the ball-park" rather than being unrelated to the target sounds. Place and manner of articulation errors predominate (e.g., substitution of a /t/ for a /p/ or substitution of a stop for a fricative), and patients are more likely to substitute voiceless consonants for voiced ones (rather than the opposite). Sequencing difficulties have long been recognized in apraxia of speech. Anticipatory errors, where a phoneme is replaced by one that occurs later in the word (e.g., "lelo" for yellow), are more common than perseverative errors (phoneme replaced by earlier one as in "dred" for "dress"). Metathetic errors (switching phoneme positions as in "tefalone" for "telephone") occur infrequently. Articulatory complexity also affects apraxic errors. Consonant errors are more likely than vowel errors, and more errors occur on consonantal clusters than on single consonants. Affricates and fricatives are more often errored than plosives, laterals, or nasals.

Prosodic disturbances in apraxia of speech have been reported by Wertz, LaPointe, and Rosenbek (1984). These include a tendency toward equal stress, inappropriate pausing between syllables, restriction or alteration of intonational and loudness contours, and an overall slower speaking rate.

Wertz, LaPointe, and Rosenbek (1984) cite other influences on apraxic error patterns that are important to remember in assessing patients, selecting treatment stimuli, and organizing a treatment hierarchy. We list some of them here.

1. Articulatory accuracy is better for meaningful than nonmeaningful utterances. In testing, then, the use of nonsense syllables may lead to spuriously high error rates. Treatment stimuli should be meaningful.

2. Errors increase as words increase in length. Assessment tasks almost always include length comparisons such as having the patient say "zip–zipper–zippering."

3. Errors increase as the distance between successive points of articulation increases. The patient, therefore, is more likely to have articulatory difficulties saying, "school" than "stool."

4. Articulatory accuracy is better for automatic-reactive than for volitional-purposive speech. In fact, the concept of "volitional" movement appears central to many definitions of apraxia and to the process of differential assessment. The patient with apraxia often exhibits many motor sequences at the involuntary level but is unable to replicate them voluntarily. (Conversely, the dysarthric patient is consistent in movement problems.) In an evaluation, comparison of error rates is often done during automatic tasks like counting and naming the days of the week, and observing spontaneous reactions such as swearing or commenting "I can't say that" versus more purposive speech such as labeling, repeating, conversing, and the like.

5. Articulatory accuracy may be better with combined auditory and visual stimulation rather than using only one modality. In working with patients, then, the instructions often begin with "Listen and watch me."

6. Imitative accuracy is better than spontaneous accuracy.

7. Articulatory accuracy often improves with consecutive attempts at production.

Oral, nonverbal apraxia can be described as problems in making volitional oral movements in the absence of significant paralysis or paresis. For example, the patient may have great difficulty when asked by the clinician to "pucker your lips" but have no difficulty kissing his/her spouse as they part for the day. Apraxia of speech and this oral, nonverbal form of apraxia may coexist or occur independently of each other.

Case History and Prognostic Factors

As with any evaluation, we collect case history information on the patient suspected of having apraxia of speech. It should be pointed out that rarely do we know ahead of time that we are going to evaluate a patient with apraxia. More often than not, we are asked to evaluate a patient who sustained brain damage and a language assessment is of foremost importance. During the testing for aphasia, we may become aware of a motor speech impairment and test further to diagnose the specific nature and extent of the impairment.

Regarding case history information, marital status, place of residence, social networks, and the like may influence treatment. Prognostic significance has been attributed to some biographical data, such as age, education, premorbid handedness, occupational status at onset and highest occupational level achieved, and premorbid intelligence (Marquardt, 1982; Wertz, LaPointe, & Rosenbek, 1984).

Medical information helpful in making a differential diagnosis includes localization evidence of damage to the third frontal convolution and the presence of right hemiplegia. Medical data suggestive of a favorable prognosis are damage from a single episode (no previous history of brain damage), a small lesion confined to Broca's area, recent onset, and absence of coexisting medical/health problems.

The Evaluation of Apraxia

As mentioned previously, seldom do we know ahead of time that a patient is apraxic. The speech-language referral merely mentions a brain-damaged adult, so a multitude of coexisting problems *could* be present: aphasia, intellectual impairment, dysarthria, apraxia, and other possibilities. The job of the speech-language pathologist is to thoroughly evaluate the patient to identify problem areas as well as strengths. In this way, a diagnosis will be arrived at based on the patient's characteristics. It is necessary, therefore, that the clinician be knowledgeable about the characteristics of various speech-language disorders. The clinician should plan a battery of measures but maintain flexibility so that as the patient's performance unfolds, planned tests can be altered and additional items can be added to the battery. A typical starting point is elicitation of a spontaneous speech sample and the administration of an aphasia test (see Chapter 8 for possibilities). As suspicions of motor problems become apparent in the patient's speech attempts, the clinician alters testing plans to investigate in detail the possibility of a motor disorder. Both formal and informal

Table 9.1 Typical Assessment Battery
for the Evaluation of Apraxia

Spontaneous speech sample
Aphasia test
Intelligence, cognitive, memory tests, as needed
Articulation test
Oral-peripheral examination
Apraxia battery

measures can be used. Table 9.1 lists areas to include in a thorough evaluation (Marquardt, 1982; Wertz, LaPointe, & Rosenbek, 1984). Diagnostic questions should unfold in the mind of the clinician: Is there a clinically significant motor speech problem? If so, is it an apraxia or a dysarthria? Which type of apraxia does the patient have? Does the patient have mixed types of apraxia? Which kind of dysarthria is present? Are coexisting motor disorders present?

Several of the aphasia tests evaluate the articulatory agility, melodic line, phonemic difficulties, and oral-nonverbal skills of patients. The *Boston Diagnostic Aphasia Examination* (Goodglass & Kaplan, 1983) and the *Western Aphasia Battery* (Kertesz, 1980) are examples. Characteristics of apraxia may become evident through such testing of a patient. A spontaneous speech sample should be analyzed and an articulation test may be given as well. Of extreme importance is the oral-motor examination. The general oral peripheral examination, which we will discuss at the end of this chapter, is supplemented with motor and articulatory tasks to reveal volitional programming deficits. Such tasks or tests should address oral, nonverbal apraxia and apraxia of speech.

Let us now walk through this evaluation process as it relates to apraxia. Although several so-called tests of apraxia exist, few have adequate psychometric properties and normative data. Only one test is commercially available; others are published in professional journals. These tools therefore should be considered informal yet insightful, rather than formal, standardized tests. The tests available for evaluating apraxia of speech are listed in Table 9.2. Let us highlight the components of a few.

Early, modern attempts to evaluate oral and limb apraxia were developed by DeRenzi, Pieczuro, and Vignolo (1966). Their test included 10 oral and 10 limb items that patients were asked to perform on command or, if necessary, on imitation. Oral items included such gestures as "stick out your tongue," "whistle," "show how you would kiss someone," and the like. A three-point scale of response accuracy was used and limited norms were available for this test.

Darley, Aronson, and Brown (1975) modified the oral apraxia portion of DeRenzi's test. The expanded version included 20 oral items, an 11-point rating scale of response accuracy, and the addition of the now-famous long words and phrases for eliciting articulatory difficulties (e.g., "gingerbread," "statistical analysis," "zip–zipper–zippering").

Rosenbek and Wertz (1976) expanded the verbal, oral, and limb battery still more. The oral and limb apraxia sections were not greatly modified;

Table 9.2 Formal and Informal Tests for Apraxia
of Speech in Adults

Test of oral and limb apraxia
   (DeRenzi, Pieczuro, & Vignolo, 1966)

Oral apraxia test
   (Darley, Aronson, & Brown, 1975)

Test of verbal, oral, and limb apraxia
   (Rosenbek & Wertz, 1976)
Apraxia Battery for Adults
   (Dabul, 1979)
An oral movement battery
   (Moore, Rosenbek, & LaPointe, 1976)
Tests of integrity and consistency of phoneme production
   (Johns & Darley, 1970)
Motor Speech Evaluation
   (Wertz, LaPointe, & Rosenbek, 1984)

---

an 11-point rating system was used. The verbal section, however, incorporated new tasks of vowel prolongation and imitation of syllable sequences, as well as the production of words and phrases. Responses were scored and analyzed for phonemic and prosodic errors.

Dabul (1979) published the *Apraxia Battery for Adults* with six subtests: diadochokinetic rate, increasing word length, limb apraxia and oral apraxia, latency and utterance time for polysyllabic words, repeated trials, and an inventory of articulation characteristics of apraxia. A variety of methods are used to score these subtests; scores are then used to complete a checklist of apraxia features and to rate the severity of the patient's impairment from mild to profound.

The *Motor Speech Evaluation* (Wertz, LaPointe, & Rosenbek, 1984) is useful in detecting the presence of apraxia of speech or dysarthria and in rating the severity of the condition. The evaluation includes the following tasks: conversation, vowel prolongation, rapid alternating movements, repetition of multisyllabic words, repeated production of the same word, repetition of words that increase in length, repetition of monosyllabic words that begin and end with the same phoneme, repetition of sentences, counting forward and backward, picture description, and oral reading. Several methods of scoring are suggested by the authors; however, severity is rated on a one to seven scale, with one being equivalent to mild and seven to severe.

The *Apraxia Battery for Adults* (Dabul, 1979) and the *Motor Speech Evaluation* (Wertz, LaPointe, & Rosenbek, 1984) are probably the most widely used instruments for the assessment of apraxia of speech. In using evaluation tools to diagnose a patient, we need to remember the important maxim: A test does not make the decision; a clinician does. There is an art to assessing the motor responses of patients on so-called tests of apraxia. Although attempts have been made to scale or rate the level of accuracy, all such scoring remains subjective.

The clinician has a responsibility to evaluate and interpret the patients' efforts competently.

Differentiating Apraxia from Other Disorders

As we stated earlier, apraxia of speech often coexists with other disorders of communication. Differential diagnosis of the many components of a patient's problem is of paramount importance.

Apraxia is often differentiated from aphasia on the basis of the patient's relatively normal auditory comprehension as compared to oral expression difficulties. In actuality, this differentiation is clear-cut for some forms of aphasia but is quite muddled for others. Recall that apraxia of speech often co-occurs with Broca's aphasia. Rosenbek, LaPointe, and Wertz explain the issue this way:

> Goodglass and Kaplan's (1983) rating scale of speech characteristics shows Broca's aphasic patients have disrupted melodic line and articulatory agility. We consider these signify disturbed prosody and the effortful, groping articulatory movements, articulatory inconsistency, and difficulty initiating utterances that constitute apraxia of speech. The short phrase length, disrupted grammatical form, tendency to produce primarily content words, word-finding problems, and mild auditory comprehension deficits represent Broca's aphasia. Thus, two disorders, apraxia of speech and Broca's aphasia, coexist. Some have difficulty in accepting the coexistence of disorders and elect to combine all symptoms into one disorder, Broca's aphasia. (1989, p. 88)

On occasion, patients with apraxia of speech have sufficient phrase length and grammatical form to appear somewhat "fluent," despite their prosodic and articulatory difficulties. Errors may mimic literal paraphasias. Table 9.3 summarizes symptoms that differentiate apraxia from fluent, conduction aphasia, as discussed by Rosenbek, LaPointe, and Wertz (1989).

Apraxia is differentiated from the language of confusion and generalized intellectual deterioration on the basis of more intact orientation, memory, and learning abilities. The reader should refer to Table 8.5 in Chapter 8 for examples of cognitive tests that might be used to make such a differential diagnosis.

Apraxia, classically, is differentiated from dysarthria by the preponderance of phonemic substitutions compared to distortion errors (Johns & Darley, 1970) and intact neuromuscular functioning with the exception of facial

Table 9.3 Differential Diagnosis of Conduction Aphasia and Apraxia

CONDUCTION APHASIA	APRAXIA
High proportion of sequencing errors	Low proportion of sequencing errors
Substitutions are unpredictable	Substitutions are predictable
Prosody intact	Abnormal prosody
Speech initiation easy	Speech initiation is difficult, often struggled
Associated with posterior brain lesion	Associated with anterior brain lesion

weakness and hemiplegia. Table 9.4 provides information useful in making a differential diagnosis of dysarthria and apraxia of speech.

Patients with apraxia of speech can generally anticipate their errors and can also recognize them once emitted. Perhaps this explains, in part, the many retrials and false starts heard in the speech of apraxics. The effortful articulatory groping and repetitive attempts may, at times, be reminiscent of stuttering secondary behaviors. This raises the question of a relationship between neurogenic stuttering (see Chapter 7) and apraxia of speech. Although we do not know the nature of this relationship, if any, it is worth considering in making a differential diagnosis.

> *Case Example.* Mr. Nils Elander was referred to the hospital-based speech-language pathologist for testing. Evidence from the neuroradiology department showed a left hemisphere thromboembolic infarct. Speech and language improvement was rapid during the two weeks postinfarct. A predischarge reevaluation

Table 9.4 Differential Diagnosis of Dysarthria and Apraxia

	DYSARTHRIA	*APRAXIA*
Definition	Distinct patterns of speech due to weakness, slowness and incoordination of speech muscles. Oral movements are disrupted and reflect different types of neuropathology	Articulation errors, in the absence of muscle slowness, weakness, incoordination, due to disruption of cortical programming for the *voluntary* production of speech sounds
Oral peripheral examination	Obvious defectiveness: slow, weak, and incoordinated. *Vegetative* functions (sucking, chewing) disturbed as well as speech movements	No obvious dysfunction except when requested to execute *voluntary* movements. Vegetative functions performed adequately
Articulation	Simplification a. distortions b. substitutions Errors consistent More complex units (clusters of consonants) are more difficult More errors in final position Errors consistent with neurological record Severity related to extent of neuromuscular involvement	Complication a. transpositions, reversals b. perseverative and anticipatory errors c. fewer distortions, more substitutions, intrusive additions Errors increase proportionate to word weight (grammatical class, difficulty of initial consonant, position in sentence and word length) Fewer errors in spontaneous performance Inconsistency is key sign
Repeated utterance	Same performance	Makes repeated attempts and may achieve correct performance. Appears to grope or struggle for correct production
Rate	Deterioration of performance with increased rate Slow rate of speech	Performance improves at faster rate Disturbances of prosody: stutteringlike struggle reactions; slow, labored speech during voluntary attempts
Response to stimulation	May alter performance slightly to match auditory-visual model. Best response to demonstration of specific articulatory gestures	Best performance if sees and hears model. Does better if provided one stimulation and given several chances to match the model

was performed by the clinician. Mr. Elander presented with mild Broca's aphasia and a moderate coexisting apraxia of speech. Numerous techniques were tried on a trial and error basis to see what stimulation and assistance aided Mr. Elander in initiating difficult words that occurred randomly, as well as at the beginning of utterances. The clinician was able to refer Mr. Elander for out-patient treatment at another facility. The report forwarded to that facility included specific recommendations as to the future direction of treatment. These recommendations included multimodality prestimulation, first phoneme cueing, and use of baton gestures or finger-tapping to impose rhythmical fluency.

DEVELOPMENTAL APRAXIA OF SPEECH

Developmental apraxia of speech is a poorly understood and controversial speech disorder in children. These children typically have little or no intelligible speech, yet they seem to possess adequate language comprehension skills and intelligence. Additionally, there is no clear evidence of muscular paresis or paralysis. The term *apraxia,* itself, emphasizes that these children have articulatory or motor programming deficits rather than any central language impairment. Presumably, the brain damage leading to these speech difficulties occurred before the onset of speech development, hence the diagnostic label of *developmental apraxia.*

Differential Diagnosis

Yoss and Darley (1974), in a classic article on the topic, reported that five predictors help differentiate developmental apraxia of speech from more typical "defective articulation " disorders. These predictors are

1. Neurologic findings, such as difficulty in fine motor coordination, gait, and alternating motion rates of the tongue and extremities (often manifested as a generalized dyspraxia)
2. Two- and three-feature articulation errors (for example, /p/ for /ð/ involves an error in place, voicing, and continuancy), prolongations and repetitions of sounds and syllables, distortions, and additions in repeated speech tasks
3. Distortions, omissions, additions, and one-place errors in spontaneous speech
4. Slower than normal rate on measurements of oral diadochokinesis
5. Poor maintenance of syllable sequences and shapes; polysyllabic words altered by addition, omission, or revision of syllables.

Yoss and Darley also reported that children with developmental apraxia of speech make more errors involving the voiced/voiceless feature than do children with defective articulation and that slower rates and equalization of stress patterns disrupt prosody. They often found coexisting oral apraxia in the children, as evidenced by difficulty performing volitional oral movements, such as puckering or biting the lower lip.

Crary (1988) elaborates on the symptomatology, stating that children with developmental apraxia exhibit slow and irregular alternating motion rates (diadochokinesis). They possess a reduced sound inventory, including vowels, and have obvious prosodic deficits, including slow rate, excess stress, prolonged sounds and pauses, postural/articulatory groping, and unusual intonational contours.

Other authors have cited nasal resonance and nasal emission as characteristics of developmental apraxia of speech (Hall, Hardy, & LaVelle, 1990; Morley, 1957). Presumably, the velopharyngeal mechanism performs inadequately during complex, rapid, sequential speech. Nasality, then, is more pronounced during conversational speech as opposed to single-word utterances.

Prognosis

Yoss and Darley (1974), after reviewing the literature and case study presentations, report that treatment involves "an inordinate amount" of time with minimal improvements being achieved. The children reportedly seldom carry over to contextual speech the level of self-monitoring attained at the syllable and single-word levels in the treatment program. Sequencing difficulties, at the heart of the disorder, appear to hinder progress in all realms.

Blakeley (1983) believes that parents should be advised of the nature and severity of their child's apraxia of speech and given an estimate of the number of years that speech habilitation may take. Blakeley states that three to 10 years of treatment are likely. As adults, these individuals may continue to have difficulty with motorically complex words.

Crary (1988) also discussed the prognosis for the future of a child with developmental apraxia of speech. He says that about 40 to 50 percent of these children are at risk for subsequent academic difficulties. Reading and writing skills seem to be particularly affected.

Case History Indicators

Square and Weidner (1981) reviewed case history information on children diagnosed as having developmental apraxia of speech and found some commonalities. Parents reported that auditory responses of the infants seemed normal but early vocal patterns were suspect. The parents often said little, if any, babbling occurred. If babbling was done by the infant, parents reported its phonetic pattern to have been undifferentiated. The infant was often described as a "quiet baby." Feeding differences were also reported by the mothers. Babies were said to prefer liquids and soft foods. Some were described as "lazy chewers." As regards general motor development, reports suggest clumsiness, developmental immaturity, and possible "soft" neurological signs. As a toddler, there remained little or no attempt to imitate sounds or words.

Assessing Developmental Apraxia

Miller (1986), recognizing the ill-defined nature of developmental apraxia, states that assessment is a process of excluding other disorders and including, or identifying, apraxic signs and symptoms. Miller calls for a multidisciplinary evaluation of the child. The medical evaluation will seek to exclude other causes of the motor impairment, such as neoplastic disease, degenerative conditions, cerebral palsy, acquired CNS damage, and the like. The psychological evaluation will exclude general mental retardation, autism, and behavioral-emotional problems (however, it is recognized that behavioral problems are often a consequence of the child's apraxia). The primary sensorimotor evaluation will exclude problems of muscular tone, strength, speed, and sensation. Miller goes on to discuss numerous subtests that may be part of an extensive assessment battery. The interested reader is referred to this detailed discussion.

Crary (1988) suggests areas important for the speech-language pathologist to tap in the assessment of developmental apraxia of speech. We have summarized these areas into a list, displayed in Table 9.5. We concur completely with his evaluation suggestions.

Let us now describe the assessment procedure advocated by Square and Weidner (1981). Pertinent topics to discuss with parents in the case history interview include the early vocal patterns used during infancy (babbling), feeding difficulties, and general motor development. The evaluation of the child incorporates both speech and nonspeech tasks. Regarding speech tasks, a spontaneous speech sample should be analyzed. A traditional articulation test may be given, as well as the spontaneous "tell a story" version available with many articulation tests. Next, the clinician engages the child in various repeated speech tasks. Have the client repeat CVC words using frequently occurring and complex consonants, such as /f, k, l, r, z, s, v, g, ʃ, θ, +ʃ, ʒ/. Sample CVC words include: lake, sack, shoes, thick, and chop. Next, have the client repeat CVC

Table 9.5 Areas to Assess in Developmental Apraxia

Motor Assessment
facial/limb praxis
oral apraxia on simple and complex tasks
lingua-mandibular and labial-mandibular synkinesis
velar function
oral reflexes
facial mimicry tasks

Motor-Speech Assessment
diadochokinesis
nasal resonance (and further tests, if noted)
standard articulation tests
phonological analysis (distinctive features and phonological error processes)

Prosody Assessment
stress patterns
intonation patterns
general fluency and articulatory flow

Language Assessment(s)
Auditory Memory Assessment

Table 9.6 Nonspeech Tasks for Assessing Developmental Apraxia

Volitional Oral Movements

    Stick out your tongue

    Try to touch your nose with your tongue

    Try to touch your chin with your tongue

    Bite your lower lip

    Pucker your lips

    Puff out your cheeks

    Show me your teeth

    Click your teeth together

    Wag your tongue from side to side

    Clear your throat

    Cough

    Whistle

    Show me that you're cold by making your teeth chatter

    Smile

    Show me how you would kiss a baby

    Lick your lips

Sequenced Volitional Oral Movements: Two Items

    Puff your cheeks, then smile

    Pucker your lips, then wag your tongue

Sequenced Volitional Oral Movements: Three Items

    Puff out your cheeks, show me your teeth, then pucker your lips

nonsense syllables using the same consonants. Using the carrier phrase, "I had a _____," have the client repeat polysyllabic words, such as butterfly, popsicle, hamburger, mosquito, basketball, firetruck, and so forth. Finally, do diadochokinetic testing, in the usual manner. The nonspeech tasks recommended by Square and Weidner are volitional oral movements and sequential volitional oral movements (both two- and three-item sequences). Table 9.6 lists some suggested nonspeech oral movements for the client to perform.

We would like to conclude this section with a reminder. In testing for developmental apraxia of speech, the clinician must, among other things, carefully observe the level of articulatory effort and the pattern of errors that the client makes. No test score will indicate a diagnosis of apraxia. The decision rests with the diagnostic skill, albeit somewhat subjective, of the speech-language pathologist.

THE ADULT DYSARTHRIAS

All the diverse structures and systems that combine to produce speech are planned and regulated by the nervous system. Any damage or disease involving this regulatory system may disrupt the processes of respiration, phonation, articulation, and resonation and thus ultimately affect the normally swift movements of the speech mechanism. Two types of motor speech disorders are apraxia of speech, which we have discussed, and dysarthria. Let us now turn our attention to a discussion of the clinical forms of dysarthria.

As defined by Marquardt (1982), *dysarthrias* are neuromuscular speech disorders arising from motor pathway damage at singular or multiple sites from the cortex to the muscle. The entire speech production mechanism, including respiratory, phonatory, articulatory, and resonatory processes may be affected (as in Parkinson's disease). Likewise, disruption may be confined to specific musculature (as in Bell's palsy of the face).

Differential Diagnosis

Novice clinicians often have difficulty differentiating the two motor speech disorders: apraxia and dysarthria. The underlying neuromotor impairment is clearly different and site of lesion knowledge will go far in sorting out the two possibilities. Yet, going only on clinical (behavioral) signs that the patient displays, the diagnosis is not clearly as clear-cut as many textbooks imply. Review Table 9.4, which lists distinguishing characteristics of patients with apraxia of speech and dysarthria. Complicating the differential diagnosis is the fact that the two disorders can co-occur.

Differential diagnosing also involves categorizing the patient's symptoms by type of dysarthria. Again, this often proves to be a difficult task for many clinicians, not just the novice student. The type of dysarthria demonstrated will depend upon the site of lesion within the motor pathways. The landmark investigation that delineated the types of dysarthria, prominent speech dimensions, and neurological disruption was conducted at the Mayo Clinic and published in the book *Motor Speech Disorders* (Darley, Aronson, & Brown, 1975). An understanding of the types of dysarthria is paramount to the assessment process and the differential diagnosis. Using the information from this book, we present a synopsis of the characteristics of each type of dysarthria. We are assuming, however, that the reader has an understanding of the nervous system and neuroanatomical terminology.

Flaccid Dysarthria. Flaccid dysarthrias result from disorders (or lesions) of the lower motor neuron system. The muscle-movement problem may be progressive, as in myasthenia gravis, or affect the bulbar motor units, as in the bulbar palsies. In bulbar palsy, a common form of flaccid dysarthria, the muscles are weak, hypotonic (flaccid), and hyporeflexive and may be atrophied. Spontaneous twitches or dimpling of the skin over the muscle may be noted (fasciculations and fibrillations). Often the bulbar palsy is due to damage of one cranial nerve, and the muscular problems are confined to the body region or group of muscles served by that nerve. For example, in facial palsy (also known as Bell's palsy), the damage to one of the facial nerves (cranial nerve VII) results in a drooping facial expression, inability to raise the corner of the mouth during a smile, infrequent blinking, lowering of the eyebrow, and inability to wrinkle the forehead on the affected side. In hypoglossal palsy, there is damage to cranial nerve XII, and the tongue becomes flabby, atrophied/shrunken, and wrinkled. The client will be unable to perform many of the tongue maneuvers asked during the oral peripheral examination. Damage may be due to multiple cranial nerve involvement as well. This type of flaccid dysarthria is known as generalized bulbar palsy. It would not be uncommon in this condition for the lips, tongue, jaw, velum, pharynx, and larynx to be affected in varying degrees.

Speech abnormalities that are often observed in the bulbar palsies include hypernasality, imprecise articulation of consonants, breathiness, monopitch, and nasal emission. Other characteristics are certainly seen in these patients. We have only attempted to highlight some of the most prominent.

Spastic Dysarthria. Spastic dysarthrias result from disorders of the upper motor neuron system, in particular, the pyramidal system. As a result, there can be whole extremity damage (as in cortical lesions) or generalized damage (as from lesions of the internal capsule). The damage may be unilateral, as often seen following a stroke where the patient has aphasia and hemiparesis, or the damage may be bilateral. If bilateral, we often use the classification *pseudobulbar palsy*, as the bulbar system is affected indirectly. Muscular symptoms include spasticity, weakness, limited range of motion, slowness of movement, and hyperreflexia.

Deviant speech dimensions include imprecise consonant articulation, monopitch, reduced stress, harsh voice quality, monoloudness, low-pitched voice, and slow speech rates. Again, we have only attempted to list some of the more prominent and severe symptoms.

Ataxic Dysarthria. Disease or damage to the cerebellum can result in ataxic dysarthria. In ataxia, there is inaccuracy of movement (affecting force, range, timing, and direction of movements), slowness of movement, and hypotonia (flabby muscles). Speech characteristics include imprecise consonant articulation, use of excess and equal stress patterns, and irregular articulatory breakdowns, among others.

Hypokinetic Dysarthria. Disorders of the extrapyramidal system, such as in the basal ganglia complex, often result in hypokinesia, a reduction of movement. A commonly encountered disease causing hypokinesia is Parkinson's. There seem to be six characteristic signs of hypokinetic dysarthria: (1) slowness of movement; (2) limited range of motion; (3) paucity of movement, where the patient may have difficulty initiating a movement and may experience false starts, arrests of movement, or even immobility; (4) rigidity or hypertonicity (may be intermittent); (5) loss of automatic aspects of movement; and (6) presence of rest tremors. Deviant speech dimensions often seen in patients with Parkinsonism highlight the movement difficulties of the hypokinetic dysarthrias. The most deviant are monopitch, reduced stress patterns, monoloudness, imprecise consonant articulation, inappropriate silences, and short rushes of speech. Other, less deviant characteristics exist as well.

Hyperkinetic Dysarthria.   Hyperkinetic dysarthrias result from disorders of the extrapyramidal system. The hallmark of these disorders is the presence of abnormal involuntary movements—some are quick movements and others are classified as slow. In the short space we have in this textbook, we cannot completely describe the numerous forms of both quick and slow hyperkinesias. The interested reader is urged to study further. We will, however, summarize some of the most distinguishing and deviant speech characteristics, averaged over the various subtypes. These include imprecise consonants, variable (or perhaps slow) rate, monopitch, harsh or strained voice quality, inappropriate silences, distorted vowels, and excess loudness variation.

Mixed Dysarthrias.   Mixed dysarthrias, as the name implies, result from involvement of several motor systems. Often mixed dysarthrias are associated with syndromes or particular diseases, such as amyotrophic lateral sclerosis, multiple sclerosis, and Wilson's disease. Due to the mixed nature of these dysarthrias, it is almost impossible to summarize characteristic speech disturbances. The reader is again urged to study this vast topic further. Books about adult dysarthrias include those by Darley, Aronson, and Brown (1975), Marquardt (1982), Perkins (1983), McNeil, Rosenbek, and Aronson (1984), and Yorkston, Beukelman, and Bell (1988).

The Appraisal of Dysarthria

As evident from the various speech characteristics associated with the types of dysarthria, the patient may have difficulty with any or all of the speech production processes. Consequently, the clinician must assess features of respiration, phonation, articulation, and resonation.

Such an appraisal follows along the lines of a voice evaluation. This topic will be dealt with more thoroughly in Chapters 10 and 12. Suffice it to say that we need to take note of any inhalatory noises, poor breath support, poor management of the airstream, abnormal vocal loudness and stress patterns, abnormal vocal pitch and inflectional patterns, and abnormal vocal-resonatory qualities.

Regarding the articulatory impairment that is often present in the dysarthrias, the clinician should analyze a sample of spontaneous speech and/or have the patient read aloud. Standard articulation tests, either single-word or sentence versions, are also useful in documenting phoneme errors. Distortion is the most common articulatory error in dysarthric speech. Unlike the difficulties seen in apraxia of speech, the imprecision of consonantal articulation is usually consistent in dysarthria.

In addition to the voice test (which includes appraisal of respiration, phonation, and resonation) and the articulatory assessment, a thorough evaluation of a patient with dysarthria should include an oral peripheral examination and a special "dysarthria test," which involves appraisal of both speech and nonspeech motor functions. So-called tests of dysarthria are helpful in assessing the severity of the disorder, as well as the type of dysarthria.

The 38 speech dimensions used in the original Mayo Clinic study may be rated by the clinician (Darley, Aronson, & Brown, 1975). A patient's speech performance is rated on each dimension using a seven-point equal-appearing interval scale of severity (1 = normal, 7 = very severe). The 38 dimensions pertain to pitch, loudness, vocal quality, respiration, prosody, articulation, and an overall or general impression of intelligibility and bizarreness.

Although there is no score or profiling system, per se, the clinician can match a patient's performance to the "standard" characteristics and thereby determine the type of dysarthria. We would add that the rating of all 38 dimensions is likely to be time-consuming.

The *Frenchay Dysarthria Assessment* (Enderby, 1980, 1983) profiles oral-motor performance for the various diagnostic categories, such as spastic—upper motor neuron, flaccid—lower motor neuron, extrapyramidal, cerebellar, and mixed neurological lesions. Clinicians may find this helpful in differential diagnosis decision-making.

The *Motor Speech Evaluation* (Wertz, LaPointe, & Rosenbek, 1984) is useful in detecting the presence of apraxia of speech or dysarthria. A severity rating is also generated on a one (mild) to seven (severe) scale. The components of this test were discussed earlier in the chapter as part of the adult apraxia section, and we will not repeat that information here.

The *Assessment of Intelligibility of Dysarthric Speech* (Yorkston & Beukelman, 1981) has the patient read words and sentences. Several measures can be derived, including intelligibility for single words, intelligibility for sentences, speech rate, rate of intelligible speech, rate of unintelligible speech, and a communication efficiency ratio. Classification by type of dysarthria is also possible with this test.

One diagnostic task to which many authorities attribute importance is that of diadochokinetic testing, also known as assessing alternating motion rates (AMRs). Darley, Aronson, and Brown (1975), in particular, state that the rhythm and speed with which alternating motion rates can be performed are helpful in sorting out the various types of dysarthrias. They acknowledge that differential diagnosis may be difficult from only a conversational sample of speech. AMRs, on the other hand, seem to "stress" the motor system and, consequently, reveal the difficulties of movement more clearly.

Diadochokinesis, or AMRs, typically involves the repetition of the sounds "puh," "tuh," and "kuh" as fast and evenly as possible. The instructions to the patient should stress this notion of "fast and even." Information that is important to the clinician includes the rate, regularity, and duration of the alternate movements of the articulators.

According to Darley, Aronson, and Brown (1975), a slow, regular diadochokinetic rate is highlighted in spasticity. For ataxia, alternate motion rates underscore the irregular breakdowns in articulatory precision. It is characteristic to hear fluctuating changes in the intervals between syllables, as well as variations in their duration and loudness. Rate of syllable production varies from normal to slow. In hypokinetic Parkinsonism, alternate motion rates may begin at a slow rate and then accelerate to a rapid, yet usually regular, rhythm. Imprecise articulation due to limited excursions of movement (i.e., hypokinesia) may produce the sound of a continuous blur. Hyperkinetic dysarthrias take on many different forms; AMRs are usually irregular, slow, and perhaps interrupted by arrests of speech.

We offer one final note about appraisal. The patient with dysarthria is not expected to have language, cognitive, intellectual, memory, or learning deficits unless such deficits are associated with the disease process that produced the dysarthria. The clinician, however, should be alert to deficits in these areas and include appropriate language-cognitive tests in the assessment battery, if necessary.

Prognosis

Marquardt (1982) states that no efficacy or prognosis studies have been completed for dysarthria. Prevailing thought, however, is that the prognosis is naturally worse when dysarthria is part of a progressive or degenerative neurological condition. Prognosis should be good when the extent of damage to the nervous system is limited. Also, prognosis would seem to be affected by the medical treatment applied. Although they do not cure the dysarthria, many pharmacological or surgical treatments can have enormous impact on the patient's motor functioning. Lastly, we believe that the emotional and environmental aspects of the patient shape treatment outcome.

> *Case Example.* A 49-year-old male was referred following a bilateral brain stem infarct with resultant quadriplegia and dysarthria. Appraisal procedures included case history, oral peripheral examination, acquisition of a speech sample, recording of a standard reading passage, and auditory testing. The oral peripheral examination revealed bilateral facial and velopharyngeal weakness and weakness of the left side of the tongue. Diadochokinetic rates, intelligibility of conversational speech, and intensity and frequency ranges were moderately reduced. Voice quality was breathy. A moderate bilateral sensorineural hearing loss was present. No cognitive or language deficits were evident from a mental status examination. Since there was no indication of hemispheric brain damage and the primary muscular deficit was weakness, the diagnosis was moderate flaccid dysarthria secondary to brain stem infarct. (Marquardt, 1982, p. 64)

CEREBRAL PALSIES AND DYSARTHRIA IN CHILDREN

Brain damage sustained before, during, or shortly after birth can produce movement disorders, known as *cerebral palsies.* Movement can be mildly affected or severely crippled. When the muscles underlying speech are affected, we may say that the person has dysarthria (a motor speech disorder) subsequent to the cerebral palsy.

Although various classification systems for cerebral palsy have been proposed, DiCarlo and Amster (1984) prefer the six principal symptom areas:

(1) Spasticity is characterized by hyperactivity of the stretch reflex. It is secondary to a lesion in the cerebral cortex that causes a loss of control and differentiation of fine voluntary movements with increased muscle tone. (2) Athetosis is involuntary writhing or squirming movements that are irregular, coarse, relatively continuous, and somewhat rhythmic. It is secondary to damage in the extrapyramidal system, often the basal ganglia complex. (3) Cerebellar ataxia is incoordination and poor balance due to cerebellar dysfunction. (4) Rigidity is a "lead pipe" characteristic of affected muscles and often resembles a severe form of spasticity. (5) Tremors, either athetoid or rigid, involve generalized trembling of the extremities. (6) Flaccidity, as a form of cerebral palsy, is due to damage to the sensorimotor cortex. Affected muscles are unable to contract except reflexively. Perhaps 90 percent of the cases of cerebral palsy are of the first three types, with spasticity overwhelmingly being the most common (DiCarlo & Amster, 1984).

Many excellent sources are available to the interested reader that thoroughly discuss the multiple aspects of cerebral palsy (Cruickshank & Raus, 1966; McDonald & Chance, 1964; Mysak, 1980).

The Assessment of a Child with Cerebral Palsy

All authorities on cerebral palsy strongly advocate the multidisciplinary approach to assessment, diagnosis, and intervention. Certainly the speech-language pathologist will not assess motor function and abnormal reflexology without the aid of a physical therapist or other health care professional. Such information, however, is necessary to shape the feeding and prespeech stimulation programs that the infant may need, the handling and positioning techniques that need to be applied, and the facilitating and inhibiting techniques that might be incorporated in the speech habilitation program.

The child with cerebral palsy typically presents with a host of impairments—orthopedic, sensory, intellectual, socioemotional, and so forth. Of interest for this chapter is the assessment of communication skills and deficits.

DiCarlo and Amster (1984) state that a review of the literature clearly documents that children with cerebral palsy (particularly athetosis) have higher auditory detection thresholds, poorer speech reception thresholds, and poor speech discrimination than do normal children. A complete audiological evaluation, then, should be part of every evaluation session.

Capute (1974) reports that about 50 to 60 percent of the cerebral palsied population show some degree of mental retardation, while the rest possess normal intellectual capabilities. Impaired language development, learning difficulties, and academic problems often occur in children with cerebral palsy. Etiological reasons may be numerous. Certainly, the speech-language pathologist must assess cognitive development and linguistic attainment in a cerebral palsied client. Procedures discussed in Chapters 4 and 5 should be utilized.

Speech is a dynamic process requiring highly skilled coordination of the articulatory movements for the production and sequencing of sounds into utterances. It is of no surprise, then, that speech impairments are common among children with cerebral palsy. Hopkins, Bice, and Colton (1954) state that about 70 percent of cerebral palsied children exhibit speech disorders; athetoid and ataxic forms seem to be particularly deleterious to speech. However, there appears to be insufficient evidence for the notion that these speech impairments are so distinctive as to justify the concept of *cerebral palsied speech.* This myth was laid to rest in Chapter 6 when we discussed articulatory and phonological speech disorders. The assessment tools discussed in that chapter are certainly applicable to the child with cerebral palsy. Respiration, phonation, and rhythm are likely to be affected as well and must be assessed by the clinician. The ultimate measure of speech effectiveness is its intelligibility; a severity rating scale may be one aspect of the assessment battery. Lastly, we would remind the clinician that an oral peripheral (oral-motor) examination be done. How to do this is the subject of our next section.

THE ORAL PERIPHERAL EXAMINATION

An examination of a client's oral cavity and surrounding area is a routine part of every speech-language evaluation. Regardless of the client's particular communication impairment, the findings of the oral peripheral examination may help shape a theory of etiology, diagnosis, and prognosis for change and provide a direction that the treatment should take. In order to avoid repetition in the chapters of this book, we thought it best to consolidate our discussion of the oral peripheral examination into one place. Since the oral peripheral examination not only looks at structures but also assesses the function of those structures from a motoric point of view, we thought it most appropriate to include our discussion in this chapter on motor speech disorders. Indeed, the oral peripheral examination is often called the oral-motor exam, a reflection of the importance of motoric integrity for normal speech production.

As we said, it is common practice to inspect a client's oral region to determine its structural and functional adequacy for speech. To provide an example of typical data gathered during an oral peripheral examination, we have included notes hastily scribbled during an evaluation of a nine-year-old boy with a hoarse voice and several articulation errors:

> Lips look okay. No asymmetry of face. Slight open bite; poor dental hygiene (lots of cavities and tartar build-up). Tongue has good mobility, no paralysis or sluggishness; can protrude, wiggle from side to side swiftly, and touch the alveolar ridge; can even curl and groove. Hard palate seems OK, no scars. Soft palate has good tissue supply; elevated fine, no asymmetry. Palatine tonsils are *really* enlarged, filling the whole isthmus between the fauces. Pharynx looks inflamed (possible postnasal drip?). Good gag reflex. Wonder why he has mandible thrust to left side on /ʃ/ and /tʃ/?

Note the systematic nature of the inspection. Although the period of observation was relatively brief—an oral examination is generally completed in less than two minutes—the clinician has a sound basis for making a referral to a laryngologist. Now we shall present a rather detailed procedure for conducting an oral examination.

Tools You Will Need

You will need a light source; a small flashlight is good (we avoid the head mirror because it makes us look like a physician). Next, we obtain a supply of wooden tongue depressors; the individually wrapped ones are best for sanitary purposes (it is curious that no one has yet invented a flavored tongue blade). Since we are living in the age of AIDS and other contagious diseases, the prudent clinician will wear sterile gloves, or at least use a finger cot, when palpating the roof of the client's mouth. Finally, your kit might include several pads of cotton gauze (for holding onto tongues), a few candy suckers, and a mirror.

For more elaborate or specialized examinations, additional materials may be needed. These might include cotton-tipped applicators, various flavor vials for taste sensation, oral stereognostic forms, bite blocks, a syringe of water, some cookies or crackers, and the like.

Areas to Be Assessed

It is important to be *systematic* and *swift* when conducting an oral examination. This demands considerable practice. Use every opportunity to scrutinize normal-speaking persons of all ages, not only to perfect your technique and observational skills but also to establish a frame of reference on the range of normal structural and functional variation. The following outline is presented as a guide for conducting a typical oral peripheral examination:

1. *Lips and Lip Movement:* Inspect the lips first for relative size, symmetry, and scars. Can the client smile, pucker his lips, and retract them? Can he close his lips tightly for the sounds /p/, /b/, /m/? Can he utter the nonsense syllable "puh" at least once per second (Fletcher, 1972)?

2. *Jaws:* Scrutinize the client's jaw in a state of rest; observe for symmetry. Can she open and close her mandible at least once per second? Does her mandible deviate to the right or the left on opening? Assess mandibular strength by having her attempt to open or move her jaw laterally against resistance.

3. *Teeth:* Inspect the client's bite during a state of rest. A normal dental bite is characterized by the upper incisors overlapping the lower incisors by not more than one half of their vertical dimension. Is there an open, under-, or overbite? Does the client have cavities, jumbled teeth, gaps between teeth, or more than the normal complement of teeth? Does he wear a dental prosthesis?

4. *Tongue:* Note the size of the tongue relative to the oral cavity. Observe for symmetry of structure and during movement. Is there any scarring,

atrophy, or fasciculations? Can the client protrude and retract her tongue, wiggle it from side to side, and touch the alveolar ridge without random movement or extraordinary effort? Inspect the tip of tongue and the frenulum for any evidence of tongue tie. (Some clients, especially those presenting with neuromuscular problems, may find it difficult to elevate the tip of their tongue to the alveolar ridge on command. We use a sucker, placing the moistened candy behind the upper incisors and encouraging the client to go after it. A spot of peanut butter or a tiny paper wedged high between the central incisors can also be used.) Can she trill her tongue when the mandible is stabilized? Test for diadochokinesis by having her utter "tuh"; can she say one per second? (Norms for diadochokinesis may be found in Bloomquist, 1950; Canning & Rose, 1974; and Fletcher, 1972. Fletcher's norms are commonly used.) Be sure to look for regularity as well as rate in any tongue movement task. Is there any evidence of tongue thrust? (An open bite might alert you to this possibility.) When she swallows does she have an exaggerated lip seal? Does her tongue protrude beyond the incisors? Is there no apparent bunching in the masseter muscle? (If the answers to these last three queries are positive, then the client may be a tongue thruster.)

5. *Hard Palate:* Note the shape (is it flat? high and arched?) and width of the hard palate. Are there any scars present? Is there any blue coloration to the palate? Can you palpate solid bone under the tissues at the palatal midline? Can the client produce /r/ and /l/?

6. *Soft Palate and Velopharyngeal Closure:* Inspect the velum for total size, scars, and symmetry of movement. Is it bifid? Look carefully for any variations in color, such as bluish borders or striations. Does the soft palate move back and up toward the posterior pharyngeal wall? What is the size of the velum relative to the depth of the pharynx (= effective velar length)? Estimate the location of the velar dimple (formed by the insertion of velar muscles) and calculate its distance along the velar length (80 percent is normal, less may indicate velopharyngeal inadequacy). Can you visualize lateral movement of the velum? Can the client whistle or puff up his cheeks? (Chapter 11 presents details of assessing velopharyngeal competency as it relates to hypernasality and nasal emission.)

7. *Fauces:* Inspect the pillars for scars, the status of the palatine tonsils, and the width of the isthmus. Check the general condition of the oropharynx.

8. *Others:* Observe the client's breathing during speech and at rest. Is there an obstruction of the nasal passages? Is the client a mouth breather? Observe the facial muscles: Is a nasolabial fold flattened? Does an eyelid droop (ptosis)? Is one side of the face smooth and devoid of normal creases? Is there anything unusual about the appearance of the individual's head or spacing of the facial features?

The preceding outline is typical of the methodical process that we do, albeit swiftly, with all clients. Several formalized procedures and recording forms have been developed to assess oral peripheral function for speech. The interested reader is referred to the popular works of Mason and Simon (1977), Dworkin and Culatta (1980), St. Louis and Ruscello (1981), Ruscello et al. (1982), and Siegel and Hanlon (1983).

There are other, perhaps less well-known, procedures that we would like to mention as well. Bosma's (1976) excellent tutorial article describes in detail the oral-motor actions necessary to speak, feed, and maintain the proper head and body positions. Bosma discusses the importance of a case history in the evaluation of oral-motor function and provides guidelines for a complete examination of the oral-motor system, including facial and suspensory muscles, tongue, pharynx, palate, submental muscles, and the craniocervical postural system.

Sonies et al. (1987) developed an oral-motor function scale that assesses three areas: oral anatomy, physiology, and speech. There are 10 categories covering these three areas and each is rated on a four-point severity scale (1 = normal, 2 = mild, 3 = moderate, 4 = severe). Some weighting of measures is done to obtain a profile of performance. Anatomy ratings include assessment of the appearance of facial bones, tissues, and oral facial symmetry. Physiology ratings include assessment of range of motion, strength, precision, and speed of lingual, labial, palatal, velar, and facial muscles along with assessment of oral sensation. Swallowing function, a subcomponent of the scale, is assessed from a questionnaire, an ultrasound visualization of the swallowing act, mealtime observations, and a medical history. Speech ratings include articulation, voice, fluency, and diadochokinetic rate.

It now may be obvious to the reader that some assessment scales are more detailed than others and that some seem to weigh heavily certain aspects of the total oral peripheral examination. This certainly is the case. If the clinician is interested in assessing swallowing function, then in addition to the scales mentioned, the works of Larsen (1972), Bell and Goepfert (1977), and Logemann (1983) should be consulted. Patients with motor speech disorders may need more indepth testing, as this chapter has pointed out. For example, oral-motor abilities of a patient with apraxia of speech may be appraised by the tests of Dabul (1979) or of Wertz, LaPointe, and Rosenbek (1984), whereas the *Frenchay Dysarthria Assessment* (Enderby, 1980, 1983) may prove useful with a dysarthric patient. Several informal assessment instruments purport to test the integrity of the cranial nerves. Examples of such cranial nerve batteries are the *Bulbar-Cranial Nerve Examination* (Rancho Los Amigos Hospital, 1966) and the example protocol provided by Marquardt (1982). Likewise, clinicians working in cleft palate centers typically have examination forms specific for oro-facial anomalies (Bzoch, 1979; Rampp, Pannbacker, & Kinnebrew, 1984).

To conclude our discussion of the oral peripheral examination, we would like to say that at some point in the not too distant future, the diagnostician may have instruments that measure tongue, lip, and other movements very precisely (Barlow & Abbs, 1983; Porter & Lubka, 1980). Remember, though, one swallow does not make a summer, and one deviancy in the oral area does not necessarily cause disordered speech.

BIBLIOGRAPHY

BARLOW, S., & ABBS, J. (1983). Force transducers for the evaluation of labial, lingual, and mandibular motor impairments. *Journal of Speech and Hearing Research, 26,* 616–621.

BELL, K. & GOEPFERT, H. (1977). Rehabilitation of head and neck cancer patients to deglutinate. *Texas Journal of Audiology and Speech Pathology, 2,* 3–5.

BENSON, D. F. (1979). *Aphasia, alexia, and agraphia.* New York: Churchill Livingstone.

BLAKELEY, R. W. (1983). Treatment of developmental apraxia of speech. In W. H. Perkins (Ed.), *Current therapy of communication disorders: Dysarthria and apraxia.* New York: Thieme-Stratton.

BLOOMQUIST, B. (1950). Diadochokinetic movements of nine-, ten-, and eleven-year-old children. *Journal of Speech and Hearing Disorders, 15,* 159–164.

BOSMA, J. F. (1976). Sensorimotor examination of the mouth and pharynx. In Y. Kawamura (Ed.), *Frontiers of oral physiology.* Basel, Switzerland: Kerger.

BZOCH, K. (1979). *Communicative disorders related to cleft lip and palate.* Boston: Little, Brown.

CANNING, B., & ROSE, M. (1974). Clinical measurements of the speed of tongue and lip movements in British children with normal speech. *British Journal of Disorders of Communication, 9,* 45–50.

CAPUTE, A. J. (1974). Developmental disabilities: An overview. *Dental Clinics of North America, 18,* 557–577.

CRARY, M. A. (1988). *A multifaceted perspective on developmental apraxia of speech.* Paper presented to the convention of the Speech and Hearing Association of Alabama, Orange Beach, AL.

CRUICKSHANK, W. M., & RAUS, G. M. (1966). *Cerebral: Its individual and community problems* (2nd ed.). Syracuse, NY: Syracuse University Press.

DABUL, B. (1979). *Apraxia Battery for Adults.* Tigard, OR: C. C. Publications.

DARLEY, F. L., ARONSON, A. E., & BROWN, J. R. (1975). *Motor speech disorders.* Philadelphia, PA: W. B. Saunders.

DERENZI, E., PIECZURO, A., & VIGNOLO, L. A. (1966). Oral apraxia and aphasia. *Cortex, 2,* 50–73.

DICARLO, L. M., & AMSTER, W. W. (1974). Communication therapy for problems associated with cerebral palsy. In S. Dickson (Ed.), *Communication disorders: Remedial principles and practices* (2nd ed.). Glenview, IL: Scott, Foresman.

DWORKIN, J. P., & CULATTA, R. A. (1980). *Dworkin-Culatta Oral Mechanism Examination.* Nicholasville, KY: Edgewood Press.

ENDERBY, P. (1980). Frenchay dysarthria assessment. *British Journal of Disorders of Communication, 15,* 165–173.

ENDERBY, P. (1983). The standardized assessment of dysarthria is possible. In W. R. Berry (Ed.), *Clinical dysarthria.* San Diego, CA: College-Hill Press.

FLETCHER, S. (1972). Time-by-count measurement of diadochokinetic syllable rate. *Journal of Speech and Hearing Research, 15,* 763–770.

GOODGLASS, H., & KAPLAN, E. (1983). *The assessment of aphasia and related disorders.* Philadelphia, PA: Lea & Febiger.

HALL, P. K., HARDY, J. C., & LAVELLE, W. E. (1990). A child with signs of developmental apraxia of speech with whom a palatal lift prosthesis was used to manage palatal dysfunction. *Journal of Speech and Hearing Disorders, 55,* 454–460.

HOPKINS, T. W., BICE, H. V., & COLTON, K. C. (1954). *Evaluation and education of the cerebral palsied child.* Washington, DC: International Council for Exceptional Children.

JOHNS, D. F., & DARLEY, F. L. (1970). Phonemic variability in apraxia of speech. *Journal of Speech and Hearing Research, 13*(3), 556–583.

JOHNS, D. F., & LAPOINTE, L. L. (1976). Neurogenic disorders of output processing: Apraxia of speech. In H. Whitaker & H. A. Whitaker (Eds.), *Studies in neurolinguistics I.* New York: Academic Press.

KENT, R. D., & ROSENBEK, J. C. (1983). Acoustic patterns of apraxia of speech. *Journal of Speech and Hearing Disorders, 26,* 231–248.

KERTESZ, A. (1980). *Western Aphasia Battery.* London, Ontario: University of Western Ontario.

LARSEN, G. (1972). Rehabilitation of dysphagia paralytica. *Journal of Speech and Hearing Disorders, 37,* 187–194.

LOGEMANN, J. (1983). *Evaluation and treatment of swallowing disorders.* San Diego, CA: College-Hill Press.

MCDONALD, E. T., & CHANCE, B. (1964). *Cerebral palsy.* Englewood Cliffs, NJ: Prentice Hall.

MCNEIL, M. R., ROSENBEK, J. C., & ARONSON, A. A. (1984). *The dysarthrias: Physiology, acoustics, perception, management.* San Diego, CA: College-Hill Press.

MARQUARDT, T. P. (1982). *Acquired neurogenic disorders.* Englewood Cliffs, NJ: Prentice Hall.

MARTIN, A. D. (1974). Some objections to the term apraxia of speech. *Journal of Speech and Hearing Disorders, 39,* 53–64.

MASON, R. M., & SIMON, C. (1977). An orofacial examination checklist. *Language, Speech and Hearing Services in Schools, 8,* 155–163.

MILLER, N. (1986). *Dyspraxia and its management.* Rockville, MD: Aspen Pub.

MOORE, W. M., ROSENBEK, J. C., & LAPOINTE, L. L. (1976). Assessment of oral apraxia in brain-injured adults. In R. H. Brookshire (Ed.), *Clinical aphasiology: conference proceedings.* Minneapolis, MN: BRK Publishers.

MORLEY, M. E. (1957). *The development and disorders of speech in children.* London: Livingston.

MYSAK, E. D. (1980). *Neurospeech therapy for the cerebral palsied: A neuroevolutional approach.* New York: Teachers College Press.

PERKINS, W. H. (1983). *Current therapy of communication disorders: Dysarthria and apraxia.* New York: Thieme-Stratton.

PORTER, R., & LUBKA, J. (1980). The linguameter: A device for investigating tongue-muscle control. *Journal of Speech and Hearing Research, 23,* 490–494.

RAMPP, D. L., PANNBACKER, M., & KINNEBREW, M. C. (1984). *VPI velopharyngeal incompetency: A practical guide for evaluation and management.* Austin, TX: PRO-ED.

RANCHO LOS AMIGOS HOSPITAL (1966). *Bulbarcranial nerve examination.* Unpublished, prepared by the Physical Therapy Department, Rancho Los Amigos Hospital, Los Angeles, CA.

ROSENBEK, J. C., LAPOINTE, L., & WERTZ, R. T. (1989). *Aphasia: A clinical approach.* Boston: College-Hill Press.

ROSENBEK, J. C., & WERTZ, R. T. (1976). Veterans Administration Workshop on Speech Motor Disorders, Madison, WI.

RUSCELLO, D. M., ST. LOUIS, K. O., BARRY, P., & BARR, K. (1982). A screening method for examination of the peripheral speech mechanism. *Folia Phoniatrica, 34,* 324–330.

SIEGEL, G., & HANLON, J. (1983). Magnitude estimation of oral cavity distances. *Journal of Speech and Hearing Research, 26,* 574–578.

SONIES, B. C., WEIFFENBACH, J., ATKINSON, J. C., BRAHIM, J., MACYNSKI, A., & FOX, P. C. (1987). Clinical examination of motor and sensory functions of the adult oral cavity. *Dysphagia, 1,* 4.

SQUARE, P., & WEIDNER, W. E. (1981). *Differential diagnosis of developmental apraxia.* Paper presented to the convention of the Speech and Hearing Association of Alabama, Birmingham, AL.

ST. LOUIS, K., & RUSCELLO, D. (1981). *The oral speech mechanism examination.* Baltimore: University Park Press.

WERTZ, R. T., LAPOINTE, L. L., & ROSENBEK, J. C. (1984). *Apraxia of speech in adults: The disorder and its management.* New York: Grune & Stratton.

WERTZ, R. T., ROSENBEK, J. C., & DEAL, J. (1970). *A review of 228 cases of apraxia of speech: Classification, etiology, and localization.* Paper presented at the convention of the American Speech and Hearing Association, New York.

YORKSTON, K. M., & BEUKELMAN, D. R. (1981). *Assessment of intelligibility of dysarthric speech.* Tigard, OR: C. C. Publications.

YORKSTON, K. M., BEUKELMAN, D. R., & BELL, K. R. (1988). *Clinical management of dysarthric speakers.* Boston: College-Hill.

YOSS, K., & DARLEY, F. L. (1974). Developmental apraxia of speech in children with defective articulation. *Journal of Speech and Hearing Research, 17,* 399–416.

LARYNGEAL VOICE DISORDERS

There were major changes in the assessment and treatment of voice disorders in the early part of this century. The speech pathologist became involved in the processes of diagnosis and remediation that were previously the province of physicians and singing teachers (Stemple, 1984). Recently, there has been increased research in the area of normal and disordered vocal physiology. Assessment and treatment are being changed further by the technological advances in microcomputers and electronics. Thus, today we possess insights into the vocal mechanism that we did not have even a decade ago. New instruments are available for diagnosis and treatment that help to objectify behaviors that were previously unobservable and fleeting. It is an exciting time for those clinicians who deal with voice disorders.

The proliferation of new instrumentation and research, however, should not obscure the fact that we have developed some very effective clinical procedures over the years that do not require equipment. Many authorities continue to believe that it is the listening skill and judgment of the well-trained clinician that are the most important tools in a voice evaluation. Voice diagnosis combines the subjective and the objective as does all clinical work, and the clinician must be able to shift from the mental set of the scientist to that of the wine taster and back again. In this chapter, we will touch upon both subjective and objective aspects of vocal assessment.

Many adults and some children are referred to the speech pathologist by their physician for voice disorders resulting from medical difficulties or surgical intervention. The clinician more frequently comes in contact with children as the result of screening large numbers of youngsters in school settings or by teacher/

parent referral. Prevalence figures for voice disorders among school-age children vary considerably. Silverman and Zimmer (1975) report that 23.4 percent of the primary-grade children they evaluated possessed chronically hoarse voices while Wilson and Rice (1977) postulate that 1 percent of the school-age population needs voice therapy. Other studies range between 4 and 6 percent. From our experience, it would appear that substantially less than 1 percent of school-age children are presently receiving voice therapy (Deal, McClain, & Sudderth, 1976). For a variety of reasons, including fear of working with voice cases and self-perceived lack of training, the practicing speech clinician is not identifying the number of voice cases that the experts predict actually exist. (Shearer, 1972).

THE NATURE OF VOCAL DISTURBANCES

The imprecision of labels, which is the bane of voice study, begins with the term *voice* itself. Some definitions restrict the term to the generation of sound at the level of the larynx, while others include the influence of the vocal tract upon the generated tone, and still others broaden the definition to ultimately include aspects of tonal generation, resonation, articulation, and prosody. In this chapter, we will limit our discussion of voice to disorders affecting the laryngeal mechanism. Cancer of the larynx, its subsequent medical treatment, and the speech rehabilitation of a person so affected is a voice disorder that warrants a chapter unto itself (see Chapter 11). Disorders of resonance will be discussed in Chapter 12.

A framework to conceptualize voice and voice disturbance is shown in Figure 10.1. The auditory characteristics of pitch, loudness, and quality constitute one dimension of our paradigm. These are the primary perceptual attributes of the voice and relate generally to the fundamental frequency, amplitude, and complexity of the signal.

Pitch that is too high, too low, too invariant, or inappropriately variant for the speaker or the circumstances constitutes a voice disorder. The loudness of the speaking voice is usually judged according to the speaking circumstance, with the aberrant ranging from the total lack of voice (aphonia) to the inappropriately loud. For our purposes, the term *quality* refers to the perceived pleasantness, or appeal, of the voice. Although this perception is linked to both the phonatory and resonatory characteristics of the speaker, we will consider only the disturbance of phonation in this chapter. Many terms have been used to describe vocal quality, yet roughness/hoarseness and breathiness seem to be the two most widely accepted.

The physical systems that most directly influence vocal production are the respiratory, phonatory, and resonatory-articulatory systems, but they are not the only systems that influence the voice. Luchsinger and Arnold (1965) discuss the impact of the endocrine and neural systems on voice production.

The respiratory system provides the motive force for voice production, and ultimately the resultant airstream becomes the vibrator that embodies all of the characteristics that the ear eventually senses. The importance of the airstream to vocal production is not really the issue at this point, but there is

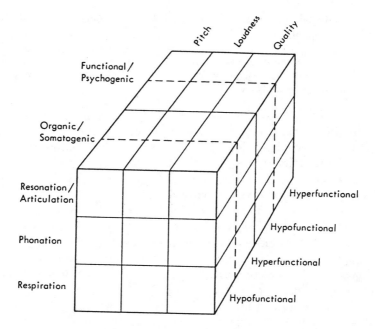

Figure 10.1 An Organizational Schema of Voice Disorders

some question as to the influence of the respiratory mechanism upon the various vocal characteristics. It appears that the respiratory mechanism must be capable of the following:

1. Providing an adequate amount of air so that the speaker can sustain speech with ease to allow for natural phrasing and prosodic factors
2. Providing adequate control of the flow of air so that the mechanism can, when necessary, either initiate or arrest the speech signal
3. Providing an airstream that is not so indebted to active muscle contraction that it encourages unnecessary muscle tension in the respiratory and phonatory mechanisms.

Knowledge of the elements of laryngeal function is crucial in guiding the diagnostic process. In order to be an efficient sound source, the larynx must perform a valving action upon the flow of air that establishes alternate, regular pressure changes within the body of air. In order to do this, the vocal folds must be

1. Capable of a wide range of valving actions, from completely open and unrestricted through closed and totally restricted
2. Able to valve completely along their entire length
3. Of approximately equal size and shape so that they can move in synchrony with one another
4. Able to close and open during phonation with just the right amount of energy to avoid extreme tension during the closing phase
5. Of appropriate size (length and mass) for the age and sex of the person

6. Capable of natural movement that is free from superimposed and undue tension
7. Capable of small, subtle, instantaneous adjustments that must be made continuously to alter the various vocal characteristics. These adjustments must allow for a variety of cyclic variations in the potential time of glottal opening and closing, from the long closing time of the glottal fry to the short closing time of the falsetto voice.

The glottal tone is complex and rich in higher harmonics, but it is only through the resonant and damping effects of the vocal tract that the speech sounds achieve their identity. In order for the resonating chambers of the vocal tract to be efficient, they must be flexible in size, shape, texture, and relationship with one another. The effect of the resonators upon the laryngeal valve has been discussed by several writers (Curtis, 1968; Wendahl & Page, 1967), but the exact nature of this relationship has yet to be determined.

The term *functional* should imply more than the simple absence of measurable organic deviation; it should imply that the diagnostician has found some active agent of etiology and that the agent is nonorganic. We agree with Powers (1971) that the term *functional* has unfortunately come to mean diagnosis by default. Voice disorders offer an interesting testing ground for the traditional organic-functional dichotomy. This separation does not stand up on almost any basis. Murphy (1964) points out the continuous nature of vocal disorder etiologies.

Figure 10.1 identified functional/psychogenic and organic/somatogenic as clinically meaningful categories. The term *functional* refers to those disorders where the learned, psychic, or maladaptive behavior has resulted in faulty vocal production, but not in physical alteration. If physical change has resulted from the functional cause, however, the proper designation is *psychogenic*. Similarly, if the original factor was physical or organic, then the term *organic* is justified; but if the physical difference results in behavioral change—that is, emotional response or faulty compensatory adjustments—the term *somatogenic* is appropriate (Murphy, 1964).

The terms *hyper-* and *hypofunctioning* refer, respectively, to an excess or insufficiency of laryngeal tension and, as such, could apply to a wide variety of organic or functional disorders.

The term *voice disorders,* then, refers to abnormal pitch, loudness, or vocal quality according to sex, age, status, temporary physiological state, purpose of the speaker, and elements of the speaking circumstances. Vocal disorders may be primarily organic or functional and may be affected by any of the primary systems.

THE PRESENTING COMPLAINT AND CASE HISTORY INTAKE

Before beginning our discussion of the diagnostic format, let us restate that this chapter will not cover the anatomy and physiology of the mechanisms of vocal production. Such information is offered in many sources and should be studied carefully before undertaking voice diagnosis (Bateman & Mason, 1984; Daniloff,

Schuckers, & Feth, 1980; Dickson & Maue-Dickson, 1982; Kahane & Folkins, 1984; Kaplan, 1971; Palmer, 1984; Perkins & Kent, 1986; Zemlin, 1988). We also cannot provide an elaborate description of each voice disorder type; this information is available to the student in several sources (Aronson, 1985; Boone & McFarlane, 1988; Greene, 1980; Luchsinger & Arnold, 1965; Stemple, 1984).

Our major focus will be on the actual planning, preparation, and execution of voice diagnoses. Diagnosis is intended to assess the parameters of the voice, determine the etiology and/or perpetuating factors, and outline a logical course of intervention, if warranted.

The diagnostic process begins with a careful scrutiny of the original statement of the problem as provided by the referral source. Four perspectives guide our evaluation of this information: who, what, why, and when.

Who Makes the Referral?

It is important to know who presents the original complaint about the client's voice. We have found that the "best" source from a motivational standpoint is the client, but any individual who might have a significant impact upon the client may be a satisfactory referral source. If the client does not consider the voice to be a problem, treatment may not be in order or, if it is, this denial may necessitate counseling and educating as precursors to the actual voice treatment.

In the schools, it is often the classroom teacher who notices a vocal difference in a student and makes a referral to the speech-language pathologist. Awareness training may be necessary in the early sessions here too. It should be pointed out, however, that without prior training, such as listening experiences during inservice programs, classroom teachers are not particularly good at recognizing and referring students with voice disorders. Several investigations have studied the classroom teacher's efficacy in referral of children with voice disorders (Diehl & Stinnett, 1959; James & Cooper, 1966).

What Problem Is Reported?

The description of the problem in the presenting complaint is important not only in helping us to understand the difficulty better, but also because it allows us to see the problem through the eyes and ears of another. When the statement comes from the person with whom we will be working, we listen not only to the actual words spoken, but also to the way in which they are presented. One of the best sources of information about the impact of the problem upon the individual is the way in which it is described. If possible, preinterview questionnaires should be completed and returned by mail to the clinician prior to the evaluation session. The submitted material is helpful in guiding the diagnostic inquiry. Questions asked on preinterview forms are important to probe further during the case history intake. Preinterview questionnaires invariably ask for a description of the voice problem: when it started and what might have caused it. Health, occupation, and family information is also typically garnered. Weinberg (1983) provides a detailed questionnaire that is a useful preinterview tool.

Why Was the Referral Made?

The reason for referral to the voice clinician may vary from something as simple as an impending trip ("I just have to sound better than this by the first of August") to fears of serious medical problems. In evaluating the reasons for referral, it is important to keep in mind that contacting a speech clinician is often seen as psychologically safer than going to medical doctors or psychologists. This points up the importance of secondary referrals.

When Was the Referral Made?

Three things are of concern here. First, it is important to know when in the sequence of development of the problem the referral was made. Is this a long-standing problem that has only recently become serious, or is it a relatively new phenomenon that has been detected early? Second, what is this person's age and maturational level? Certain vocal changes are to be expected before puberty (Curry, 1949) and would be considered normal, but a similar vocal quality at a later maturity level may be abnormal. Third, does this problem appear in cycles? For example, the client may suffer from this vocal change only during "hay fever" season. The time of year of the referral may provide some important diagnostic information.

Referral by the Speech Pathologist

Laryngologists often refer clients to speech-language pathologists for behavioral vocal intervention. Equally often, persons with voice problems seek the help of SLPs without first seeing a doctor. In most cases of phonatory voice disorders, some type of referral for medical or psychological evaluation will be necessary. We must remember that speech-language pathologists diagnose the voice and its characteristics whereas medical doctors—particularly laryngologists—diagnose the vocal mechanism per se. It is not within the province of the SLP to diagnose nodules, inflammation, cancer, or the like; we do assess the parameters of the voice that may or may not reflect such structural changes. Voice disorders may be caused by life-threatening situations such as carcinoma of the larynx or something as simple as vocal misuse. The importance of medical referral, then, is obvious. Structural changes such as ulcers, polyps, tumors, or nodules may be detected by the laryngologist through laryngeal examination (and confirmed by tissue biopsy). Auditory symptoms such as hoarseness or harshness of the voice and/or sensory complaints (e.g., laryngeal pain, lumps, and the like) should prompt the clinician to make the referral. Hoarseness lasting beyond 14 days, particularly in persons over the age of 40, should be referred on suspicion of being a serious, life-threatening condition until proven otherwise (Pracy et al., 1977). The need for a medical diagnosis cannot be underestimated because of the life/health implications for the client, the legal implications for the practicing clinician, and the requirement of third-party reimbursement agencies that services provided be "medically necessary."

It is widely accepted that the speech pathologist and the laryngologist should ideally cultivate a close working relationship when dealing with voice cases (Aronson, 1985; Boone, 1980, 1982). Each professional can provide significant information to the other and *voice treatment* that attempts to alter one or more parameters of the voice, such as pitch, should not begin without a laryngological examination. A *vocal hygiene* program, which does not alter the voice but teaches care of it, can begin with many clients prior to laryngoscopic examination. Thus, waiting for medical examination in cases of vocal abuse should not be used as a reason to postpone enrollment in an intervention program.

During an examination by a medical specialist, indirect laryngoscopy will be accomplished via a mirror or fiberoptiscope. In cases of infants or preschool children, for whom indirect procedures are difficult, the laryngologist may use direct laryngoscopy under anesthesia. Other sophisticated methods are available for observing the condition and function of the vocal folds and will be discussed later in the chapter. The speech-language pathologist will be interested in the findings of the laryngeal examinations for several reasons and may wish to personally view the folds to better understand the reported findings and diagnosis. First, the examination can document any physical alteration to the vocal mechanism (e.g., nodules, polyps) that may account for vocal differences. Second, the speech pathologist will want to have the extent of any vocal fold pathology documented as baseline information if voice therapy is indicated so that alterations in the client's voice over time, as the result of treatment, might be correlated with concomitant organic changes that show in future laryngological examinations. Forms containing drawings of the vocal apparatus have been recommended so that the physician can make notes indicating the size and location of abnormalities (Boone, 1980, 1982; Stone, Hurlbutt, & Coulthard, 1978; Weinberg, 1983). This could become part of the client's record and be used for comparisons over time with other examinations. A third reason the speech pathologist will be interested in the laryngeal examination is that surgical intervention may be recommended as the treatment of choice for a particular patient. A dialogue between the clinician and the doctor may be necessary to discuss this decision and to discuss recommendations regarding the appropriateness of follow-up voice therapy. Finally, the absence of organic deviations on the laryngoscopic examination may suggest more functional bases for the client's disorder. Such knowledge would have direct implications for the direction of voice treatment and may also indicate that other referrals by the speech pathologist (e.g., to a psychologist) are in order.

A general medical evaluation or specific neurological or endocrinological examination may be indicated in certain cases. When dysfunction of the peripheral or central nervous system appears to be a possible contributing factor to the voice disorder, as in dysarthria (see Chapter 9), referral is indicated.

During a routine screening of all college students entering the teacher education and certification program, Susan came to our attention. Susan's voice was weak and she had difficulty projecting it louder or trying to shout when requested to do so. On questioning, it was revealed that her voice tires easily throughout the day and a slight hoarseness is typical. This prompted us to inquire further—trying to unravel the mystery of Susan's voice problem and wondering about a possible endocrinological basis. Suspicions of a hyperactive thyroid gland became stronger when Susan complained of nervousness and irritability, generalized muscle weakness, and fatigue—making it difficult for her to complete her aerobics routine at the local gym (one day her legs trembled and were so weak she could not rise from a squat), excessive sweating, weight loss—which she was happy about even though she still ate lots of food, insomnia, and irregular menstrual periods. Her once-radiant skin had turned sallow in recent months. Referral to a physician was made and hyperthyroidism (Grave's disease) was diagnosed.

The Case History Interview

There are many excellent sources for guidance in taking an adequate case history with an emphasis on voice disorders and many of these sources provide forms for the clinician's use (Aronson, 1985; Boone & McFarlane, 1988; Fox & Blechman, 1975; Greene, 1980; Johnson, Darley, & Spriestersbach, 1963; Moncur & Brackett, 1974; Murphy, 1964; Wilson, 1987). Table 10.1 lists sample case history questions that we routinely ask during a client interview. Table 10.2 may be used as a checklist on which clients may indicate any coexisting sensory symptoms (Cooper, 1973; Pindzola, 1987). In the following section, we will elaborate on those case history topics most relevant to vocal diagnosis and subsequent intervention.

Family Data.   Information regarding parental occupation, number of siblings, history of family adjustment, other voice problems within the family,

Table 10.1   Sample Questions to Ask in the Case History Intake

1. In your own words, describe the problem.
2. When did the voice problem begin?
3. Did the problem begin suddenly or develop slowly?
4. What conditions surrounded the onset of the voice problem (colds, illness, surgery, personal problems, etc.)?
5. When is your voice better? When is it worse?
6. Describe the daily use of your voice (typical weekday behaviors and job demands on the voice; typical weekend activities).
7. Are there specific situations when abuse occurs? Inquire about the frequency of common misuses and abuses such as excessive crying, throat clearing, coughing, smoking, screaming, and so forth.
8. Describe your general health (sinus problems; allergies; illnesses; injuries to head, neck, or scrotum; endocrine disorders; heart disease; surgery; use of medications; fatiguability; smoking/drinking habits; etc.).
9. What has your doctor told you about your voice?

Table 10.2 Checklist of Sensory Symptoms

Mark (X) all symptoms associated with the voice problem

_____ 1. Frequent throat clearing

_____ 2. Frequent coughing

_____ 3. Vocal fatigue which progresses with use of the voice

_____ 4. Irritation or pain in the voice box or throat

_____ 5. Strain or bulging of neck muscles

_____ 6. Swelling of veins and/or arteries in the neck

_____ 7. Feeling of a foreign substance or "lump" in throat

_____ 8. Ear irritation, tickling, or earache

_____ 9. Frequent sore throats

_____ 10. A tickling, soreness, or burning sensation in the throat

_____ 11. Scratchy or dry throat

_____ 12. Tension and/or tightness in the throat

_____ 13. A feeling that talking is an effort

_____ 14. Pain or difficulty swallowing

_____ 15. Pain or burning sensation at the base of the tongue

and general health pattern of the family tells us a great deal about the young client's social and physical milieu. Generally, the following characteristics may be considered potentially remarkable and should be explored further: (1) too much or too little structure and organization to the home; (2) premium placed on verbal competition; (3) interparental friction; (4) unusual sibling competition; (5) history of voice disorders; (6) poor parental adjustment; (7) history of extended recurrent health problems; and (8) general level of concern for physical and health problems. For the adult client, we are interested in many of the same issues, particularly occupation, number of persons living in the home, and health problems or communication disorders among those living in the home.

> Barbara was a 32-year-old mother of twins. Both four-year-old boys were described as rambunctious and Barbara was the archetypical housewife. She also cared for her mother-in-law who was hard-of-hearing, a bit senile, and lived in the same home. Barbara just could not understand why she had developed bilateral vocal nodules and why the doctor insisted on her enrolling in voice therapy. Clearly, family information of this type suggests etiological factors of vocal abuse and provides behavioral change as a direction for treatment.

Onset of the Problem.   In many instances, the beginning of the voice problem will have great diagnostic significance. It is important to investigate not only the nature of the onset, but also the circumstances surrounding it. Physical or psychological trauma may have equally instant effects upon voice production. In some cases, extended questioning may be necessary because it is common for clients to repress uncomfortable incidents of the past. Aronson (1985) indicates that a sudden onset within hours suggests the high probability of a conversion vocal disorder or a neurological origin (such as stroke), whereas many other types of vocal disturbances develop gradually (mass and approximation lesions, degenerative disease, etc.).

Although the abrupt onset of a vocal disorder is traumatic and startling, most voice disorders are of insidious origin. Many people cannot pinpoint the exact date of the onset and tend to indicate when people first noticed or remarked about their voices. Since a gradual onset is not necessarily specific to organic or functional etiologies, the examiner must look to other data for final answers. Probably more important than the rate of development is information on coincident factors such as the client's general health and emotional state.

Course of Development. A careful description of the developmental stages of the voice disturbance may provide helpful diagnostic information. The course of the development of the voice disorder may be found to parallel a chronic medical problem, cumulating vocational stress, certain periods of physical maturation, changes in family relationships, or developing financial crises. We want to know how the problem has changed since its onset and any circumstances surrounding variability of the voice disturbance. For instance, were there changes in the voice disorder during its development that might be correlated with changes in personal habits (e.g., smoking, use of alcohol), work conditions (e.g., excessive noise, stress), or medical conditions (e.g., sinus, allergy). The clinician will want to keep in mind that once a voice disorder has been firmly established, only a minimal amount of tension, misuse, or abuse will be necessary to perpetuate the problem.

Description of Daily Vocal Performance and Problem Variability. While the course of development questions seek a historical perspective, we need information on factors that influence the voice at the time of the evaluation. For instance, we might ask the client to describe his/her daily routine and relate it to talking. Does the problem become worse through the day? Does it become better as the day progresses? Boone and McFarlane (1988) suggest having the patient identify any situations that seem to be consistently related to good and poor vocal performance. It is especially important in cases of childhood vocal pathology to obtain an accurate picture of the youngster's typical use of voice and instances of misuse or abuse (Wilson, 1987).

Social Adjustment. Assessment of the personality characteristics of the individual may assist the diagnostician in interpreting other information. Formal personality testing is not within the jurisdiction of the speech pathologist, but each clinician is expected to be perceptive and sensitive to clues about the client's basic adjustment of life. The notion that the voice is closely related to the individual's self-concept and reveals inner conflict has been carefully examined by several researchers. Moses (1954) and Rousey and Moriarty (1965) present interesting views of the interaction of the personality and voice production. Classification of voice characteristics with specific personality types has not provided overwhelming evidence of definite relationships; but the personality and the voice interact in a complex fashion, and this results in many symptomatic characteristics.

Vocation. We are interested in the vocation of our voice client for two reasons. First, we must determine if the occupation demands a great deal of talking and if that talking is under adverse conditions. Not all teachers develop "teacher's nodules," however, and the vocation must be judged in relation to the person. Several writers have postulated that there is a personality type that develops vocal nodules (Green, 1989; Jackson, 1941; Withers, 1961). We have found many of these people to be tense, energetic, high strung, and verbally aggressive. Place this type of person in an occupational setting that demands a great deal of speaking under tension, and a bit of poor judgment in choosing adaptive procedures, and the chances of finding an individual with vocal nodules could be greatly enhanced.

A second factor in our evaluation of the vocation of an individual is to assess the possibility of changing aspects of the client's job routine or behavior at work if the vocation has a deleterious effect on the voice disorder.

> We worked with a college professor who taught several large lecture classes to groups of over 150 students. His vocal abuse and misuse during these presentations had resulted in small nodules for which voice therapy was recommended. In an effort to be audible, dynamic, and authoritative, he had been speaking loudly, with a lower pitch, and with excessive tension. We explored the possibility of his using a lavalier microphone in the large lecture rooms, and this effectively eliminated an abusive situation that was vocationally related.

Health. Realizing that the voice is influenced by many physiological systems, a complete medical history and examination are necessary in many instances. A history of the general health and physical development of the client should be obtained, along with information about specific illnesses, surgeries, and medications. The clinician should also obtain data concerning the general energy level and health-related habits such as smoking, drinking, and drug usage. Luchsinger and Arnold (1965) present a particularly comprehensive discussion of vocal disorders of organic etiology. Referral of a client to a physician may uncover a medical problem of which vocal quality is a symptom:

> Sherry was identified in the speech and hearing screening program. Her voice was described as breathy, low in pitch and volume, expressionless, and varying in degrees of nasality. The more she talked the more noticeable these symptoms became. Shouting while counting was particularly difficult for her and articulatory slurring became evident at the higher numbers. Sherry complained of excessive fatigue by the end of the day and frequently found chewing steak dinners more of a chore than a pleasure. Subsequent medical referral indicated specific muscle weakness and a medical diagnosis of myasthenia gravis. It should be noted that the speech clinician's alertness to the accumulation of medical danger signs in addition to the speech characteristics resulted in a proper referral and subsequent identification of the problem.

INFORMAL EVALUATION: A LISTENING AND RATING PROCESS

The first step in voice analysis is simply listening to the client in an analytical manner. Obviously, this listening process is largely judgmental. Much of what we do in a routine voice assessment is perceptual and subjective. The "craft" of vocal evaluations is augmented with informal tasks, ratings scales, and the like. Often we consider what we do in the diagnostic session as constituting a formal evaluation, but we must recognize the informal, perceptual basis of our techniques and observations. In recent years, instrumentation to objectify our perceptual methods has become more readily available in medical and research settings. However, the evaluation remains, for most clinicians, a listening process. As such, rating scales, profiles, checklists, and assessment outlines are the order of the day.

A checklist, such as the simple one shown in Table 10.3, may guide the clinician in a cursory appraisal of the various characteristics of the voice. Many voice assessment tools (rating scales, profiles, checklists, open-ended observation forms, and the like) are available; Table 10.4 lists some of the more commonly used resources. Let us highlight a few of them here.

Profiles and assessment instruments typically include scales that rate a variety of vocal aspects in terms of severity of deviation from the norm. The *Buffalo III Voice Profile* (Wilson, 1987) rates on a five-point scale laryngeal tone, pitch, loudness, nasal resonance, oral resonance, breath supply, muscles, voice abuse, rate, speech anxiety, and speech intelligibility and provides for an overall voice rating. The *Voice Profile System* by Wilson and Rice (1977) has received wide acceptance. It rates the laryngeal cavity, resonating cavity, intensity, vocal range, and overall severity using numbered scales. Ratings of these types should be a helpful starting point in the voice evaluation; the clinician who notes disturbance in any parameter of vocal production can move on to more specific analysis techniques that illuminate further the affected aspect of the voice.

A detailed analysis of vocal parameters is typical in clinical practice. The critical listening, previously described, combined with estimates or measurements of the voice, using little or no specialized equipment is perhaps a blending of the informal-formal dichotomy. An assessment tool illustrative of this type of appraisal is the *Voice Assessment Protocol for Children and Adults* (Pindzola, 1987). The protocol facilitates quick interpretations of vocal parameter normalcy by use of a Likert scale, or grid-marking system. Five parameters of the voice are assessed: pitch, loudness, quality, breath features, and rate/rhythm. Analysis of a client is best done using a conversational speech sample supplemented with phoneme prolongation tasks, singing the scale, diadochokinetic testing, reading, and similar tasks of one's choosing. A high-quality tape recording of the voice is suggested. Perceptual judgments are adequate or the clinician may choose to supplement estimations with instrumental measurements, such as a piano or other musical instrument, pitch pipe, sound spectrography, loudness indicators, and the like.

Let us now turn our attention to a discussion of the vocal parameters and how they are routinely assessed. As in evaluating other communication

Table 10.3 Checklist of Vocal Characteristics

PITCH

| 1 | 2 | 3 | 4 | 5 | 6 | 7 |

Description				Severity			
—Too high	1	2	3	4	5	6	7
—Too low	1	2	3	4	5	6	7
—Invariant	1	2	3	4	5	6	7
—Pitch breaks	1	2	3	4	5	6	7
—Diplophonia	1	2	3	4	5	6	7
—Repetitive pattern	1	2	3	4	5	6	7

LOUDNESS

| 1 | 2 | 3 | 4 | 5 | 6 | 7 |

Description				Severity			
—Excessive	1	2	3	4	5	6	7
—Inadequate	1	2	3	4	5	6	7
—Uncontrolled variation	1	2	3	4	5	6	7
—Repetitive pattern	1	2	3	4	5	6	7
—Invariant	1	2	3	4	5	6	7
—Tremulous	1	2	3	4	5	6	7

QUALITY

| 1 | 2 | 3 | 4 | 5 | 6 | 7 |

Description				Severity			
—Hoarseness	1	2	3	4	5	6	7
—Harshness	1	2	3	4	5	6	7
—Breathiness	1	2	3	4	5	6	7
—Hypernasal	1	2	3	4	5	6	7
—Hyponasal	1	2	3	4	5	6	7
—Other (describe)	1	2	3	4	5	6	7

JUDGMENT OF VOCAL TENSION

- —Aphonia/whisper
- —Breathy phonation
- —Normal
- —Hypertension
- —Hypertension/intermittent phonation

OVERALL JUDGMENT OF VOICE

| 1 | 2 | 3 | 4 | 5 | 6 | 7 |

Note: 1 = normal; 7 = severely disordered

disorders, the clinician must realize that the type of sample obtained affects how "ecologically valid" it is. For instance, in the case of a child with vocal nodules who is suspected of being a vocal abuser, it would be ideal to observe the youngster in a play situation with others, during school activities, and in the home environment. Most often, a variety of sampling activities are used in the evaluation, ranging from conversation, counting, coughing, singing the scale, and prolonging isolated speech sounds. The point here is that the

Table 10.4   An Annotated Listing of Some of the Available Rating Scales and Evaluation Materials

Remediation of Vocal Hoarseness
(Blonigen, 1980)
> Although primarily a treatment guide, this booklet will prove useful in the appraisal stage where abuses and misuses must be identified.

The Boone Voice Program for Children
(Boone, 1980)
> Screening, evaluation, and referral instructions are included in a manual with this remediation kit. Also provided are the necessary forms and stimulus materials.

The Boone Voice Program for Adults
(Boone, 1982)
> Both diagnosis and remediation procedures for vocal disorders are contained in this kit.

Voice Patient Case History
(Fox & Blechman, 1975)
> A detailed listing of case history questions is presented. Testing of vocal function is also described and presented in a concise format. Pitch, loudness, quality, time, and breathing are tested.

General Voice Quality Examination,

Supplementary Examination for Harshness,

Supplementary Examination for Breathiness,

Supplementary Examination for Nasality
(Johnson, Darley, & Spriestersbach, 1963)
> The detailed examination form is dominated by case history questions and clinical observations. Three supplementary forms provide for detailed observations of vocal quality. The effects of phonetic context, loudness, pitch, rate, and other factors are investigated.

Voice Assessment Protocol for Children and Adults
(Pindzola, 1987)
> This protocol directs and quantifies clinical observations of voice. The following vocal parameters are assessed: pitch, loudness, quality, breath features, and rate.

Symptomatic Voice Therapy
(Polow & Kaplan, 1980)
> This detailed notebook describes the differential diagnosis, possible etiologies, management decisions, and therapy techniques for disorders of pitch, loudness, phonation, and resonance.

Voice Profile System
(Wilson & Rice, 1977)
> This *Programmed Approach to Voice Therapy* includes two methods of treatment for voice disorders in children and adults (tension increase and tension decrease). It also contains a profiling system useful for vocal assessment. Sample recordings (on cassette) accompany the program with training instructions for severity judgments.

Buffalo III Voice Profile

Buffalo III Voice Screening Profile

Buffalo III Group Behavior Profile

Buffalo III Voice Abuse Profile

Buffalo III Speech Anxiety Profile

Buffalo III Voice Recording Profile

Buffalo III Voice Diagnostic Profile
(Wilson, 1987)
> The Buffalo system consists of 10 profiles for various purposes (7 pertinent here) with the "Voice Profile" being a general, overall rating scale.

clinician should be aware that a broad sampling of vocal performance is needed in order to make correct judgments on any parameter of the voice.

Pitch Assessment

Clinicians routinely evaluate various pitch characteristics of the client's voice. Pitch is a perceptual phenomenon that correlates with the valving rate of the vocal folds. Rightly or wrongly, clinicians interchange the terms *pitch* and *frequency* when talking about a client's voice. *Pitch determination* of the speaking fundamental frequency, also known as habitual pitch, can be accomplished with musical-matching methods or by instrumental analysis (e.g., Visi-Pitch). The client's speaking fundamental frequency can then be compared to normative data, based on age and sex. Table 10.5 shows average fundamental frequencies for a representative sample of ages, synthesized from the literature (Hollien & Shipp, 1972; Kelley, 1977; Wilson, 1987).

Pitch determination methods can also be used to locate a client's optimal pitch. *Optimal pitch* is a controversial concept that supposes each person has an optimal or natural pitch range at which he/she *should* be speaking. If we accept the premise of optimal performance, then, when optimal pitch does not match habitual pitch, habitual pitch may need to be raised or lowered in treatment. The determination of optimal pitch is by no means precise. Also, it should be emphasized that optimal pitch is not a single note, but a range of notes where the vocal mechanism appears to function best with the least muscular tension. Various vegetative (natural, involuntary, and nonspeech sounds) and range singing techniques have been proposed for eliciting optimal pitches from clients; once elicited and recorded, the value of the optimal pitch can be determined musically or instrumentally. The following sources can be consulted regarding procedures for determining optimal pitch: Fairbanks (1960), Murphy (1964), Moncur

Table 10.5 Average Fundamental Frequencies for Selected Ages

AGE	SEX	MEAN FUNDAMENTAL
1–2	either	445 Hz
3	either	390 Hz
6	either	320 Hz
10	male	235 Hz
15	male	165 Hz
20–29	male	120 Hz
50–59	male	118 Hz
60–69	male	112 Hz
80–89	male	146 Hz
10	female	265 Hz
15	female	220 Hz
20–29	female	227 Hz
50–59	female	214 Hz
60–69	female	209 Hz
80–89	female	197 Hz

and Brackett (1974), Polow and Kaplan (1980), Pindzola (1987), and Boone and McFarlane (1988). Table 10.6 summarizes some of the more commonly used methods for eliciting a client's optimal pitch. Later in the chapter, we will discuss how these techniques are useful as probes or facilitators of voicing abilities.

The normal voice is characterized by *pitch variability,* also known as *intonation* or *inflection.* The voice is abnormal when there is a lack of pitch variability or when pitch fluctuations are excessive. Dysarthrias may be characterized by monopitch where a limited range of notes are used monotonously (Darley, Aronson, & Brown, 1975). Monopitch and restricted pitch ranges are also associated with superior laryngeal nerve paralysis (Luchsinger & Arnold, 1965), additive lesions (Boone & McFarlane, 1988), and other disorders. Excessive pitch variability or prosodic excess may be heard in the dysarthrias, particularly spastic, ataxic, and hyperkinetic forms (Darley, Aronson, & Brown, 1975). Hearing-impaired and deaf speakers also often utilize excessive pitch fluctuations (Martony, 1968).

Diplophonia refers to the presence of two or more simultaneous pitches or tones in the voice and may be caused by separate or unequal vibratory sources.

Table 10.6 Some Techniques for Determining Optimal Pitch

1. *Resonance-Swell Method*

   Have client hum at the same intensity up the scale and note whether his voice becomes louder or swells in a given range of pitches. Client and/or clinician should listen for this swell in loudness.

2. *Loud-Audible Sigh*

   Client should take a deep breath and produce /a/ as a loud sigh. Listen most carefully for the pitch at the onset of the sigh because one tends to lower the pitch during the sound. Optimal is said to be the onset tone.

3. *Yawn-Sigh*

   The client should yawn and sigh audibly in a relaxed manner. Yawning opens the throat and minimizes the constriction around the larynx.

4. *Vegetative Techniques*

   Listen to the natural, spontaneous laugh, cough, throat clearing, or grunt of the client. These vegetative forms of phonation may be representative of optimal pitch.

5. *Inflection Methods*

   Have the client say "um hum" using a rising inflection with lips closed, as though she were spontaneously and sincerely agreeing with what was just said. Also, the clinician could have the client say "hello" in a natural, spontaneous, and sincere way. An automatic affirmative utterance often approximates optimal pitch. A related method is to have the client say "hello" with rising inflection, as though asking a question. The slight inflection may reveal a more optimal voice.

6. *Pushing or Pulling Techniques*

   The client should attempt to phonate /a/ of optimal quality while pushing down or pulling up on his chair. This method may be particularly useful for clients with disordered closure of the vocal folds.

7. *Pitch Range Methods*

   The type of phonation may be do-re-mi or ah-ah-ah or one-two-three, and so on. The client phonates her entire vocal range from the lowest sound that can be produced to the highest, excluding falsetto. One-third of this range should represent optimal pitch. An alternate, and popular, method is to have the client phonate her entire vocal range from the lowest note to the highest, including falsetto. The total range is then divided by one-fourth to locate the optimal. For example, calculate the number of full-step notes in the client's range and then locate the note that is one-fourth of the way from the bottom.

Possible causes include a paralyzed vocal fold vibrating at a rate different from the healthy one, a vibration of a growth or lesion, simultaneous adduction of the ventricular folds and true folds, and even an innocuous saliva globule.

Pitch breaks most often occur in a person using an inappropriately low-pitched voice. Intermittently, the pitch will suddenly break upward toward a more optimal level. Any condition that adds to the mass or size of the vocal folds may alter their vibratory characteristics. Pitch breaks may be one symptom of additive lesions such as but not limited to nodules, polyps, and tumors.

To summarize our discussion of pitch, the clinician must observe the client and seek answers to the following questions: What is the client's habitual pitch (speaking fundamental frequency) and is this appropriate for the person's age, sex, and body stature? What is an optimal level for the client to use? Is a normal amount of pitch variability present in the speaking voice or is it monotoned or widely varying and sing-songed in pattern? Are pitch breaks present? Is diplophonia present?

Loudness Assessment

Perceptual judgments of vocal loudness are sufficient for appraisal purposes. Instrumentation is available for measuring intensity and may prove useful in providing feedback to the client during intervention. Of interest during the assessment is whether the *loudness level* is appropriate for the speaking situation. In normal conversational speech, some three feet from the speaker, the average sound intensity is 65 dB (range 55–75 dB) (Van Bergeijk, Pierce, & David, 1960). Typical loudness levels may be abnormal in various pathologies. Adults with dysarthria may speak too softly (as in Parkinsonism) or with a booming voice (as in some spasticities and dystonias) (Darley, Aronson, & Brown, 1975). Lack of vocal loudness is characteristic of paralyzed cords and psychogenic disorders. Vocal abuse cases often speak with excessive effort and loudness, at least in some situations; the end result however may be hypofunctional loudness.

The clinician should also note if the typical loudness level can be maintained comfortably, without trailing off, or whether there is a *degree of effort*. Listen for loudness that trails off at the end of a sentence, which may be typical in vocal fold paralysis, dysarthrias, or obstructive lesions (Darley, Aronson, & Brown, 1975; Wilson & Rice, 1977). *Phonation breaks* or momentary skips of loudness are abnormal and may indicate difficulty maintaining vocal fold adduction and vibration.

A certain amount of *loudness variability* is normal and is reflected in the stress patterns of the language. In addition to critically listening to conversational speech, we often ask the client to read "with feeling" sentences such as the following:

> Get out of here, get out of here!
> I don't know, I said I don't know!
> I need more money, Dad, I'm broke!
> Where did she go? I can't find her.
> Will you cut that out!

Other vocal variety drills are available in the drillbooks of Fairbanks (1960) and Hanley and Thurman (1970). We have observed that lack of loudness variability may take two differing forms of monoloudness: excess and equal stress patterns are typical of many dysarthrias (Darley, Aronson, & Brown, 1975), whereas the monoloud but weak and "bland" voice is typically seen in affective disorders (Leff & Abberton, 1981; Weintraub, Mesulam, & Kramer, 1981) and some forms of dysarthria (Darley, Aronson, & Brown, 1975).

The clinician may wish to have the client demonstrate his/her *loudness range,* from soft to maximal levels. Whispering and shouting can be requested. One method is to ask the client to count, beginning softly and increasing loudness with higher and higher numbers. Restricted loudness range is often seen in clients with respiratory involvement, particularly the dysarthrias (Darley, Aronson, & Brown, 1975).

Loudness abuses may be situation-oriented. For instance, conversational levels may be appropriate but frequent loud talking or screaming (as in lectures, sermons, playground activities, etc.) may be perpetuating a vocal disorder. Questions asked in the interview should probe the client's daily uses of the voice with the purpose of discovering situational abuses.

After appraising the client's voice, the clinician should then have answers to the following questions about loudness: Is the loudness level used appropriate for the speaking situation? Can the level be maintained comfortably without undue strain? Can the level be maintained throughout the entire utterance or does it begin to trail off? Are loudness breaks present? Is loudness variable to reflect stress and emphasis patterns of English or is the client monoloud? Can loudness vary from minimal (whispered) to maximal (shouted) levels? What, if any, situations are frequently encountered in which loudness abuse occurs?

Quality Assessment

The descriptive terminology used with disorders of vocal quality reflects the perceptual nature of the judgments. It can be argued that the clinician's ear is the best tool for describing the quality of a voice—and many clinicians use just that. However, rather sophisticated equipment is also available to study, categorize, and "objectify" acoustical parameters of the voice. For example, Isshiki, Yanigahara, and Morimoto (1966) provide some spectrographic guidelines for classifying four severity levels of hoarseness. Technology is available to measure periodicity of vocal fold vibrations, changes in amplitude (shimmer), changes in frequency (jitter), and opening-closing characteristics. Still, deciding whether a voice is breathy, harsh, or hoarse is done most efficiently by critical listening.

Vocal quality is affected by the manner of vocal fold vibration. Many terms of vocal quality appear in the literature. Most disorders are classified as breathy, harsh, or hoarse; hoarseness is the most prevalent. Designations such as strident and husky are used less frequently.

The breathy voice is characterized by an audible escape of air through partially closed folds. The lack of firm adduction may be due to obstruction by a mass or lesion, a paralyzed cord, or muscular incompetence.

The voice displaying effort and force is the harsh voice. Harshness is usually perceived in a phonatory milieu of hard glottal attacks, low pitch, intensity problems, and overadduction of the vocal folds. Equivalent terms are roughness and unpleasantness, although strident, coarse, grating, rasping, rough, metallic, and gutteral have been used as synonyms for harshness (Murphy, 1964).

The hoarse voice incorporates the features of both breathiness and harshness. As such, turbulent air flow, rough/aperiodic vibrations, low pitch, and neck muscle strain may be evident. Hoarseness is a common symptom of many vocal pathologies and should be recognizable by all speech-language pathologists. In particular, the public school clinician should be familiar with the auditory symptoms of hoarseness as a warning sign of vocal abuse and related lesions in children. The clinician must make medical referrals as appropriate. Also, the clinician must educate teachers through inservice programs to recognize voice disturbances in students so that teacher referrals to the SLP will be accomplished.

The perception of vocal quality is also affected by *glottal approximation*. The hard glottal attack refers to an abrupt impact or strong initiation of speech. Extra effort is used to start the vibrations of tightly adducted folds. Presumably, then, prior to phonation there is too much tension in laryngeal muscles. Conversely, soft attack is an abnormally weak glottal approximation. Breathiness usually precedes this phonation. The astute clinician is listening for symptoms of an inappropriate glottal approximation.

Quality can also be affected by resonance imbalances; however, these problems will be discussed in Chapter 12.

Assessment of Breath Features

Breathing variables affect laryngeal function in general, and vocal loudness and rate of speech in particular. Several features of the respiratory system and breath management are typically assessed in a voice evaluation. The clinician may first want to observe the *predominant region* used for breath support. The diaphragm is the principal muscle of inhalation and various thoracic muscles assist when needed in expanding the lung-thoracic unit (Zemlin, 1988). Diaphragmatic breathing involves descent of the diaphragm and expansion of the abdomen during inhalation. Although quite normal—and a preferred way of breathing for both song and speech—it is difficult if not impossible to observe in a clothed, seated client. Expansion of the chest, not the shoulders, in a slight heaving motion is more observable; this type of thoracic breathing is used by many people. Clavicular breathing, in contrast, is characterized by shoulder elevation, upper thoracic tension (in the area of the clavicle or collar bone), and neck muscle strain. Clavicular breathing is an inefficient method of lung expansion for inhalation as it involves too much effort for too little breath. The clinician should try to observe the region predominately used for breathing by clients; many hyperfunctional voice cases employ this inefficient form of breathing.

The maximum amount of air that can be exhaled following maximal inhalation is called *vital capacity*. The relationship of vital capacity to speech production is somewhat a matter of conjecture at this point. Vital capacity is apparently related to several factors, such as body size, physical condition, and sex (Gray & Wise, 1959; Van Riper & Irwin, 1958). There is little or no research to vindicate those who have worked to increase the vital capacity of their voice clients. On the other hand, it is logical to assume that an individual with an extremely small amount of available air would find it difficult to sustain phonation and might resort to increased laryngeal tension and forcing to maintain normal or near-normal phrasing. It is probably not so much the volume of air as it is the individual's ability to control the airflow (Hardy, 1961).

Equipment, such as the spirometer, is necessary to measure vital capacity. Clinically, however, we have found that a vital capacity insufficient for normal speech purposes was so obvious from normal observation that further formal testing was not necessary. Vital capacity measurements may be of particular concern in cases of emphysema, later stages of Parkinson's disease, and cerebral palsy in children. Related to lung volume are indications of the client's tidal volume, inspiratory reserve volume, expiratory reserve volume, and air flow rates, which some authorities recommend measuring clinically (Boone & McFarlane, 1988; Hirano, 1981).

Inhalation for speech should be quick and quiet. The clinician should listen for *associated noises* such as gasps and vocalizations during inhalation as the client speaks. Rating scales may also prompt the clinician to judge their conspicuousness or severity. *Inhalatory stridor* refers to noticeable phonatory sounds during inhalation and may be common in cases of vocal fold paralysis and dysarthrias (Darley, Aronson, & Brown, 1975).

When respiratory support is inadequate for normal speech, clients may breathe more frequently. In addition, fewer words (or syllables) may be spoken per breath group. These two factors contribute to the perception of "choppy" speech. The clinician should assess *words per breath;* a patient who can only utter six or so words per air charge is displaying poor breath support. Occasionally, a patient may say an excessive number of words per breath group. Research as to what is excessive is, however, lacking. Perhaps upwards of 12 or 13 words per breath group is typical of normal speakers. Increased speaking rates and loss of intelligibility may be the negative by-products of too many words per breath.

Of interest in a voice evaluation is the maximum duration that a client can sustain sound plus air. *Maximum phonation time* (MPT) is typically measured with a stopwatch as the client prolongs certain voiced phonemes, such as /a/ or /z/. A similar measure is that of *maximum exhalation time* (MET), where a voiceless phoneme such as /s/ is used. The clinician should provide several trials, instruct the client to use a deep breath, and record the longest sustained attempt. Wilson (1987) presents data on average maximum phonation times for /a/, /i/, and /u/ for ages three to 29 years. Hirano (1981) also provides normal MPT values for adults. Distilling down this information, we find the following rules of thumb to be clinically useful: Elementary school-age children (six- to 10-years-old) should be able to prolong /a/ for at least nine seconds, regardless of sex; adult males average 25 to 35 seconds MPT; and adult females average 15 to 25 seconds MPT. Coleman, Michel, and Lynn (1987) caution against using normative data collected from healthy, young to middle-aged adults when evaluating geriatric clients. They encourage collection of local norms by practicing clinicians. Values for maximum exhalation time (MET) that they report as clinically useful are 35 seconds for clients who are trained singers or actors; 20 seconds for a typical young adult; and 12 seconds for persons over age 65.

Related to the measures of MPT and MET is the clinical procedure of computing the *S/Z ratio*. The S/Z ratio as proposed by Eckel and Boone (1981) and Tait, Michel, and Carpenter (1980) is a quick screening device used to determine how much of a voice problem may be related to respiration control and how much may be the result of laryngeal problems. Clients who have laryngeal pathology will have less control of the air stream during the production of a prolonged /z/. Using a stopwatch, two trials are given for the prolongation of both the voiceless /s/ and the voiced /z/ phonemes. The best or longest /s/ and the longest /z/ are used in calculating the S/Z ratio. If the S/Z ratio is greater than 1.2 for a child or 1.4 for an adult, a laryngeal pathology may exist (Eckel & Boone, 1981).

Assessment of Rate and Rhythm

Although it is not a traditional part of vocal evaluations, the *rate* at which a client talks should be assessed, since rate can affect or be affected by other variables of speech and the voice. Excessive rates are often related to poor breathing features and improper phrase groupings. The client may try to say too many words on one breath, giving the perception of an excessive rate of speech, such as in Parkinsonism. The converse may also occur. Frequent air intakes may give the perception of choppiness—the client may only be able to say a few words, then breathe, then a few more words, then breathe, and so forth. The result is not only a choppy *rhythm* but an overall slowness of speech due to the increased pause time. Rate changes may also interfere with intelligibility, as is so typical of the dysarthrias (Yorkston, Beukelman, & Bell, 1988).

Rate is typically expressed as words per minute or syllables per minute. It can be quite cumbersome to measure an entire speech sample for the determination of rate. Therefore, we offer the following efficient and clinically useful estimation method (tape recording for later playback is recommended): Count the number of words in a 60-second sample of "connected" speech. If no connected 60-second samples are available on the tape recording, then count the number of words in whatever connected sample is available and mathematically calculate words per minute. For example, if a 20-second speech sample contains 50 words then, on the average, the person is talking at 150 words per minute (60 seconds divided by 20 seconds = 3 and 3 times 50 words = 150 wpm). An alternative method, useful for determining rate of speech during reading, has been suggested by Fox and Blechman (1975). Give the client a reading passage with prenumbered words. Allow the client to read aloud for one minute, as timed with a stopwatch, and note how many of the words were read.

Conversational speech rates typical of young children have only recently been published. Ryan (1984) found that normal-speaking children (ages 2:10 to 5:2) converse at 195 syllables per minute or 157 words per minute. A slightly slower rate was reported by Pindzola and colleagues in that normal three-, four-, and five-year-olds average 148 syllables per minute of talking with a range between 109 and 183 syllables (Miller & Pindzola, 1985; Pindzola, Jenkins, & Lokken, 1989). During an oral reading task, normal adult speakers, speak at a mean rate of 167 words per minute (Darley, 1940), yet conversational rates may be higher at 195 words per minute (Walker, 1979). As rate norms were collected from young, healthy adults, caution is advised in assessing speech rates of geriatrics. Preliminary studies suggest that older adults speak slower than younger adults. Persons over age 65 average about 141–144 words per minute or 186–289 syllables per minute (Duchin & Mysak, 1987; Leeper et al., 1990). At the present time, we do not know what constitutes "too fast" or "too slow" a speech rate and so the clinician's judgment of normalcy is important. Rate determinations may be most necessary with neurological voice disorders (Darley, Aronson, & Brown, 1975; Yorkston, Beukelman, & Bell, 1988).

OBJECTIVE AND SOPHISTICATED MEASURES

Great strides have been made in the last decade to advance our knowledge of voice science. Technological advances have permitted us to study laryngeal function and much of this technology is now ready for clinical application. Ludlow and Hart (1982) concluded from a conference involving voice scientists, speech pathologists, and laryngologists that fiberoptic, electromyographic, airflow, acoustic, and laryngographic techniques are useful in the assessment of neurologic dysfunction, vocal fold lesions, morphologic changes of the folds, and abnormal phonatory function.

Hirano (1981) has done much to standardize the clinical examination of the voice and feels that proper instrumentation is essential to a thorough assessment. The following section of this chapter will outline equipment-dependent techniques and provide a framework for interpretation of the data generated from such instrumentation.

Electromyography

Electromyography, or EMG, permits direct assessment of the laryngeal muscles. Hirano (1981) describes the necessary apparatus and electrode insertion techniques. EMG has not been used routinely in this country except in major research centers with medical affiliations. Yet, EMG is important to the diagnosis of vocal fold paralysis; true paralysis may be differentiated from other forms of vocal fold immobility. Also, EMG can indicate the degree and extent of paralysis, which may suggest recovery potential in that the presence of action potentials induced by voluntary activity indicates a favorable prognosis. It can also be useful in shaping the course of surgical procedures, as in lateral fixation of a fold for cases of bilateral paralysis.

Aerodynamic Tests

Aerodynamic tests can assess the aerodynamic properties of phonation, including subglottal pressure, supraglottal pressure, glottal impedance, and the volume velocity of the airflow at the glottis. Hirano (1981) states that the values of these four parameters vary during the opening and closing maneuvers of the glottis and may be difficult to measure. For example, the determination of subglottal pressure necessitates an invasive approach (such as a tracheal puncture) and glottal resistance must be mathematically calculated as it cannot be measured directly. The measure of *mean flow rate* (MFR), however, is often done as an office procedure.

The mean flow rate of a sustained vowel, such as /a/, spoken at a natural pitch and loudness level, has been used clinically to evaluate phonatory function. The patient sustains the vowel for a maximum period of time while wearing a mask fitted tightly to the face or using a mouth piece with the nose clamped. The mask or mouth piece is coupled to a spirometer, pneumotachograph, or hot-wire anemometer. The mean flow rate is obtained by dividing the total volume of air used during phonation by the duration of phonation.

As reviewed by Hirano (1981), numerous studies suggest that normal values of the mean flow rate range from 40 to 200 ml/sec in adult males and females. The work of Shigemori (1977) suggests that similar values hold true for children. MFR values greater than 200 ml/sec or less than 40 ml/sec obtained at habitual pitch and loudness levels should be regarded as abnormal.

MFR is greater than normal in cases of recurrent laryngeal nerve paralysis. MFR values in cases of nodules, polyps, polypoid swelling (Reinke's edema), and neoplastic tumors also exceed the normal range but are not as marked as with recurrent laryngeal nerve paralysis. In contrast, MFR values are typically within normal limits for the conditions of laryngitis, contact granuloma, and spastic dysphonia. Hirano (1981) concludes that MFR is not only diagnostically important, but it may be used to monitor treatment as well.

Another aerodynamic measure that may be calculated is that of *phonation quotient.* Hirano (1981) calculates the phonation quotient (PQ) by dividing the vital capacity (VC) by the maximum phonation time (MPT):

$$PQ = \frac{VC}{MPT}$$

He also reports that the phonation quotient has a high positive relationship to the MFR and therefore is a reasonable, clinical substitute for MFR when no equipment for airflow measurement is available. Normal values of the PQ in adults and children are typically between 120 to 190 ml/sec. High phonation quotients are associated with recurrent laryngeal nerve paralysis and additive lesions of the folds, such as nodules, polyps, polypoid swelling, and neoplasms.

Subglottal pressure measures are also aerodynamic, yet invasive, tests. To measure air pressures below the vocal folds, a tracheal puncture needle, transglottal catheter, or esophageal balloon may be used. Clinicians working in nonmedical settings do not typically measure subglottal pressure in their clients. Normal values of subglottal pressure during habitual phonation are typically 5 to 10 cm H_2O, but this varies with variations in vocal intensity and fundamental frequency (Hirano, 1981). Subglottal pressure values are abnormally high in laryngeal carcinoma, recurrent nerve paralysis, laryngocele, and perhaps even in functional dysphonias.

Examination of Vocal Fold Vibration

By observing the vibrating vocal folds, clinicians and researchers can better understand both healthy and pathological laryngeal characteristics. Special equipment is needed to view movements occurring 100 to 300 times per second, as is typical during conversational speech. Stroboscopy and glottography are clinically useful methods; other, more elaborate research methodologies are also available. The serious student will want to consult Hirano (1981) for a detailed account of examination techniques and the numerous behaviors that can be assessed by such vibration studies (e.g., horizontal excursion of the vocal fold edge, glottal width, glottal area, frequency of vibration, symmetry of movements, closure phase information).

Acoustic Measures

Acoustic measures, according to Perkins (1985), are the most frequently employed, and perhaps preferred, objective or formal techniques for assessing the voice. This is because acoustic measures are nonintrusive; easily gathered, analyzed, and quantified; and applicable to a wide range of normal and abnormal laryngeal conditions. The serious student will want to consult the works of Davis (1979, 1982) regarding the applications of acoustic measures to the assessment of voice. Research has shown that acoustic measures are useful in both the detection of laryngeal pathologies and the assessment of voice quality. Perkins states:

> Pathology that affects vocal fold mass, elasticity, stiffness, or length will affect fundamental frequency. Paralysis of respiratory or laryngeal musculature will reduce sufficiency of subglottal pressure and, accordingly, of vocal intensity. The traditional early warning sign of laryngeal pathology, hoarseness, is heard as a deviant quality but can also involve fundamental frequency and intensity. A tumor or paralysis of one cord that produces asymmetric mass, stiffness, or elasticity will cause asymmetric cord vibration with consequent breathiness, reduced intensity, pitch perturbation (jitter) and amplitude perturbation (shimmer). (1985, p. 82)

The measures of jitter and shimmer are becoming more commonplace because of their utility at early detection of pathology, even when the laryngologist sees no obvious lesion or tissue change. Speech pathologists working in concert with laryngologists will be called upon to obtain measures of jitter and shimmer on their patients. There are several methods of computation for jitter and shimmer values; the serious student is urged to study this topic further.

The sound spectrogram has long been a favorite piece of equipment for the voice scientist and clinician. Isshiki, Yanigahara, and Morimoto (1966) proposed that narrowband analyses can provide measures of hoarseness. They described four types:

- Type 1—shows the slightest degree of hoarseness where the distinct harmonic component is mixed with the noise component which is limited within the formant region of the vowels; vowels to use are /u, o, a, e, i/.
- Type 2—shows a slight noise component in the high frequency region (3000–5000 Hz). The noise components predominate over the harmonics, most noticeable for the vowels /e/ and /i/.
- Type 3—shows only noise in the second formant of /i/ and /e/; there is also a further intensification of noise above 3000 Hz.
- Type 4—is characterized by noise in the second formant of /e/, /i/, and /a/ and in the first formant of /a/, /o/, and /u/. In these formant regions, the harmonic components are hardly noticeable.

The clinician can use the typing system of Isshiki, Yanigahara, and Morimoto for baseline, objective documentation of a patient's hoarseness. Spectrographic reassessments and retyping could be used as a barometer of improvement through treatment.

INFORMAL ASSESSMENT PROBES

We have now explained both the perceptual-informal and the technological-formal methods of voice appraisal. Clearly, most speech-language pathologists operate in work settings with limited instrumentation available. Over the years, then, clinicians have developed effective behavioral techniques for assessing, probing, treating, and reassessing laryngeal voice disorders. Indeed, the process of voice therapy is behavioral; that is, we as clinicians use strategies, techniques, devices, and even psychological "tricks" to change or alter a client's voice. Of course this presupposes that the changes are somehow better for the client—the voice sounds better, less effort is expended in its production, further damage is not being inflicted on their vocal mechanism, and so forth. But just completing a voice evaluation, where deviant vocal parameters have been analyzed, in and of itself does not suggest how to proceed clinically. As clinicians, we want to know what we can do to make the client's voice "better." Here we enter the world of trial therapy and the use of facilitating techniques to probe the client's potential to alter his/her voice for the better. Let us now highlight some of these probe techniques in hopes that clinicians will try out the client's ability to modify and improve parameters of the voice during the initial diagnostic evaluation. By doing so, the clinician will be able to accomplish two important things: a meaningful prognosis and a direction for intervention.

Patients with hypofunctional voice problems often show improved phonatory abilities by increasing glottal tension. Indeed, Wilson and Rice (1977) have developed a clinical approach termed *tension increase therapy*. The clinician should probe which maneuvers, if any, are successful in improving the voice. Do any of the so-called optimal pitch techniques help, such as grunting, pushing, pulling, throat clearing, or coughing (see Table 10.6)? An intentional hard glottal attack, even if accompanied by increased tension in the arms and trunk while pushing forcefully, may facilitate approximation of the vocal folds. Used this way, these may be thought of as hypertonic techniques rather than as techniques to achieve optimal pitch. Table 10.7 presents a useful sampling of techniques that may facilitate, or improve, voice production. The works of the following authorities should be consulted for more in-depth discussions of facilitating techniques: Van Riper and Irwin (1958), Johnson, Darley, and Spriestersbach (1963), Moncur and Brackett (1974), Prater and Swift (1984), Boone and McFarlane (1988).

Two case examples may illustrate how the use of hypertonic probe techniques in the evaluation affected treatment recommendations.

> Mrs. Hernandez was involved in a rather messy divorce settlement after 22 years of marriage. Over the past few months, she has experienced periodic losses of voice—sometimes during heated conversations but occasionally for an afternoon or an entire day. Mrs. Hernandez indicated that the voice was reduced to a whisper during these episodes and was not hoarse like in laryngitis. The current episode of voice loss, and the reason she was seeing a speech-language pathologist, had lasted over a week. The clinician was not able to get

Table 10.7 Some Facilitating Techniques for the Improvement of Voice

To improve adduction and phonatory abilities
    Gutzmann lateral compression of thyroid lamina
    Head turning or tilting
    Pushing or pulling concomitant with voicing
    Hard glottal attacks

To alter pitch and/or quality
    Gutzmann frontal compression of thyroid prominence
    Any/all of the optimal pitch techniques (Table 10.6)
    Change in loudness
    Change in speech rate
    Soft glottal attacks
    Relax musculature/reduce tension
    Alter respiratory patterns

Mrs. Hernandez to speak above a whisper in the evaluation; she showed no potential to talk, sing, or shout. The clinician was able to elicit, rather quickly, a cough and a throat-clearing maneuver that contained true phonated sound. A diagnosis of hysterical aphonia was made and, because of the rehabilitation potential displayed for phonation, treatment was recommended immediately. After three sessions of behavioral shaping, beginning with vegetative eliciting techniques, the client was speaking normally. Referral was then made for psychological support services.

Mrs. Osborne, age 42, presented with unilateral vocal fold paralysis subsequent to thyroid surgery. The laryngologist referred the patient for voice improvement therapy. Teflon injection was contraindicated as it would further compromise the reduced glottal airway. The patient presented with stridor during physical exertion; the speaking voice was hoarse and of limited loudness. Hoarseness diminished and loudness improved when the speech-language pathologist exerted medical pressure against the thyroid lamina on the side of the paralyzed fold (a rendition of the Gutzmann medial compression technique). Other hypertonic facilitating techniques were helpful, as well, in improving Mrs. Osborne's voicing abilities. With medical management contraindicated, the clinician felt compensatory strategies involving increased muscular effort and glottal attack were appropriate and realistic. Treatment was recommended along these lines.

Vocal quality improvements can also be brought about by changes in the manner of speaking. Adjustments in the respiratory, phonatory, and articulatory processes impact on the overall perception of the voice. We provide one case example here.

Greg was a college student referred to us by the university infirmary. Greg had gone to see the doctor with general complaints of not feeling well, simply in an effort to get a medical excuse for missing a class exam for which he had not studied. The doctor could find nothing wrong with Greg but was concerned by his "gravel-sounding, hoarse voice." Indirect laryngoscopy revealed normal structures and referral was made to our speech clinic. Greg's voice was pitched abnormally low and the quality was indeed abnormal. The aberrant quality was the more conspicuous problem. He indicated that his voice always sounded like this and gave him no trouble other than fatigue after any day of heavy talking. Part of our evaluation session was spent with "trial and error" attempts to change Greg's voice. Some things we tried had no effect, others made him sound more harsh, and a few techniques seemed to bring out a "better" voice. In particular, raising Greg's pitch slightly decreased the harshness. The higher pitch, he assured us, felt comfortable. We hypothesized that Greg was using an inappropriately low and harsh voice, perhaps to project a more masculine image, and that the functional disorder would remediate quite well. Treatment was recommended to improve the harsh quality by raising pitch.

PROGNOSIS

Prognosis has several aspects. First, there is the question of spontaneous remission of the presenting symptoms. Will this individual display an improvement in voice without intervening therapy? Second, how much improvement can be expected following the prescribed clinical program? That is, to what degree is the voice therapy, as projected, going to be effective? Third, how permanent are the gains shown in therapy going to be? Is the vocal improvement such that continuous therapy will be necessary to maintain optimal voice performance? (Medicare and most third-party reimbursement agencies will not fund "maintenance therapy.") Finally, would some other clinical procedure be of greater benefit to the client?

A variety of factors have potential prognostic value in voice cases. Some of the variables are directly observable and subject to quantification; others are much more subjective. The factors appear to fall into three broad categories: characteristics of the disorder, the person, and the environment. Those factors include:

1. Duration of the problems. Generally disorders of long standing have greater resistance to clinical treatment.
2. Etiological factors. Two factors are relevant here. First, is the cause of the problem identifiable? Second, is the cause of the problem alterable? And if so, is the type of habilitating service required available?
3. Degree of secondary psychological components. Generally, the greater the degree of psychological disturbance, the poorer the prognosis.
4. Variability and general flexibility of the voice. Generally, the more the client is able to alter his/her vocal behavior the better the prognosis. This underscores the importance of probing for vocal change with facilitating techniques during the initial session.
5. Auditory and imitative skills. The better the client is at hearing differences in quality, pitch, and loudness, coupled with the ability to imitate these differences, the more favorable the prognosis.
6. Impact or degree of disability. The greater the impact of the voice difference upon the individual, the better the chances for cooperation and motivation. Generally, too, if the family of the client is supportive, the outlook is more favorable.
7. Structural integrity of the vocal mechanism. Clearly, the more the speech mechanism is disrupted anatomically or neurologically, the more limited the prognosis will be.

CONCLUSION

The evaluation of voice disorders is a challenge to the speech pathologist. It requires the ability to deal with older adults as well as young children. The clinician must often work closely with medical personnel and other allied health workers which necessitates knowing procedures and terminologies that are peripheral to speech-language pathology. The clinician must also remain abreast of current technological developments in electronics, surgery, and medical technology. Finally, the clinician must keep interpersonal clinical skills finely honed so that psychological aspects of vocal disorders can be detected and dealt with through treatment or referral. Beginning students are encouraged to read widely about voice disorders, seek out clients with vocal problems, and gain as much clinical experience as they can in this interesting area.

BIBLIOGRAPHY

ARONSON, A. (1985). *Clinical voice disorders* (2nd ed.). New York: Thieme-Stratton, Inc.

BATEMAN, H. E., & MASON, R. M. (1984). *Applied anatomy and physiology of the speech and hearing mechanism.* Springfield, IL: Charles C Thomas.

BLONIGEN, J. A. (1980). *Remediation of vocal hoarseness.* Hingham, MA: Teaching Resources Corp.

BOONE, D. (1980). *The Boone voice program for children.* Austin, TX: PRO-Ed.

BOONE, D. (1982). *The Boone voice program for adults.* Austin, TX: PRO-Ed.

BOONE, D., & MCFARLANE, S. C. (1988). *The voice and voice therapy* (4th ed.). Englewood Cliffs, NJ: Prentice Hall.

COLEMAN, R. F., MICHEL, J., & LYNN, P. (1987). *Use and misuse of instrumental analysis in clinical voice practice.* Paper presented at annual convention of the American Speech-Language-Hearing Association, New Orleans, LA.

COOPER, M. (1973). *Modern techniques of vocal rehabilitation.* Springfield, IL: Charles C Thomas.

CURRY, E. (1949). Hoarseness and voice change in male adolescents. *Journal of Speech and Hearing Disorders, 14,* 23–24.

CURTIS, J. (1968). Acoustics of speech production and nasalization. In D. Spriestersbach & D. Sherman (Eds.), *Cleft palate and communication.* New York: Academic Press.

DANILOFF, R., SCHUCKERS, G., & FETH, L. (1980). *The physiology of speech and hearing: An introduction.* Englewood Cliffs, NJ: Prentice Hall.

DARLEY, F. L. (1940). *A normative study of oral reading rate.* M. A. Thesis, University of Iowa.

DARLEY, F. L., ARONSON, A. E., & BROWN, J. R. (1975). *Motor speech disorders.* Philadelphia, PA: W. B. Saunders Co.

DAVIS, S. (1979). Acoustic characteristics of normal and pathological voices. In N. Lass (Ed.), *Speech and language: Research and theory.* New York: Academic Press.

DAVIS, S. (1982). Acoustic characteristics or normal and pathological voices. In *Proceedings of the Conference on the Assessment of Vocal Pathology. ASHA Reports, 11,* 97–115.

DEAL, R., MCCLAIN, B., & SUDDERTH, J. (1976). Identification, evaluation, therapy and follow-up for children with vocal nodules in a public school setting. *Journal of Speech and Hearing Disorders, 41,* 390–397.

DICKSON, D., & MAUE-DICKSON, W. (1982). *Anatomical and physiological bases of speech.* Boston: Little, Brown.

DIEHL, C., & STINNETT, C. (1959). Efficiency of teacher referrals in a school speech testing program. *Journal of Speech and Hearing Disorders, 24,* 34–36.

DUCHIN, S. W., & MYSAK, E. D. (1987). Disfluency and rate characteristics of young adult, middle-aged, and older males. *Journal of Communication Disorders, 20,* 245–257.

ECKEL, F., & BOONE, D. (1981). The S/Z ratio as an indicator of laryngeal pathology. *Journal of Speech and Hearing Disorders, 46,* 147–150.

FAIRBANKS, G. (1960). *Voice and articulation drillbook* (2nd ed.). New York: Harper & Row.

FOX, D. R., & BLECHMAN, M. (1975). *Clinical management of voice disorders.* Lincoln, NE: Cliffs Notes, Inc.

GRAY, G., & WISE, C. (1959). *The bases of speech* (3rd ed.). New York: Harper & Row.

GREEN, G. (1989). Psycho-behavioral characteristics of children with vocal nodules: WPBIC ratings. *Journal of Speech and Hearing Disorders, 54,* 306–312.

GREENE, M. (1980). *The voice and its disorders.* Philadelphia, PA: J. B. Lippincott Co.

HANLEY, T., & THURMAN, W. (1970). *Developing vocal skills.* New York: Holt, Rinehart and Winston.

HARDY, J. (1961). Intraoral breath pressure in cerebral palsy. *Journal of Speech and Hearing Disorders, 26,* 309–319.

HIRANO, M. (1981). *Clinical examination of voice.* Vienna, Austria: Springer-Verlag.

HOLLIEN, H., & SHIPP, T. (1972). Speaking fundamental frequency and chronological age in males. *Journal of Speech and Hearing Research, 15,* 155–159.

ISSHIKI, N., YANIGAHARA, N., & MORIMOTO, H. (1966). Approach to the objective diagnosis of hoarseness. *Folia Phoniatrica, 18,* 393–400.

JACKSON, C. (1941). Vocal nodules. *American Laryngological Association, 63,* 185.

JAMES, H., & COOPER, E. (1966). Accuracy of teacher referral of speech-handicapped children. *Exceptional Child, 30,* 29–33.

JOHNSON, W., DARLEY, F., & SPRIESTERSBACH, D. (1963). *Diagnostic methods in speech pathology.* New York: Harper & Row.

KAHANE, J., & FOLKINS, J. (1984). *Atlas of speech and hearing anatomy.* Columbus, OH: Charles E. Merrill.

KAPLAN, H. (1971). *Anatomy and physiology of speech.* New York: McGraw-Hill.

KELLEY, A. (1977). *F₀ measurements of female voices from 20–90 years of age.* Unpublished manuscript, University of North Carolina at Greensboro. Cited in Aronson, A. (1980). *Clinical voice disorders: An interdisciplinary approach,* pp. 52–53. New York: Thieme-Stratton.

LEEPER, L. H., CULATTA, R. A., PINDZOLA, R. H., & CESKA, S. (1990). *Elderly speakers' rate/fluency: What we know, what it means.* Paper presented at annual convention of the American Speech-Language-Hearing Association, Seattle, WA.

LEFF, J., & ABBERTON, E. (1981). Voice pitch measurements in schizophrenia and depression. *Psychological Medicine, 11,* 849–852.

LUCHSINGER, R., & ARNOLD, G. (1965). *Voice-speech-language.* Belmont, CA: Wadsworth.

LUDLOW, C., & HART, M. (1982). Preface. *Proceedings of the Conference on the Assessment of Vocal Pathology. ASHA Reports, 11,* v.

MARTONY, J. (1968). On the correlation of the voice pitch level for severely hard-of-hearing subjects. *American Annals of the Deaf, 113,* 195–202.

MILLER, M. K., & PINDZOLA, R. H. (1985). *The development of speaking rates in preschool children.* Paper presented at the annual convention of the American Speech-Language-Hearing Association, Washington, DC.

MONCUR, J., & BRACKETT, I. (1974). *Modifying vocal behavior.* New York: Harper & Row.

MOSES, P. (1954). *The voice of neurosis.* New York: Grune & Stratton.

MURPHY, A. (1964). *Functional voice disorders.* Englewood Cliffs, NJ: Prentice Hall.

PALMER, J. (1984). *Anatomy for speech and hearing.* New York: Harper & Row.

PERKINS, W. H. (1985). Assessment and treatment of voice disorders: State of the art. In J. M. Costello (Ed.), *Speech disorders in adults: Recent advances.* San Diego, CA: College-Hill Press.

PERKINS, W. H., & KENT, R. D. (1986). *Functional anatomy of speech, language, and hearing: A primer.* San Diego, CA: College-Hill.

PINDZOLA, R. H. (1987). *A voice assessment protocol for children and adults.* Austin, TX: PRO-Ed.

PINDZOLA, R. H., JENKINS, M. M., & LOKKEN, K. J. (1989). Speaking rates of young children. *Language, Speech and Hearing Services in Schools, 20*(2), 133–138.

POLOW, N. G., & KAPLAN, E. D. (1980). *Symptomatic voice therapy.* Austin, TX: PRO-Ed.

POWERS, M. (1971). Functional disorders of articulation: Symptomatology and etiology. In L. Travis (Ed.), *Handbook of speech pathology and audiology.* Englewood Cliffs, NJ: Prentice Hall.

PRACY, R., SIEGLER, J., STELL, P. M., & ROGERS, J. (1977). *Ear, nose and throat surgery and nursing.* New York: John Wiley.

PRATER, R. J., & SWIFT, R. W. (1984). *Manual of voice therapy.* Boston: Little, Brown.

ROUSEY, C., & MORIARTY, A. (1965). *Diagnostic implications of speech sounds.* Springfield, IL: Charles C Thomas.

RYAN, B. P. (1984). *Stuttering in preschool children: A comparison and longitudinal study.* Paper presented at the annual convention of the American Speech-Language-Hearing Association, San Francisco, CA.

SHEARER, W. M. (1972). Diagnosis and treatment of voice disorders in school children. *Journal of Speech and Hearing Disorders, 37,* 215–221.

SHIGEMORI, Y. (1977). Some tests related to the air usage during phonation: Clinical investigations. *Otologia, 23,* 138–166.

SILVERMAN, E., & ZIMMER, C. (1975). Incidence of chronic hoarseness among school-age children. *Journal of Speech and Hearing Disorders, 40,* 211–215.

STEMPLE, J. (1984). *Clinical voice pathology: Theory and management.* Columbus, OH: Charles E. Merrill.

STONE, E., HURLBUTT, N., & COULTHARD, S. (1978). Role and laryngological consultation in the intervention of dysphonia. *Language, Speech and Hearing Services in Schools, 9,* 35–42.

TAIT, N., MICHEL, J., & CARPENTER, M. (1980). Maximum duration of sustained /s/ and /z/ in children. *Journal of Speech and Hearing Disorders, 45,* 239–246.

VAN BERGEIJK, W. A., PIERCE, J. R., & DAVID, E. E. (1960). *Waves and the ear.* Garden City, NY: Anchor Books, Doubleday and Co.

VAN RIPER, C., & IRWIN, J. (1958). *Voice and articulation.* Englewood Cliffs, NJ: Prentice Hall.

WALKER, V. G. (1979). *Speech durations of young adults during speaking and reading.* Unpublished doctoral dissertation, The Florida State University, Tallahassee, FL.

WEINBERG, B. (1983). Phonatory based voice disorders. In I. Meitus & B. Weinberg (Eds.), *Diagnosis in speech-language pathology.* Baltimore: University Park Press.

WEINTRAUB, S., MESULAM, M., & KRAMER, L. (1981). Disturbances in prosody: A right hemisphere contribution to language. *Archives of Neurology, 38,* 742–744.

WENDAHL, R., & PAGE, L. (1967). Glottal wave periods in CVC environments. *Journal of the Acoustical Society of America, 42,* 1208.

WILSON, D. K. (1987). *Voice problems in children* (3rd ed.), Baltimore: Williams & Wilkins.

WILSON, F., & RICE, M. (1977). *A programmed approach to voice therapy.* Austin, TX: Learning Concepts, Inc.

WITHERS, B. (1961). Vocal nodules. *Eye, Ear, Nose and Throat Monthly, 40,* 35–38.

YORKSTON, K. M., BEUKELMAN, D. R., & BELL, K. R. (1988). *Clinical management of dysarthric speakers.* Boston: College-Hill.

ZEMLIN, W. (1988). *Speech and hearing science* (3rd ed.). Englewood Cliffs, NJ: Prentice Hall.

chapter

11

ASSESSMENT AND REASSESSMENT OF THE LARYNGECTOMEE

Laryngeal excision is done primarily to preserve the life of the patient, most often because of the presence of cancer. However, the surgeon, in removing the malignant tumor and a healthy margin of tissue, is also conscious of the need to provide as great a chance for continued vocal function as is possible. Surgery may include excision of the total larynx, half of the larynx, one vocal fold and part of the other, removal of the anterior section of the thyroid cartilage and both vocal folds, or various other combinations. In cases of early detection, subtotal laryngectomies are becoming more routine and the surgeon is often able to reconstruct a serviceable larynx and preserve voice. It is important that the speech-language pathologist know exactly what procedures were undertaken since the rehabilitation program will vary relative to the type of surgery and the condition of the remaining structures. This chapter, however, will focus on the assessment process following total laryngectomy.

The assessment of a person who has undergone a total laryngectomy is inherently different from the initial assessment of persons with other communication disorders. We do not approach the initial session to solve the problem–no problem issue. When we get a referral to see a laryngectomee we immediately know that the ability to speak has been lost—there is a problem and the diagnosis is obvious—we also know that some form of intervention will be necessary to re-establish a means of communication for the patient. What needs to be assessed is the current status of the patient (physically, psychologically, and the like), the potential for rehabilitation, and the direction (or directions) that the intervention program should take. Questions floating around the clinician's mind are likely to include: Is the patient psychologically ready to begin rehabilitation in earnest?

What is the physical health of the patient like, both in general and as relates to the laryngeal surgery? Are there educational or intellectual limitations that may affect the short- and long-term courses of treatment? And, most importantly, for which avenues of communication does the patient show potential or preference (e.g., gestures, artificial devices, esophageal speech, tracheoesophageal speech)?

From this overview, it should be clear that the evaluation process involves the collection of background information, current status indicators, and trial therapy, among other things. There really are no formal "tests" to administer, and so the clinician's insights, judgments, and competencies with trial therapy techniques are crucial. The evaluation session is truly the initial treatment session as well.

In this chapter, then, we will discuss the process of informally evaluating a newly laryngectomized patient. Since standardized tests do not exist, it could be said that formal diagnostic procedures also do not exist. We will include, however, the screening-testing procedures used to evaluate a patient's candidacy for tracheoesophageal puncture techniques. Also, we will discuss the on-going assessment of a patient enrolled in the various alaryngeal speech rehabilitation programs. Once the patient is talking, it is important to subjectively and objectively appraise the quality of the speech. Research has provided us with many yardsticks on which to measure the progress of our patients. Many re-evaluation materials are available for this purpose.

THE COUNSELING PROCESS

The evaluation will seek to determine a patient's rehabilitation potential and to provide information necessary to shape the direction of treatment. But the evaluation process also has the goal of providing information, support, and emotional release for the patient and the patient's family. The clinician must wear many hats. In this section, let us explore the clinician's role in the preoperative visit, family and spouse counseling, arranging or assisting with the visit by another laryngectomee, and postoperative counseling of the patient.

The Preoperative Visit

Ideally, the surgeon requests that a preoperative visit be made by the speech-language pathologist. When the physician informs the patient of the cancer, a thousand thoughts must surge through the patient's mind: Will I die? Will I be disfigured? Will my family be able to look at me? Will I talk again? Will I lose my job? Private thoughts, such as these, may happen so forcefully and quickly that the patient does not absorb much of what else the physician says. We often see patients with only a small understanding of the surgery and its many consequences for daily living. Explanations offered by the physician, then, can be supplemented at a later meeting by the speech pathologist. A preoperative visit is an ideal time to meet the patient, who can still talk, ask questions, express feelings and fears, and so forth. The clinician must be emotionally and professionally capable of dealing with the issues of this meeting. It can be a time when grown men cry, when grown women react with such anger as to order you out of their room, when denial is apparent, and/or when the patient desperately needs to hear some words of hope and optimism.

One goal of the first meeting, then, is to provide emotional release and support. The clinician must remember in the preoperative visit that the patient is facing a trauma unparalleled in his/her lifetime. Fears of death, loss of communication, loss of job, and social and marital adjustments plague such patients. The first confrontation is no social chat and may well demand all of the professional proficiency the clinician can muster. Occasionally, the clinician might find that the patient is not capable of dealing rationally with the topic immediately before surgery and, in these cases, it may be preferable to postpone detailed discussion until after recovery.

Another major goal of the first meeting is to provide some information about the operation and the implications for speech. After consultation with the physician, every attempt should be made to present a clear discussion of the anatomical changes. Charts and diagrams are often helpful. We often give the patient some booklets or pamphlets, available from the International Association of Laryngectomees of the American Cancer Society (contact the IAL for a list of available materials). The one entitled *Helping Words for the Laryngectomee* (IAL, 1964) contains a positive emotional message, some information of interest, as well as sketches of the vocal tract before and after total laryngectomy. We make sure the patient understands, among other things, that the vocal folds will be removed (consequently no speech will be possible) and that a stoma will be cut permanently into the neck for a breathing passage. We mention these two items here because so many patients have been misinformed and fully expect to be able to talk or whisper and that the "hole in their neck" is only temporary.

Duguay (1966) interviewed more than 50 preoperative laryngectomy candidates who had been counseled by their surgeons about the impending surgery. Their confusion and lack of understanding are reflected in their verbatim comments. We provide a few examples here.

> A 62-year-old housewife: "When they operate, they put in a switch. I don't know—like a little box. I never saw it."
>
> A 63-year-old retired steel plant foreman: "They put something in there, don't they? You draw breath in some way into your lungs—develop some kind of pressure. The sound comes from your lungs. The words are formed down there too."
>
> A 59-year-old automobile factory foreman: "You can talk from the stomach. It comes all the way up—take a deep breath."

While we are explaining the stoma to the patient, using language that can be easily comprehended, we stress the notion that "breathing for breathing and breathing for speech" will be different in the future (unless tracheoesophageal puncture is planned). We find that planting this idea early will help later in teaching esophageal speech and minimizing associated noise.

We explain that many communication avenues exist. At this time, we decide on an appropriate short-term method (e.g., writing, gesturing, pointing to pictures), depending on literacy, vision, and manual dexterity abilities or limitations. We arrange for the hospital, family, speech services, social services, or other department or agency to make the necessary supplies available immediately after surgery (e.g., paper/pencil, wipe-off writing boards, picture communication boards, synthetic speech devices, and so forth). We also introduce other methods that the patient may learn to use, such as esophageal speech and speech with an artificial larynx. The introduction must offer the optimism that he/she may actually speak again, but care must be taken not to overwhelm the patient with too many details at this point.

A brief explanation of the methods and some of the novel terminology may be all that is appropriate at this time. Showing and demonstrating an artificial larynx, playing a tape of an esophageal speaker, and/or showing a film about alaryngeal rehabilitation (available from IAL) certainly can be done in this initial meeting, but we typically do not. These aids seem more fitting for a subsequent session. Other authorities do recommend presurgery speech instruction, such as initiating esophageal air charging and vibration. The works of Green (1980) and Gardner (1971) can be consulted in this regard.

The speech pathologist might enhance the future clinical rapport by making short, daily visits before and after the surgery. This would spread the information into smaller bits so that the patient could better absorb it and ask pointed questions. In summary, we agree with Vallencien et al. who state that

> To give a new voice to the laryngectomized is a good thing, but to give him a normal life is better. It is necessary, before and after surgery, to supply him with information to help himself and his family accept his new situation. (1971, p. 369)

Family-Spouse Counseling

Providing adequate information to the family can have far-reaching clinical implications. The spouse and immediate family must also understand the anatomy of the operation. Often, clinicians stress what the laryngectomee will be unable to do, and although this information is important, it is also important to stress to the family what the patient will be able to do. We generally attempt to have a frank discussion with the spouse about the typical reactions of the family. If a problem can be identified before it develops, it may be easier to control. The tendency to dominate the silent mate (or parent) must be controlled, as must the inclinations to infantilize, overindulge, and pity. Often we have to warn the family not to shout at the patient—they may think that someone who cannot talk also does not hear well. Some families readily admit to feelings of repulsion because of the physical changes; this can be easily conveyed to the patient. The silent mate is sometimes excluded from conversation and decision-making in the family. The clinician must be sensitive to the fact that the spouse will have significant concerns. The fear of death, reduced income, new responsibilities, social changes, and alterations in the marital (and sexual) relationship may be topics for discussion. One of the primary purposes of the clinician's visit with the family is to let them know that their feelings are understood. It is expected that the clinician will be warm, sincere, and insightful, but we resist the temptation to dictate any specific attitude beyond this because each patient will require a somewhat different approach. Some need to be dealt with gently, others straightforwardly and frankly. Find the level and type of interaction your patient and his/her family respond to best and use it.

Materials available from the International Association of Laryngectomees are useful in spouse-family counseling. Many different pamphlets can provide the family with information and inspiration. We also like to arrange a viewing of one or more films; the patient should attend with the family. The IAL film list should be consulted for something appropriate. *To Speak Again* is well suited for families and new patients still in the hospital; we also like *A Second Voice*, which is an overview of the total rehabilitation of the laryngectomee. At a subsequent spouse-family session, after the surgery but ideally before the patient is discharged home, we like to show a film about first-aid. *Check the Neck* or *Three Critical Minutes: Emergency Air for Neck-Breathers* are available from the IAL. The IAL also has pamphlets describing "mouth-to-neck" resuscitation techniques that we like to provide families. Family counseling, then, seeks to ensure that the family is emotionally and physically ready to assist in the rehabilitation program and care of their loved one.

Laryngectomee Visitation

It is ideal when the surgeon and/or the speech-language pathologist can arrange for the patient to be visited by a laryngectomee either before or after the surgery. The laryngectomee visitor, by his/her sheer presence, offers the patient hope: He/she sees a person who survived cancer, survived the operation, learned to talk, perhaps returned to work, and generally has gotten back into life. The laryngectomee can offer the patient sincere understanding of the emotional turmoil—he/she has been down that road—and may be the best paraprofessional to offer advice and empathy. The laryngectomee visitor is, however, first and foremost a model for the patient. Patients who adopt the attitude "if they could do it, I can do it too" will probably be the successful and motivated ones for a rehabilitation program. The modeling of the visitor's speech is also of prime importance. The patient hears first-hand what practiced esophageal speech and/or artificial larynx speech sounds like. Visitors are also great at explaining the importance of personal drive and daily practice. They come prepared with self-help items, information, and advice; the visitor's kit may include such things as stoma covers (hand-made crocheted bibs), emergency decals, and IAL reading materials.

Visits by laryngectomees are becoming less casual and more organized. The American Cancer Society offers a *Laryngectomee Visitor Program Manual* (1985) as a training program for these paraprofessionals. The speech-language pathologist should become familiar with the guidelines and procedures of the visitor program. Opportunities abound for mutual cooperation and help in the assessment and intervention program.

Postoperative Counseling

When preoperative referrals were not made, the postoperative meetings offer the opportunity for emotional release, support, and information-sharing. All that we have described in the previous sessions needs to be accomplished now. If preoperative visits were done, then postoperatively the speech clinician is ready to move forward with the rehabilitation program, which involves a balance between treating and reassessing the patient's emotional, physical, and speech status.

The first few postoperative days may be the emotional low point for the patient. Frequent and brief visits may provide the support needed. The speech pathologist should also ensure that the patient has a means to communicate. Earlier we mentioned planning for written messages, picture communication boards, and the like. Patients with limited reading and writing abilities may benefit from the book of pictures depicting daily needs entitled *Communication for the Laryngectomized* (Bradley & Ormond, 1970). The clinician, with physician knowledge, may introduce artificial larynx devices for immediate speech. The interested student is urged to consult any of the many excellent sources describing the available devices, their types, and how to begin training a patient in their use. In addition to the usual voice disorders textbooks, we would like to suggest the specialized book by Salmon and Goldstein (1978).

The use of artificial larynx devices early in the rehabilitation has long been debated because of their supposed deleterious effects on the subsequent learning of esophageal speech. Current thinking seems to be supportive of colearning both methods of esophageal and artificial larynx speech. What we wish to stress in this section on postoperative work is that artificial devices do offer a means of immediate speech. Let us also summarize some of our experiences with the use of the devices immediately after surgery. We tend not to get a good seal between the stoma cup of the pneumatic devices and the protruding steel or plastic tracheostomy tube. Electric neck-type devices may work, and a variety of placement sites may be tried, but generally neck tenderness is such that the patient seems not to like using the device. Electric intraoral devices, or neck-type devices adapted temporarily for intraoral use, seem to be best in those first few days or weeks following surgery. We acknowledge that intraoral tubes adversely affect intelligibility and overall speech acceptability, and so we strive to switch the patient over to a neck-type device when possible (Moffet & Pindzola, 1988; Pindzola & Moffet, 1988).

After a certain amount of counseling and information-sharing, the speech-language pathologist may wish to administer the *Inventory for the Assessment of Laryngectomy Rehabilitation* (La Borwit, 1981). The purpose of this inventory is to assess the patient's functional knowledge of his/her overall condition. The more functional information a laryngectomee possesses, the greater will be the capacity to act upon that information and achieve rehabilitation goals. As stated by La Borwit:

> . . . scores serve as an index of the level of rehabilitation likely to be attained. Results of scores and the specific responses . . . can expedite the therapeutic process by denoting to the clinician the type and quantity of information (or misinformation) upon which the patient may be relying. Awareness of these responses on the clinician's part can facilitate such decision making as the need for counseling intervention, utilization of artificial larynges or other devices, a modification of clinical teaching or reiteration of necessary concepts, influencing family support, and consultation with the physician. (1981, p. 2)

Using a multiple-choice format, 72 questions are posed in seven categories: speech, family, vocation, attitudes, anatomy, first aid, and support groups.

Efforts to begin esophageal speech training await clearance by the physician. Some physicians refer for treatment once the patient is moved out of intensive care, perhaps two or three days postoperatively. Others wait for removal of the nasogastric feeding tube and resumption of chewing and swallowing, typically four to 14 days postoperatively. Prior to the go-ahead for initiating esophageal speech training, the physician's orders for a speech consult include the pre- and/or postoperative counseling (emotional support and information-sharing), establishment of a temporary means for communication, and the evaluation proper.

One final comment as to what we do for the patient and family postoperatively. We provide or assist the family in ordering detailed reading material. The pamphlets, given earlier, surely have served a useful purpose, but the patient may further benefit from books such as *Self-Help for the Laryngectomee* (Lauder, 1989) or *Looking Forward: A Guidebook for the Laryngectomee* (Keith et al., 1984).

BACKGROUND AND CURRENT STATUS INFORMATION

The evaluation of the newly laryngectomized patient truly began with the first preoperative meeting and has continued through all subsequent contacts. Where the patient is psychologically, physiologically, and intellectually is important to know, and these places keep changing. Dynamic assessments, rather than static evaluations are the order of the day. Yet, as in traditional evaluations of a patient, we need to collect background as well as current status information. We begin by reading the patient's hospital chart with particular emphasis on the initial (admitting) medical report, the surgical report, the daily notes by the nursing staff, and the family history critique provided by the social worker.

In determining the potential for speech, a thorough case history is helpful with laryngectomized patients. Three facets are particularly crucial. It is important to know the extent of the surgery, the degree of involvement of related structures such as the tongue or pharynx, general health of the patient, and medical prognosis. The second critical area is the individual's vocation and interests. We find it most helpful to plan our clinical work about the patient's preferred activities. It is also important to know if the person will be able to continue in those vocations and hobbies that involve communication. A third variable related to the patient's potential for learning esophageal speech is attitude and motivation. Some patients are depressed, discouraged, and unmotivated while others evidence a high level of interest in recovering their communication abilities. This is a subjective judgment on the clinician's part, but it is one of those intangible variables that certainly relates to the potential of the patient to speak again.

Knepflar (1960, 1962) has compiled an extensive list of the necessary medical and background information helpful in planning a rehabilitation program. Case history forms have also been published by Johnson (1960), Snidecor (1962), Travis (1971), and Kelly (1983). Table 11.1 lists questions that guide us in the thorough collection of information on a patient. In addition to shaping the treatment program, such information provides prognostic insights.

A necessary part of the evaluation concerns the current status of the patient's oral-motor abilities. Chapter 9 provided details on an oral examination; suffice it to say that we thoroughly evaluate the tongue, lip, and jaw mobility. Articulation may be affected if surgery involved the hyoid bone, which is an anatomical connection for many muscles of the tongue, mandible, and

Table 11.1 Laryngectomee Case
History Outline

1. *Surgical Factors*

   Date of surgery
   Extent of surgery
   Postoperative complications
   Irradiation/other treatment procedures

2. *Physical-Mental Factors*

   General physical condition
   Upper respiratory health
   Status of oral structures
   Hearing acuity
   Other physical factors or conditions
   Cognitive-mental clarity
   Educational background

3. *Emotional Factors*

   Level of negative emotion—depression
   Level of motivation
   Degree of dependency on spouse-family
   Other personality traits or problems

4. *Social Factors*

   Home-family situation
   Occupational aspects
   Hobbies–pastimes
   Smoking and drinking habits
   Social network–sociability
   Family attitudes and acceptance

pharynx. Also, it is not uncommon that surgical alterations were necessary to contain concomitant oral, lingual, or lymph node cancers. Table 11.2 summarizes some of the more common anatomical alterations to nerves and tissues. Some information about the previous articulation, speech, and language patterns of the patient is also helpful. For example, we have had poor success with alaryngeal speech intelligibility in cases where, premorbidly, the patient was edentulous and seldom wore dentures.

An assessment of the patient's hearing acuity is desirable. Since a high percentage of laryngectomees are above the age of 55, it is common to find a presbycusic hearing loss. A moderate-to-severe hearing loss may hinder the learning process and, of necessity, shape the direction of the rehabilitation program. Artificial larynx speech, which is typically about 7 dB more intense than normal speech, may prove to be the treatment of choice for cases with significant hearing loss; in contrast, esophageal speech averages 6 to 10 dB below normal speech levels (Goldstein & Rothman, 1976; Hyman, 1955; Robbins, Fisher, & Blom, 1984).

Case Example. Mr. Wayne Johnson, a 61-year-old white male, was admitted with a six-month history of hoarseness. Examination by otolaryngologist revealed a hard mass in the neck at the angle of the jaw (at the area of the middle one-third of the left anterior lymphatic chain), and dysplasia involving the left aryepiglottic fold, false fold, and true fold. Biopsy confirmed locations with the finding of

Table 11.2 Some Common Anatomical Alterations in Laryngectomy

---

Removed in a Total Laryngectomy

    All laryngeal cartilages

    All intrinsic muscles and membranes

    Hyoid bone (optional)

    Upper two or three tracheal rings (typically)

Typically Removed in a Radical Neck Dissection
(often done unilaterally, for cervical metastasis)

    Sternocleidomastoideus muscle

    Omohyoid muscle

    Internal jugular vein

    Spinal accessory nerve (cranial nerve XI)

    Submaxillary salivary gland

Removed for More Extensive Cancer
(any or all may be removed)

    Same structures as in radical neck dissection

    External carotid artery

    Strap muscles of the neck

    Vagus nerve (cranial nerve X)

    Hypoglossal nerve (cranial nerve XII)

    Lingual branch of trigeminal nerve (cranial nerve V)

---

squamous cell carcinoma. A left radical neck dissection and total laryngectomy were performed.

Background information, contained in the report from social services, included mention that Mr. Johnson was a salesman and lived in an affluent resort community on a lake and golf course. He and his wife golfed several times a week and enjoyed all water sports, including skiing.

The speech pathologist, after reading the medical chart, began to wonder about the quality of life for Mr. Johnson following laryngectomy. Being a salesman, communication and meeting the public are necessary parts of his job. Will he return to work? Will he experience a loss of earnings from lost commissions (the public might not buy from an unusual-sounding person)? Will the company "urge" him to take early retirement? Could the company shift his duties from sales force to office work? To be sure, questions such as these were not only going through the mind of the speech pathologist but also of the patient and his wife. The clinician felt that an impending return to work would be a strong motivator for Mr. Johnson to speak. The clinician also had thoughts concerning his avocations and knew future counseling would have to deal with these issues. Mr. Johnson almost certainly would play golf again, but with a reduction in general strength, head-neck rotation abilities, and a less effective golf swing because of the radical neck dissection. The lake life style posed particular dangers. Stoma breathers are generally advised to stay clear of water. Skiing is out for Mr. Johnson, as is swimming; riding in a motor boat carries a certain risk (accidents do happen). Will Mr. Johnson adjust to these restrictions? He could wade in the water and even try to snorkel with a special breathing device for laryngectomees, but clearly his life style is in for a drastic change. Of prime importance, however, is the containment of cancer, his survival, and a return of the ability to communicate.

CANDIDACY FOR TRACHEOESOPHAGEAL PUNCTURE

The evaluation may proceed differently with patients planning to have a tracheoesophageal puncture (TEP), also known as tracheoesophageal fistulization. Since this is a relatively new, but ever more popular procedure, we will first provide some background.

The surgeon places a hole (puncture or fistula) in the membraneous wall between the trachea and the esophagus, thus providing a route or connection between these two structures. A prosthesis placed in this opening will allow for pulmonary air to be routed into the top of the esophagus under certain conditions. Breathing is still done through the stoma. Aspiration of saliva, liquids, and foods is minimized by the one-way directionality of the prosthetic device. The conditions that allow for diverting exhaled air into the esophagus, rather than out the stoma, are digital occlusion of the prosthesis opening, located in the stoma, or the use of a valving device to reroute the airstream.

Upon muscular effort, air diverted into the esophagus will be compressed and forced through the top of the closed esophagus, thereby setting the pharyngoesophageal segment into vibration. This segment is the sound source or pseudoglottis; articulation of the sound is accomplished in the usual manner in the upper vocal tract. In essence, tracheoesophageal speech (TE speech) is esophageal in nature, yet supported by the pulmonary system. TE speech obviates the need to learn esophageal speech via injection or inhalation methods and is therefore easily mastered. Furthermore, the use of lung air provides acoustic and perceptual advantages over traditional esophageal speech.

Hospitalization for healed laryngectomees who come back for only the TEP procedure is less than 10 days; some surgical procedures can even be done on an outpatient basis or as an office procedure. Punctures can also be done on newly laryngectomized patients; still, many surgeons prefer the patient to convalesce for a period of weeks or months before puncture. Screening for candidacy, fitting of the device, and instructing in the care and use of the device are often done solely by the speech pathologist, sometimes in concert with the nurse and doctor. Fluent conversational speech is typically acquired rapidly. The speech-language pathologist, then, has a brief but vital role to play in the rehabilitation of TEP patients.

The success of any method depends, in part, on the proper selection of candidates for that method. Patient selection criteria and contraindications for tracheoesophageal puncture include the following (Singer & Blom, 1980):

1. Motivation to undergo the procedure and sustained motivation to care for the prosthesis on a daily basis.
2. Absence of physical or mental limitations to the daily care and fitting (insertion) of the prosthesis. In particular, the patient should have adequate vision and eye-hand coordination to place the prosthetic device while in front of a mirror. Manual dexterity (e.g., absence of arthritis) is necessary for the handling of the prosthesis and all associated materials (particularly if a tracheostoma valve is also used).
3. Good general health. Weak, feeble persons do not do well with TEP; however, conditions such as chronic pulmonary disease, diabetes, and alcoholism do not necessarily rule out candidacy.
4. Concern for hygiene in cleansing of the device, in neck tissue care (adhesives used with the valve can be irritating to sensitive skin), and in touching/handling all materials.
5. Adequate stoma characteristics. In particular, the stoma must not be retracted behind the manubrium. Size of the opening should be a minimum of 1 cm across the axis, but for some procedures 2 cm are needed. An excessively large stoma can be corrected somewhat by tape.
6. Recovery from postsurgical radiation treatment, if any.
7. Absence of chronic tracheitis or ulceration.
8. Absence of a history of unplanned fistulas, pharyngoesophageal stricture (spasm), or flap reconstruction. The presence of any of these conditions, however, does not necessarily rule out TEP candidacy but suggests the need for a more detailed assessment. A barium esophagram may yield findings suggesting that dilation may be necessary to maintain an adequate opening for airflow and voice.

In this regard, we need to explain that the primary reason for failure with tracheoesophageal speech is spasms of the pharyngoesophageal segment. Spasms make the vibration and production of sound difficult, if not impossible. The spasms can usually be relaxed by surgically cutting some of the muscle fibers in the pseudoglottis. The need for this surgical procedure, called a myotomy, can be predicted with a simple screening test. The speech-language pathologist, or surgeon, or both perform an air insufflation procedure, where air is introduced into the esophagus and the patient is asked to phonate. Good phonation, of course, indicates that the patient's pharyngoesophageal segment is capable of vibration and so a myotomy would not be needed. Such a patient is considered an excellent candidate for TEP. Brief, unusual, or absence of phonation suggests that spasms are interfering with vibratory attempts; further testing and a myotomy may be considered for such a patient. Often, administration of this air insufflation test falls under the purview of the speech pathologist, and so we present details of how to administer this assessment "test" and interpret the results.

Air Insufflation Test.   We would like to point out that the validity of this test has been questioned, yet Drs. Blom and Singer, who pioneered TEPs, strongly recommend that it be done to identify potential failures of TE speech. To do the test, the speech pathologist should pass a catheter tube (such as the size #14 French) through the patient's nares, down the pharynx, and into the top of the esophagus. As a guide to the depth of placement, the distance from nares to the top of the esophagus in an adult male is approximately 25 cm. The speech pathologist should then insufflate the patient's esophagus by blowing about 80 cc of air into the free end of the tube. A gentle blow of about one second duration is usually sufficient. Immediately have the patient try to count aloud. The patient passes this test if he/she can count aloud, vibrating the pharyngoesophageal segment. The ideal patient can count to 15 or 20, about 8–10 seconds, on the insufflation test. Lack of voice or voice cutting off before the patient counts to 10 suggests failure. Failure can occur for three reasons: (1) If speech is whispered, then the catheter is not placed deep enough into the top section of the esophagus. Insert more tubing and repeat the insufflation test. (2) In testing, take care not to blow too much air into the esophagus. The top of the esophagus is an antireflux barrier that will forcefully close if overinsufflated. Also, air that does not come out the mouth enters the stomach and may cause a sense of fullness or gas. The esophageal closure or pharyngoesophageal spasmodic contraction is due in this case to improper test procedures. Repeat the insufflation using less air. (3) Some patients show this forceful closure or spasmodic contraction even when the proper amount of air is blown to distend the esophagus. No esophageal speech will be heard on attempts to count aloud. This failure represents a contraindication for TEP, unless corrective surgery for esophageal constrictures is first done. The surgeon can pretest the need for myotomy with a nerve block.

An alternative way to do the insufflation test is marketed by the American V. Mueller Corporation; it is the *Blom-Singer Esophageal Insufflation Test Set.* The disposable test set consists of a 50-cm long, #14 French, imprinted latex catheter with an insertable tracheostoma adapter. A flexible housing and adhesive discs are included to attach this adapter to the tracheostoma skin. The catheter, imprinted with centimeter measurements, simplifies placement for the speech pathologist. By using the insertable stoma adapter, the patient's exhaled air is used to insufflate the esophagus. This "self-test" feature elimi-nates the need for the clinician to breathe into the catheter.

THE PROCESS OF GETTING STARTED

The scope of this book does not allow for a discussion of alaryngeal treatment options nor the training methods used. Many excellent texts on laryngectomee rehabilitation are available to the serious student. Typically, the postoperative evaluation session is also the "let's get started in treatment" session. The ease or difficulties encountered in the initial learning attempts with an artificial lar-ynx, or in trying to inject air and get sound back out, or in diverting lung air through a prosthesis are diagnostically important.

Artificial Larynx Attempts

A patient should not just be given an artificial larynx; instructions on its use and training in its use are essential. With a neck-type device, help the patient seek out its best placement. How quickly will the patient learn to return the vibrating head precisely to that spot—five trials or 50? Are other feedback cues necessary to learn this skill? If so, things such as tactile stroking of the spot by the clinician before each attempt at placement may prove beneficial. Also, marking an "X" on the skin with a washable marker and having the patient practice placement drills in front of a mirror may be just what is needed. Explain and demonstrate the noisy effects of poor contact of the vibrating head with the skin. How efficiently will the patient absorb this knowledge and learn to consist-ently place the device in the correct spot with *firm* contact? Advise the patient to exaggerate articulation movements, especially in opening the mouth and moving the tongue. Will the patient quickly adjust to such pantomiming actions or persist in trying to "breathe for speech" only to have a noisy exhalation out the stoma? Explain and demonstrate the on–off mechanism and the precise timing needed to coordinate phrasing. How agile or clumsy will the patient be in manipulating the switch concurrent with phrases? Slow learners make one or more mistakes here: having the device continuously on and not stopping at grammatical junctures; turning the device off and on excessively and creating choppy speech; or turning the device on or off in a poorly timed fashion at the beginning and ending of utterances. The result is that sounds or syllables are chopped off or buzzing noises occur when speech is not being mouthed.

In training the use of artificial devices with intraoral tubes, how quickly can the patient learn proper placement? Efficient and accurate placement are necessary for speech spontaneity and intelligibility. The tube's orientation must minimize interference with articulation and saliva build-up and must radiate the tone well.

The point here is that during the early training in the use of an artifi-cial larynx device, the clinician should constantly be evaluating the learning skills of the patient. Some patients can speed quickly through your teaching units and others will progress with painful slowness. Observations, such as those just presented, therefore, shape the prognosis and course of treatment.

Esophageal Speech Attempts

Regardless of the technique being taught, be it inhalation or any of the variants of the injection method, the essence of learning esophageal speech involves getting "air in and sound out." As baseline data, the clinician can rate the client's esophageal production abilities. Some fortunate patients will be successful in eructating simple words or sounds in the first session, others may occasionally get out a "burp," and still others may remain mute—unable to get any sound out and needing much practice in performing air intake maneuvers appropriately. A scale, such as that suggested by Wepman et al. (1953) may be useful for a baseline rating. Wepman's self-explanatory seven points are

1. Automatic esophageal speech
2. Esophageal sound produced at will with continuity; word grouping
3. Esophageal sound produced at will; single-word speech
4. Voluntary sound production most of the time; vowel sounds
5. Voluntary sound production part of the time; no speech
6. Involuntary esophageal sound production; no speech
7. No esophageal sound production; no speech.

Certainly, the baseline data for most patients would be a Wepman score of 7 or 6. This same scale can be used periodically to reassess and document the progress of the patient in producing esophageal sound and speech.

Of interest in these early sessions is the learning skill and potential displayed by the patient following adequate instruction and demonstration. Early eructation abilities suggest a favorable prognosis for acquiring esophageal speech and perhaps a speedy trek through the treatment stages.

Early Speech Attempts with a Tracheoesophageal Prosthesis

Getting a patient started in the use of tracheoesophageal speech is a complex issue. We will attempt to subdivide the tasks and provide an overview of each.

Prosthesis Fitting. The speech pathologist is often responsible for fitting the patient with a prosthesis of proper size. Brands differ in size, features, and design to optimize individual patient fit. The Panje Voice Prosthesis and the Storz Henley-Cohn Laryngeal Prosthesis both come in one universal size. The Blom-Singer Voice Prosthesis and the Blom-Singer Low Pressure Voice Prosthesis (both marketed by American V. Mueller) are available in the following sizes: 1.8 cm, 2.2 cm, 2.6 cm, 3.0 cm, 3.3 cm, and 3.6 cm. The Bivona Duckbill Voice Prosthesis is available in the following lengths: 2.2 cm, 2.6 cm,

3.0 cm, 3.3 cm, 3.6 cm, 4.0 cm, and 4.3 cm. The Bivona Low Resistance Voice Prosthesis is available in the same lengths, except for 4.3 cm.

Following typical TEP surgery, a catheter is left in place for 24 to 72 hours to prevent closure of the puncture site. After that, a prosthesis should be fitted and voice will be possible. The speech pathologist should recheck the patient in four to five weeks and refit the prosthesis, if necessary. Occasionally, after the edema subsides, a shorter prosthesis is more appropriate. The majority of patients seem to need the 2.2, 2.6, or 3.0 cm size.

The process of fitting the prosthesis is as follows: Instruct the patient not to swallow. Remove the catheter that has been in place since the surgery. Insert the Dummy Prosthesis Depth Gauge (from Bivona, Inc.) or the Fistula Measurement Probe (from American V. Mueller) through the stoma and into the puncture; feel it "pop" into place. Pull out slightly until the retention collar is firmly against the puncture opening and read the distance on the imprinted probe. This indicates the length of prosthesis needed.

An alternative to using a depth gauge or measurement probe is to use the stick end of a long cotton-tipped applicator. Insert the stick through the stoma, exploring carefully to find the puncture opening. Then, mark the depth on the stick with a pencil and withdraw it. The distance on the stick may now be measured with a ruler. Yet another alternative, for those experienced in fitting, is to shine a light in the stoma and "eyeball" the distance to the puncture site.

Once the size of the needed prosthesis has been determined, insert one, applying double-faced tape on the flanges, if necessary (depending on design). Once in place, have the patient drink some water to make sure there is no leakage around or through the prosthesis. Demonstrate digital occlusion for the patient and instruct him/her to try to talk on exhalation while the stoma/prosthesis opening is occluded with the clinician's thumb or finger. If voice is not produced, assess the reason(s) why (see next section). If successful, continue talking practice. Later, allow the patient to do his/her own digital occlusion.

During the fitting process and placement of the prosthesis, do not be alarmed by blood-tinged mucous. Also, it is important that either a catheter, a prosthesis, or some sort of dummy device be inserted in the puncture at all times (even during sleep) to prevent its closure. The patient must remember this as well.

Voice Failure Assessment. If the patient is unable to produce voice, the speech pathologist should try to determine whether the problem lies with the prosthetic device or with the patient. The speech pathologist should try troubleshooting with and without the prosthesis in place.

Common problems of voice failure, due to patient factors, include the following: (1) The patient may be using excessive finger pressure against the stoma. (2) The patient may be using inadequate expiratory pressure. A weak, feeble patient is a poor candidate for TE speech because of the energy necessary to overcome the air resistance of the plastic devices. Alternately, perhaps the patient simply needs to be instructed to use more effort and more air in speech attempts. Other devices (styles and brands) may be tried as well; each model differs in its airflow resistance. An ultra-low resistance model may work for the patient. (3) Salivary secretions may have accumulated, blocking the pharynx. In this case, the speech will sound "gurgly." Expectoration should solve the problem. (4) A most likely reason for the absence of voice is the presence of pharyngoesophageal spasm. Perhaps the air insufflation pretest was not done prior to TEP. At any rate, do the insufflation test to see if voice is possible with the prosthesis removed. A myotomy may be necessary to counteract the spasms.

Voice failure may be due to problems with the prosthetic device. These problems are often easily identified and rectified. In these cases, the patient would have voice without the prosthesis (using stoma digital occlusion or with the air insufflation test), but no voice with a faulty prosthesis in place. (1) The patient may be unable to produce voice because the prosthesis is inserted upside down. Remove and reinsert the prosthesis. (2) The valve slit may be stuck together on devices with a slit (duckbill) design. (3) Incorrect prosthesis length could be the reason for lack of voice. A device that is too long, particularly a device with a slit design that would be so impeded, may be touching the posterior wall of the esophagus. Refitting the patient with a shorter device and/or changing to a different design (nonslit, flap-door) is in order. A prosthesis that is too short would not have the tip residing in the lumen of the esophageal tube. A slit designed tip would be impeded from passing its air into the esophagus. Try rotating the placement a bit. A longer prosthesis may be necessary. (4) Occlusion of the port may block airflow and hence voice. Clearing of saliva (or other matter) is in order.

If the patient has used TE speech for a period of time and begins to experience a change in the voice, or loss of it, troubleshooting to find and eliminate the cause is necessary. We recommend the work of Bosone (1986) for troubleshooting ideas.

Tracheostoma Valve.   Talking with the voice prosthesis requires digital occlusion (finger or thumb). This may be an unnecessary inconvenience for users of the Blom-Singer (American V. Mueller) or Bivona brands of prostheses. After a few weeks' experience with the voice prosthesis, the patient may be a candidate for using a Blom-Singer Tracheostoma Valve (marketed through American V. Mueller), the Bivona Tracheostoma Valve, or the Bivona Tracheostoma Valve II. More and more often, the patient is trained with a valve at the same time the prosthesis is introduced. The valve is fitted into the stomal opening; naturally, the patient still wears the voice prosthesis. Again, these are tasks that are within the purview of the speech-language pathologist responsible for assessing and rehabilitating the laryngectomee.

Tracheostoma Valve Contraindications.   The valve fits into a flexible circular housing that is attached to the skin area surrounding the stoma with nonirritating adhesive. When positioned over the stoma, the valve diaphragm remains in a fully open position during quiet breathing and routine physical activity. For speech, a slight increase in exhalation causes the valve diaphragm to close and divert air into the esophagus. The valve automatically reopens when exhalation decreases at the completion of an utterance.

A tracheostoma valve must be maintained by the patient; it is easily disassembled for cleaning. The diaphragm can be replaced by the patient without return to the manufacturer.

Four contraindications to using a valve seem to exist: (1) Patients with high phonatory pressure may blow the seal often. (2) A very recessed or irregular stoma may not accommodate the valve. (3) Patients with excessive tracheal discharge may occlude or dangerously hinder the operation of the valve. (4) Inadequate pharyngoesophageal segments preclude usable speech, even with a valve.

Valve Fitting. The diaphragm is available in several thicknesses or sensitivities. Bivona, Inc., markets four valve diaphragms: ultra light, light, medium, and firm. American V. Mueller markets three diaphragm thicknesses: ultra light, light, and medium. Select the diaphragm thickness that does not inadvertently close on the patient during routine physical exertion or heavier than usual exhalation. Conversely, do not select one too thick as to require excessive exhalation for the generation of voice. A practical method for fitting involves the "stair-step" test. Have the patient try out a diaphragm sensitivity while going up and down some stairs. The speech pathologist and patient should carefully watch for valve closure as breathing deepens during this exertion. If the valve closes, remove it and try the next thicker size. Repeat the stair-step test until the proper diaphragm size has been determined. Some patients may wish to purchase two diaphragms: one for general use and a thicker one for use while dancing, exercising, and the like.

Patients should be instructed not to sleep with the tracheostoma valve in place. Also, patients may find it helpful to remove the valve from its housing when they feel an urge to cough or forcefully exhale. This prevents blowing the seal and the necessity of cleaning and reapplying the adhesive. The Tracheostoma Valve II, by Bivona, contains a spring action valve (rather than the usual butterfly valve) with a cough relief valve that is said to eliminate blowout from a cough or instance of high airway pressure production.

To summarize the placement procedure, the prosthesis is first inserted. Next, the valve housing is glued over it and to the neck/stoma skin with an adhesive. The valve assembly is then placed into the housing.

Voice Treatment Sessions. Treatment begins with prosthesis fitting, usually done by the speech pathologist, as described previously. Once fitted, demonstrate digital occlusion for the patient. Instruct the patient to try to talk (on exhalation) while the prosthesis opening is digitally occluded. If voice is not produced, assess reasons why. If successful, continue talking practice. Later, allow the patient to do his/her own finger occlusion. It is simple, yet the coordination needs to be practiced.

Concomitant with speech practice, the patient should be trained in the placement of the prosthesis and the valve, if applicable. Instructions as to taping and/or gluing should be detailed for some types of devices, allowing for much supervised practice. Care and cleaning of the devices should be taught as well.

Usually by the third session, the patient is independent in talking with the prosthesis and in its placement, adhesion, and daily care.

We would like to offer a few observations about these first few sessions. One aspect of treatment may involve the unlearning of esophageal speech techniques in the patient who spoke esophageally prior to TEP. The two forms of speech are incompatible. Patients using esophageal speech must break whatever habits they have developed and return to what amounts to their prelaryngectomy form of speaking with lung air. This is usually easily achieved; yet, patients may require the speech pathologist to guide and monitor their unlearning or deconditioning of the esophageal speech habit.

Train the patient to use the proper amount of finger pressure on the prosthesis opening at the stoma. There is a tendency to push too forcefully at first. Similarly, patients may need the speech pathologist to assist in learning the minimal amount of expiratory pressure needed to drive the system. Some begin learning TE speech with the valve, using an excessive amount of air pressure. This can result in "blowing a seal" or loosening of the valve housing. If the housing develops a broken seal, it becomes difficult to close the valve and utilize the prosthesis for voice production. Instead, the air leak becomes audible and speech breakdown occurs. When this happens, the patient must manually hold the housing down while speaking, until there is an opportunity to reapply the housing. This is less of a problem with low-resistance prostheses. Regular prostheses have a higher resistance to opening and to air flowing through them. A greater air pressure build-up is required of the speaker with the danger of straining the glued seal of the housing.

In addition to learning the minimal amount of pressure needed on which to speak, the patient must learn proper ways to adhere the device to prevent blowout. Applying the proper amount of glue is important, as is getting the taped collar onto the housing without wrinkles in it, and applying it to the neck evenly. This is highly individualistic and must be learned by each patient with the help of the speech pathologist and sheer practice.

Treatment should also focus on articulatory intelligibility, such as distinguishing between voiced-voiceless cognates (e.g., face/vase) and between easily confused sounds (e.g., ship/chip), as is done in traditional esophageal speech rehabilitation.

ONGOING ASSESSMENTS: A DYNAMIC PROCESS

Assessing the proficiency of alaryngeal speech and refining that speech in treatment sessions are two intertwined processes. The direction that treatment should take is directly related to how well the patient is doing in the various components of speech. Ideally, the patient's status changes for the better on a daily or weekly basis, making frequent reassessments a necessity. Dynamic, ongoing assessments, then, suggest to the clinician (1) what to work on, (2) how much therapeutic time needs to be devoted to certain tasks, and (3) what tasks or steps in the program may be skipped or bypassed. This last item points out that reassessments serve as probes as to what the patient can already do without training, as well as measures of achievement.

Assessing Artificial Larynx Speech

Rothman (1978) consolidated much of the research information concerning acoustic characteristics of artificial larynx speech and perceptual ratings of what comprises "good" and "poor" users. Information of this kind is useful in setting goals toward which patients can strive. That is, we want our patients to acquire characteristics typical of "good" speakers. The information also serves as a useful barometer of patient progress. The clinician should frequently reassess the patient to see the current level of achievement and how that compares to the norms.

Information of this type collected by Rothman (1978) and others (Fleming, Simpson, & Weaver, 1983; Gandour & Weinberg, 1983; Moffet & Pindzola, 1988; Pindzola & Moffet, 1988; Weiss, Yeni-Komshian, & Heinz, 1979; Williams & Watson, 1985) seems to cluster into six categories. We will summarize them here.

Frequency Range.   "Good" speakers using neck-type devices acquire a variety of techniques to alter the frequency output, such as "riding" the device on the neck using different pressures. They exhibit a frequency range, or pitch variability, between 13 and 20 Hz, with an average range or fluctuation of 16 Hz. In contrast, "poor" speakers range from 6 to 15 Hz with a mean of 11 Hz.

Speech Rate.   Speech rate is the best variable to differentiate "good" from "poor" users of artificial larynges (Rothman, 1978). "Good" users speak test sentences faster than "poor" users. Research also indicates that a mean rate of speech with an electric larynx is 125 words per minute (Moffet & Pindzola, 1988).

Intensity Variations.   Intensity variations, which contribute to perceptions of linguistic stress or emphasis, are greater in "good" speakers. "Poor" users tend toward monoloudness.

Extraneous Noise.   "Poor" users frequently fail to achieve firm coupling of the vibrating head with their neck tissues. "Good" users do not generate leaked, extraneous noises.

Inappropriate Pauses.   Instances when the electric device is shut down during utterances occur more frequently with "poor" users. "Good" speakers are adept at timing and phrasing.

Consonantal Differentiation.   "Good" users employ buccal air and precise timing of device activation to more effectively produce stops, fricatives, and affricates. Voiced-voiceless distinctions are also achieved by careful manipulation of buccal air and/or by varying the coupling pressure of the device with the neck tissue. "Poor" users have yet to master the nuances of consonant production with artificial larynges.

Assessing Esophageal Speech

Once a patient has begun learning esophageal speech, some measure of current performance level is necessary. Most authorities would agree that a clinician with critical listening ability is the most effective means for evaluating esophageal productions. It is perhaps best to judge the overall effectiveness of the patient's speech and then focus on more specific parameters. The clinician can rate the patient's esophageal speech production on one of many scales available for this purpose (Barton & Hejna, 1963; Berlin, 1963; Robe et al., 1956; Shipp, 1967; Snidecor, 1969; Wepman et al., 1953). We will discuss several assessment instruments here.

Earlier we mentioned the Wepman et al. (1953) seven-point scale for establishing baseline esophageal proficiency. In addition to a baseline rating, the clinician should periodically rescore the patient to document improvement. Little to no time is necessary to do this rating.

A patient's learning curve should continuously shape the clinician's prognostic statement and modify the treatment program and pace. Berlin (1963) described four skills and their clinical measurement for use in assessing the acquisition efficiency of patients' learning esophageal speech. Berlin's classic criteria have recently been resurrected and modified by Dabul (1981). Table 11.3 displays information from Berlin and Dabul regarding the four skills, their

Table 11.3 Four Classic Skills in the Acquisition of Esophageal Speech

1. Consistency: Ability to phonate reliably on demand

   Patient makes a single inflation and phonates /a/. Allow 20 trials. Clinician scores each attempt with plus or minus scoring. Compute final score as a percentage of correct attempts. Goal is 100 percent.

   Good speakers phonated 100 percent of the time on demand after 10 to 14 days of daily speech treatment. Poor speakers averaged 68 percent after 20 days of treatment.

2. Latency: Short latency between inflation and vocalization

   Patient phonates as quickly as possible after inflation. Have the patient signal the clinician at the start of inflation; clinician engages a stopwatch. Clinician stops the watch at vocal onset. Allow 10 trials and compute an average latency time. Goal is 0.5 seconds or less.

   Good speakers maintained latency of 0.2 to 0.6 seconds by the 20th day of treatment; poor speakers 1.3 seconds.

3. Duration: Duration of phonation of /a/

   Patient makes a single inflation and a single phonation of /a/, sustaining it as long as possible. Allow 10 trials and compute an average duration. Goal is 1 to 2 seconds.

   Good speakers sustained the vowel for 2.2 to 3.6 seconds by the 24th day of treatment.

4. Syllables: Sustaining phonation during articulation of /da/

   Patient makes a single inflation and repeats the syllable /da/ as many times as possible. Allow 5 trials and compute an average number of syllables spoken. Goal is 5 to 7 syllables.

   Good speakers phonated 8 to 10 syllables after 25 days of treatment; poor speakers averaged 2.3.

elicitation procedures, patient criteria, and comparative acquisition data from "good" and "poor" speakers.

Rigrodsky and Lerman (1971) suggest the following treatment outline for acquiring competent esophageal speech: Learn an air intake method; practice esophageal speech on basic sounds, short words, polysyllabic words and phrases, then sentences and connected speech; improve articulation, phrasing, inflection, pitch, and loudness. A similar progression was suggested by Snidecor (1971). The final level in Snidecor's six-level program calls for practice on articulation, stress, pitch, quality, loudness, and time in a conversational situation.

We mention these two treatment programs as being typical; both stress that getting the patient talking does not mean discharge from treatment is at hand. Rather, patient and clinician must strive to perfect the esophageal speech— there is almost always room for improvement. The clinician's responsibility, then, includes frequent monitoring of the patient's conversational speech for adequacy in the more sophisticated areas of speech, such as rate, pitch and loudness variability, consonantal differentiation, and the like. Many assessment checklists, whether published or not, seem to be in the possession of most speech pathologists. A good many have been acquired through convention presentations, lost cord clubs, or college courses.

The *Alaryngeal Speech Proficiency Evaluation* (Knepflar, 1962) has the clinician rate 10 areas of speech using a five-point scale of proficiency. "Highly proficient, normal or near normal" is a rating of one while "generally inadequate for basic communicative needs" is a five. The 10 areas assessed are loudness, pitch, quality, inflection, rate/rhythm/fluency, articulation proficiency, linguistic proficiency, acoustic distractions, visual distractions, and overall proficiency.

The factors on which we rate our patients are shown in Table 11.4. These 11 factors are taken from the literature on characteristics of esophageal speech, in particular, the differences between "superior" users of esophageal speech and "poor" users. Such information can be used in setting treatment goals for patients. The information is also useful as a yardstick for measuring progress over time. The early research of Snidecor and Curry (1959, 1960), among others, is acknowledged in our overview of the characteristics of esophageal speech as they relate to our clinical ratings.

Pitch Level.   According to Martin (1979), an average male esophageal speaker will have a fundamental frequency of about 65 Hz, which is about half that of a normal speaking male. Weinberg and Bennett (1972) reported esophageal speech in males to average 58 Hz, and in females to average 87 Hz. Perceptual ratings seem to suggest that esophageal speech is more acceptable at higher, rather than lower, fundamental frequencies.

Inflection.   Pitch variation is difficult to achieve with the pseudoglottis. Rate of frequency movement varies over a range of 7.9 tones per second in esophageal speakers as compared to normal values of 17.7 tones per second. Kelly (1983) notes that listeners will perceive a change in pitch through control

Table 11.4 Factors on Which to Rate Esophageal Speech

1. Pitch Level

   Estimate or measure fundamental frequency.

   Is a higher pitch possible and comfortable?

2. Inflection or Pitch Variability

   Rate degree of inflection: absent/monotoned; present, needs improvement; present, typical of good user.

3. Quality

   Note degree of tension or strain.

   Is degree of roughness excessive or typical?

   Other comments:

4. Excess Noise

   Note presence or absence of noticeable klunking.

   Note presence or absence of stoma noise.

   Note conditions that improve or worsen the excess noises.

5. Visual Distractors

   Note and comment on types observed.

6. Rate of Speech

   Measure rate as words per minute or syllables per minute.

   Comment on perceptual impact (e.g., choppiness).

7. Words per Charge

   Average words (or syllables) per air charge.

   Compare between reading and conversation.

8. Latency of Air Charge

   Measure average time between start of air maneuver and onset of voice.

   How easily is the air charging accomplished (relaxed versus effortful)?

9. Latency of Phrasal Pauses

   Does patient pause at linguistically appropriate junctures?

   For how long?

   Compare durations between items 8 and 9.

10. Articulatory Intelligibility

    Comment on perceptual confusions noted (e.g., ship–chip).

    Rate intelligibility:

    poor

    requires careful listening and topic knowledge

    generally good but errors noted

    good-to-excellent

11. Intensity and Intensity Variability

    Comment on ability to display stress and emphasis on key words.

    Rate overall loudness:

    Adequate in quiet environment

    Adequate against normal background noise

    Adequate in noisy situations

of loudness, rate, length of time spent on a word, and the use of pauses. For example, an esophageal speaker should use a greater volume to raise the pitch but less intensity to lower the pitch.

Quality.   Speech quality is not normal and never will be; a certain amount of hoarseness or roughness is typical. Strain and tension, however, adversely affect the quality of the speech produced. The clinician should take note of the ease with which the patient can charge air into the esophagus.

Excess Noise.   Esophageal speakers exhibit some problems unique to their disorder. All distracting noises should be diagnosed early because they are more easily eradicated before a great deal of practice occurs. Excess noise can be associated with air intake or it can occur at the level of the stoma. When a patient injects air too rapidly into the esophagus, a "klunking" sound can occur. Some patients exhibit multiple "klunks" when they attempt more than one inflation before phonation. Another distracting behavior is stoma noise, or stoma blast, which is caused by the patient's forcing exhalations through the stoma at the time he/she is phonating esophageally. The patient has not adequately learned that "breathing for breathing and breathing for speech" are two separate functions. Sometimes the stoma noise masks the esophageal speech to the point of affecting intelligibility.

Visual Mannerisms.   Other, nonvocal aspects of communication can be distracting to the listener. Facial grimaces, including eye squinting, and head movements often occur when a patient is trying to learn an air intake method such as injection. The clinician should note these types of behaviors in patients and seek to eliminate them early in the treatment program before they become habituated.

Rate of Speech.   Perceptual studies suggest that rate of speech is the most important aspect that differentiates superior from poor esophageal speech. According to Snidecor and Curry (1960), superior esophageal speakers average 113 words per minute, with a range of 85 to 129 words per minute. This is also a rate that can be achieved by "good" patients, and we should point out that this rate is approximately 80 percent as fast as for normal (laryngeal) speakers, who average about 166 words per minute. Rate of speech declines as a function of air charging. The more frequently a patient charges, the slower the overall rate becomes. Superior esophageal speakers charge air less often than do poor speakers. Although the clinician should encourage proficiency at charging and increasing speech rates, we should point out that undue emphasis on increasing speech rates may be at the expense of loudness and suitable phrasing.

Words per Charge.   In the study by Snidecor and Curry (1960), superior esophageal speakers used 30 air charges to read a paragraph that took normal speakers 11 breaths to complete. Esophageal speakers, therefore, recharged air 3 times more often. Superior esophageal speakers utilized their charge for 1 to 1 1/2 seconds during which they averaged 2.8 to 6.3 words. This is compared to normal speakers who utilized a breath for 4.19 seconds and spoke 12.5 words. A satisfactory number of syllables on a single insufflation is 11 to 12. During connected speech, 4 to 9 syllables may be more typical.

Latency of Air Charge. Superior esophageal speakers gulp air at a rate of 0.42 to 0.80 seconds. Some patients can even get as low as 0.17, which is as fast as normal speakers. A good rule of thumb for setting treatment goals is a latency of 0.5 seconds or less. It is easier for patients to take air in quickly than it is to take in large amounts of air. Also, we should point out that a 0.5 second charge is more rapid than the time most normal speakers pause for a phrasal juncture.

Latency of Phrasal Pauses. Phrase-limiting pauses are longer than the pauses for air charging—approximately 1.41 times longer. Both normal and esophageal speakers pause for phrases, but the superior esophageal speaker pauses longer than the normal person in order that such pauses contrast with air charge pauses. In other words, practiced esophageal speakers have learned to use silent times differentially, thus aiding the listener in linguistic comprehension. For example, a patient who charges air in 0.5 seconds would use a phrase-limiting pause of 0.7 seconds ($0.5 \times 1.41 = 0.7$).

Articulatory Intelligibility. Removal of the larynx and hyoid bone disrupts the muscular connections of the tongue and so articulatory mobility may be affected. Most patients, however, compensate quite well. The surgery also shortens the effective length of the vocal tract, altering format frequencies, and perhaps affecting vowel intelligibility. The pseudoglottis is not equipped for abductor-adductor coordinations, and so the voicing of cognate phonemes is often a problem and the glottal fricative /h/ is impossible for a laryngectomee to produce. Clearly, then, articulation and speech intelligibility are of concern to the speech-language pathologist.

Treatment should involve practice with strategies to differentiate similar phonemes, and periodic assessments of how well the patient is doing are in order. For example, can a listener distinguish between "jip–chip–ship"? We feel strongly that intelligibility testing should be done in a regular fashion and treatment exercises be assigned for any deficiencies noted. Kelly (1983) recommends daily intelligibility testing by a family member. Kelly also suggests a four-step process:

1. Speaker and listener stand close together. Stimuli can involve lists of sounds, words, phrases, or sentences.
2. Speaker and listener stand across the room from each other.
3. Listener looks away while speaker is speaking.
4. Speaker stands four to six feet away from the listener and turns with back to the listener.

Table 11.5   Self-Administered Esophageal Checklist

NOTE: The following list comprises a few areas that contribute to effective esophageal communication. Others can and should be added. It is hoped that these will provide some assistance in helping you evaluate your esophageal speech and communication.

	YES	NO
DISTRACTORS		
1. Eyes		
a. I close my eyes as I try to produce esophageal tone.	___	___
b. I blink my eyes as I speak.	___	___
c. I look away from my listener as I speak.	___	___
2. Shoulders		
a. I move my shoulders as I try to produce speech.	___	___
3. Hands		
a. I move my hands as I try to speak.	___	___
4. Arms		
a. I move my arms as I try to speak.	___	___
5. Chin		
a. I move my chin, bob it up and down as I take in air for esophageal speech.	___	___
6. Mouth		
a. I twist or stretch my mouth as I try to speak.	___	___
7. I have watched myself in the mirror as I speak.	___	___
8. I look "ill at ease" or "tense" when I speak.	___	___
9. I sometimes lose saliva from my mouth as I speak.	___	___
10. I sometimes fail to cover my stoma when I cough or sneeze.	___	___
11. I make audible noises as I breathe when I speak. (I hear noises as I breathe in and out.)	___	___

OTHER NOISES

	YES	NO
1. I use the air in my mouth to make sounds such as "p" and "t," by moving the air in my mouth with my tongue against the roof of my mouth or by moving my cheeks or lips against my teeth. (Buccal speech)	___	___
2. I use the air in my mouth to produce a "Donald Duck" type of speech. The sounds come from the back of my mouth and sound "slushy" and are short. (Pharyngeal speech)	___	___
3. I make "clunking" noises in my throat just before I produce an esophageal tone.	___	___
4. I breathe heavily as I produce the esophageal tone, to "get it out" and I hear a rush of air coming out of my stoma. It sometimes covers up the esophageal speech sounds I've produced.	___	___

PHONATION

	YES	NO
1. I produce belches but do not have control over them when they come. They are produced by the air that has gone to my stomach and is coming up without my control. (Gastric speech)	___	___
2. I produce short esophageal speech sounds most of the time when I try to produce the sounds.	___	___
3. I can produce 1–2 syllable-length words using esophageal phonation (e.g., pop, popcorn).	___	___
4. I can produce 3–4 syllable-length words using esophageal phonation (e.g., policeman, constitution).	___	___

Table 11.5 *(Continued)*

	YES	NO
5. I can produce words of 5 syllables or more using esophageal speech (e.g., hospitalization).	___	___
6. I can, after producing a word or short phrase, get another charge of air and produce the next word very rapidly without a long pause.	___	___
7. I can judge how much air I have in my esophagus so that I do not complete each word and phrase without running out of phonation or tone.	___	___
8. I can be heard in most speaking situations where there is not an unusual amount of noise.	___	___
9. I can vary the loudness of my esophageal speech.	___	___
10. I can change the pitch of my esophageal speech by 1 tone.	___	___
11. I can change the pitch of my esophageal speech by 2 or more tones.	___	___
12. I can clearly articulate the final sounds of words in my speech.	___	___
13. I do not "over articulate" the sounds of words making my speech sound "stilted" or "formal."	___	___
14. I can produce all the consonants and vowels of speech clearly.	___	___
15. I can produce all but "h."	___	___
16. I can produce all but "m," "n," and "ng."	___	___
17. I can clearly produce "p" and "b," "k," and "g" and "t" and "d" so that each sound is clearly distinctive one from the other.	___	___
18. I pace my rate of speech so that each sound is clearly articulated.	___	___

COMMUNICATION

	YES	NO
1. I check to see that the person I am speaking to truly understands what I have said.	___	___
2. If I am asked to repeat what I said, I rephrase what I have said.	___	___
3. I try to give my listener as much information as possible so I try to speak in full sentences as opposed to single words or short phrases.	___	___
4. I direct my listener to watch my mouth as I speak to give him/her further help in understanding what I have said.	___	___
5. I use an amplifier or artificial larynx		
a. If my listener has a hearing loss and cannot hear my esophageal voice.	___	___
b. If I'm tired and my esophageal voice is not adequate.	___	___
c. If I'm emotionally upset and I cannot adequately obtain a charge of air for esophageal speech.	___	___
d. If I am not feeling well physically and cannot produce esophageal speech readily.	___	___
e. If I'm speaking in a situation where there is a great deal of noise and I cannot produce adequate volume with my esophageal voice to be heard above the noise.	___	___
f. If I'm speaking or have used my esophageal voice for a long period of time.	___	___

Intensity.   Intensity is approximately 6 to 10 dB softer in esophageal speech than in normal speech (Hyman, 1955). The intensity range is also more restricted: Esophageal speakers exhibit a range of about 20 dB and normal speakers 45 dB. Lack of loudness is often an early concern for patients. We like to discourage this concern as attempts to speak louder may be counterproductive. In trying to talk louder, patients adopt patterns of strain and effort, develop more noticeable klunking noises, and have longer injection latencies as they try to take in more air. We explain that loudness will improve over time. When appropriate, we also teach techniques for projecting louder, such things as digital pressure on the throat or using a handkerchief tied about the neck (Snidecor, 1971). We monitor loudness subjectively in our patients, although objective measures could be made.

We would also like to mention that assessment checklists can be useful for the patient to complete, as well as for the clinician. Self-ratings provide an opportunity for the patient to "take stock" of his/her progress and often serve as motivating devices. Table 11.5 displays an *Esophageal Communication Checklist* that we acquired at a Greater Atlanta Voice Masters Meeting in 1976. The author is unknown to us. We have often found this self-administered checklist useful to the patient.

ASSESSING TRACHEOESOPHAGEAL SPEECH

Since TE speech is produced with exhaled lung air, we need not concern ourselves with latency of air charging, klunking noises, or stoma blasts. Yet, using lung air does not mean that TE speech will be equivalent to normal, laryngeal speech. More air will be expended in TE speech because of the resistance of the prosthetic device and routing passage. Hence, duration of sustained phonation and number of words spoken per breath will be shorter than normal. Lung air will permit variety in pitch and loudness, but the pseudoglottis may tend to restrict it. The result of all this is that TE speech is generally superior to esophageal speech but inferior to normal speech on most measures (Pindzola & Cain, 1989; Robbins, Fisher, & Blom, 1984).

Many of the characteristics that clinicians use to rate esophageal speech can be used with the TE patient, but with some obvious exceptions, as previously noted. A prime area of dynamic assessment is that of articulatory intelligibility. TE speakers need to constantly monitor and improve articulation proficiency with voiced-voiceless cognates and phonemes that pose perceptual confusion. Again we mention "jip–chip–ship" as an example of potential difficulties. The intelligibility testing by family members, as suggested by Kelly (1983) for esophageal speakers, would certainly be a useful clinical exercise for TE speakers as well.

Regarding specific data pertinent to the assessment of TE speech, we would like to mention the work of Robbins, Fisher, and Blom (1984) and Pindzola and Cain (1989). Both studies show good agreement in their data. Pindzola and

Cain compared TE speakers, esophageal speakers, and normal speakers on certain criteria, including the following points:

1. Speech rate differed among the three groups of speakers. Normal talkers averaged 170 words per minute; TE speakers averaged 152 wpm; and esophageal speakers averaged 94 wpm.
2. The fundamental frequency of the TE speakers was slightly lower than expected of normal males of the same age. TE speech averaged 108 Hz. Esophageal speech was much lower, with an average of 84 Hz. Lung air offers advantages here, even though the pharyngoesophageal segment acts as the pseudoglottis in both forms of alaryngeal speech.
3. The range of fundamental frequency, or pitch variability, was equivalent among the three groups. This indicates that both TE and esophageal speakers can achieve use of intonation with the pseudoglottis.
4. The number of words spoken per breath, or per air charge, showed the expected pattern: Normal speakers averaged 12 words per breath, TE speakers averaged 8 words per breath, and esophageal speakers averaged 3.5 words per air charge.

We would also like to remind the reader of the troubleshooting suggestions provided by Bosone (1986). Although most TE patients begin speaking immediately and need speech treatment only for a brief while, problems do arise. The speech pathologist will be called upon for reassessments and troubleshooting.

PROGNOSIS

At the end of the evaluation sessions, we should have obtained pertinent case history data, as well as provided information to the patient and the family about the anatomical changes and potential communication methods. We should also have a good idea about the patient's current method of communication and potential for treatment. As a review of much of what we have said in this chapter, we offer the following list of prognostic indicators for success.

1. The patient should have competent anatomical structures for the method or methods of speech chosen. The pharyngoesophageal segment must be adequate for development of esophageal or TE speech. The tendency for esophageal spasms (as pretested with air insufflation) is contraindicative for both forms of speech. Obesity and thick, scarred neck tissues may interfere with the use of neck-type artificial larynges.
2. The severity, extent, and type of surgery seem not to be related to the acquisition of speech. Yet, this assessment may be highly individualistic.
3. Patients should be of good general health. Feeble patients generally do not do well in learning esophageal or TE speech. These speech forms require energy to persist in the rehabilitation process. Artificial larynges, on the other hand, seem well suited for the more feeble patient.
4. The date of the surgery relative to the enrollment in the speech rehabilitation program is important. Gardner (1971) reviewed the literature and concluded that the chances for attaining adequate speech diminish with the passage of time

since surgery. He was referring to esophageal speech but the dictum probably holds true for all speech forms. The prognosis for speech after waiting one or two years postsurgery is extremely poor. By that time, other habits (such as total dependency on the spouse) have developed and are difficult to break.

5. Patients with a positive attitude and motivation to practice often throughout the day tend to be the successful ones, no matter which form of speech they are learning.
6. Those planning to return to work seem to have an extra ounce of motivation to master speech and to do so more quickly than those staying home or in an institution.
7. Patients who have family support at home, willing communication partners, and people willing to participate in the rehabilitation program and help with daily practice generally do quite well.
8. Patients who are literate and willing to read and study materials about laryngectomy rehabilitation seem to make good progress. They make good use of workbooks, stimuli lists, and the like in daily practice.
9. Patients who were able to burp preoperatively or who have quickly acquired this ability postoperatively are good candidates for esophageal speech.

To conclude, then, we have shown the multitude of complex issues involved in the assessment, counseling, prognosing, and reassessment of persons with laryngectomies. The speech-language pathologist must be well versed in the three main avenues of rehabilitation: artificial larynx, esophageal speech, and tracheoesophageal speech.

BIBLIOGRAPHY

American Cancer Society (1985). *Laryngectomee Visitor Program Manual.* Available from IAL National Office, c/o American Cancer Society, 90 Park Avenue, New York, N.Y. 10016.

BARTON, J., & HEJNA, R. (1963). Factors associated with success or nonsuccess in acquisition of esophageal speech. *Journal of the Speech and Hearing Association of Virginia, 4,* 19–20.

BERLIN, C. (1963). Clinical measurement of esophageal speech: I. Methodology and curves of skill acquisition. *Journal of Speech and Hearing Disorders, 28,* 42–51.

BOSONE, Z. T. (1986). Trouble-shooting after tracheoesophageal fistulization for voice restoration. *Seminars in Speech and Language, 7,*(1), 43–51.

BRADLEY, R. C., & ORMOND, T. F. (1970). *Communication for the laryngectomized.* Chicago, IL: Interstate Printers.

DABUL, B. (1981). *Early assessment of progress in esophageal speech.* Paper presented at the annual convention of the American Speech-Language-Hearing Association, Los Angeles, CA.

DUGUAY, M. J. (1966). Preoperative ideas of speech after laryngectomy. *Archives of Otolaryngology, 83,* 69–72.

FLEMING, S. M., SIMPSON, M. L., & WEAVER, A. W. (1983). *A comparison of four types of laryngectomized speech rehabilitation.* Paper presented at the annual convention of the American Speech-Language-Hearing Association, Washington, DC.

GANDOUR, J., & WEINBERG, B. (1983). Perception of intonational contrasts in alaryngeal speech. *Journal of Speech and Hearing Research, 26,* 142–148.

GARDNER, W. H. (1971). *Laryngectomee speech and rehabilitation.* Springfield, IL: Charles C Thomas.

GREENE, M. (1980). *The voice and its disorders.* Philadelphia, PA: J. B. Lippincott Co.

GOLDSTEIN, L. P., & ROTHMAN, H. B. (1976). *Analysis of speech produced with an artificial larynx.* Paper presented at the annual convention of the American Speech and Hearing Association, Houston, TX.

HYMAN, M. (1955). An experimental study of artificial larynx and esophageal speech. *Journal of Speech and Hearing Disorders, 20,* 291–299.

JOHNSON, C. L. (1960). A survey of laryngectomee patients in Veteran's Administration hospitals. *Archives of Otolaryngology, 72,* 768–773.

KEITH, R. L., SHANE, H., COATES, H., & DEVINE, K. (1984). *Looking forward: A guidebook for the laryngectomee.* Rochester, MN: Mayo Foundation.

KELLY, L. S. (1983). *A guide for rehabilitation and assessment of the total laryngectomee.* Tucson, AZ: Communication Skill Builders.

KNEPFLAR, K. J. (1960). *Individualized speech therapy for laryngectomized patients.* Paper presented at the annual convention of the American Speech and Hearing Association, Los Angeles, CA.

KNEPFLAR, K. J. (1962). *Therapy approaches for the improvement and refinement of pseudovoice in laryngectomized speakers.* Paper presented at the annual convention of the American Speech and Hearing Association, New York.

LA BORWIT, L. J. (1981). *Inventory for the assessment of laryngectomy rehabilitation.* Tigard, OR: C. C. Publications, Inc.

LAUDER, E. (1989). *Self-help for the laryngectomee.* San Antonio, TX: E. Lauder Pub.

MARTIN, D. (1979). Evaluating esophageal speech development and proficiency. In R. Keith & F. Darley (Eds.), *Laryngectomee Rehabilitation.* Houston, TX: College Hill Press.

MOFFET, B., & PINDZOLA, R. (1988). Acoustic properties of artificial larynx speech. *Journal of NSSLHA, 16,* 1–9.

PINDZOLA, R. H., & CAIN, B. H. (1989). Duration and frequency characteristics of tracheoesophageal speech. *Annals of Otology, Rhinology, and Laryngology, 98,* 12, 960–964.

PINDZOLA, R., & MOFFET, B. (1988). Comparison of ratings of four artificial larynges. *Journal of Communication Disorders, 21,*(5), 459–467.

RIGRODSKY, S., & LERMAN, J. (1971). *Therapy for the laryngectomized patient: A speech clinician's manual.* New York: New York Teachers College Press.

ROBBINS, J., FISHER, H., & BLOM, E. (1984). A comparative acoustic study of normal, esophageal, and tracheoesophageal speech production. *Journal of Speech and Hearing Disorders, 49,* 202–210.

ROBE, E. Y., MOORE, P., ANDREWS, A. H., & HOLINGER, P. H. (1956). A study of the role of certain factors in the development of speech after laryngectomy: 1. Type of operation. *Laryngoscope, 66,* 173–186.

ROTHMAN, H. B. (1978). Analyzing artificial electronic larynx speech. In S. J. Salmon & L. P. Goldstein (Eds.), *The artificial larynx handbook.* New York: Grune & Stratton.

SALMON, S. J., & GOLDSTEIN, L. P. (1978). *The artificial larynx handbook.* New York: Grune & Stratton.

SHIPP, T. (1967). Frequency, duration and perceptual measures in relation to judgments of alaryngeal speech acceptability. *Journal of Speech and Hearing Research, 10,* 417–427.

SINGER, M., & BLOM, E. (1980). *An endoscopic technique for restoration of voice after laryngectomy.* Paper presented at the annual meeting of the American Laryngologic Association, Palm Beach, FL.

SNIDECOR, J. C. (1962). *Speech rehabilitation of the laryngectomized.* Springfield, IL: Charles C Thomas.

SNIDECOR, J. C. (1969). *Speech rehabilitation of the laryngectomized* (2nd ed.). Springfield, IL: Charles C Thomas.

SNIDECOR, J. C. (1971). Speech without a larynx. In L. E. Travis (Ed.), *Handbook of speech pathology and audiology.* Englewood Cliffs, NJ: Prentice Hall.

SNIDECOR, J. C., & CURRY, E. T. (1959). Temporal and pitch aspects of superior esophageal speech. *Annals of Otology, Rhinology and Laryngology, 68,* 1–14.

SNIDECOR, J. C., & CURRY, E. T. (1960). How effectively can the laryngectomee expect to speak? *Laryngoscope, 70,* 62–67.

TRAVIS, L. E. (Ed.). (1971). *Handbook of speech pathology and audiology.* Englewood Cliffs, NJ: Prentice Hall.

VALLENCIEN, B., BOUCHIERE, D. M., GACHES, L., & CABIROL, F. (1971). Social and familiar readaptation of laryngectomees. *Folia Phoniatrica, 23,* 365–370.

WEINBERG, B., & BENNETT, S. (1972). Selected acoustic characteristics of esophageal speech produced by female laryngectomees. *Journal of Speech and Hearing Research, 15,* 211–216.

WEISS, M. S., YENI-KOMSHIAN, G. H., & HEINZ, J. M. (1979). Acoustical and perceptual characteristics of speech produced with an electronic artificial larynx. *Journal of the Acoustical Society of America, 65,* 1298–1308.

WEPMAN, J. M., MACGAHAN, J. A., RICKARD, J. C., & SHELTON, N. W. (1953). The objective measurement of progressive esophageal speech development. *Journal of Speech and Hearing Disorders, 18,* 247–251.

WILLIAMS, S. E., & WATSON, J. B. (1985). Differences in speaking proficiencies in three laryngectomee groups. *Archives of Otolaryngology, 111,* 216–219.

chapter

12

ASSESSMENT OF RESONANCE IMBALANCE

Disorders of voice, particularly disorders of vocal quality, may be due to the defective transmission of sound through the vocal tract. Sound generation at the level of the larynx occurs normally and so these are not the laryngeal disorders discussed in Chapter 10. Problems of resonance may be classified as hyponasality, hypernasality, nasal emission, cul-de-sac resonance, or thin/effeminate resonance. The assessment of resonance imbalance will be the focus of this chapter.

CATEGORIES OF ABNORMAL RESONANCE

The *denasal* or *hyponasal* voice lacks the normal nasal resonance expected on /m/, /n/, and /ɔ/ in English. Often these articulatory distortions resemble /b/, /d/, and /g/, respectively. The vocalic elements may also take on the characteristics of "talking with a head cold." Hyponasality usually results from some blockage or obstruction in the nasopharynx or nasal cavity. This may stem from congestion, nasal polyps, or various structural deformities.

    Hypernasality is an excessive amount of nasal resonance during the production of vowels and vocalic elements. The nasal cavity is not adequately separated from the oral cavity during speech. Such velopharyngeal incompetence, or VPI, may stem from neuromuscular deficits or structural defects. Congenital clefts of the hard or soft palate are obvious examples of structural defects frequently leading to hypernasality, and we will discuss these conditions later in the chapter. Not only can hypernasality result from clefts of the hard or soft palate, but also from submucous clefts, velums with inadequate length, or pharyngeal dimensions that are too large. A neuromuscular deficit, such as a paralyzed or paretic velum, or dysfunction of the pharyngeal constrictor muscles may be attributed to trauma-induced dysarthria or disease-related dysarthria. Diseases such as myasthenia gravis, muscular dystrophy, and poliomyelitis often affect velopharyngeal functioning.

Hypernasality may be pronounced or only slightly apparent; also, it can be continuous or intermittent. In mild, intermittent cases, the excess nasality on vowels may be most noticeable in the context of nasal consonants. This represents assimilation nasality and indicates a velum that can function but moves too slowly during connected speech.

Nasal emission is an audible escape of air through the nares during the production of pressure consonants, such as plosives, fricatives, and affricates. Implicated in this condition is an incompetent velopharyngeal mechanism. Nasal emission is different from the resonance imbalance of hypernasality, although the two problems may co-occur. It has been argued that nasal emission is more of an articulatory problem than a vocal resonance disorder (Peterson, 1975); however, we will discuss it here because of convention.

Cul-de-sac resonance typically occurs in the oropharynx, largely due to posterior tongue retraction. This resonance imbalance is heard as a muffled and hollow-sounding voice with a pharyngeal focus. Also, Peterson-Falzone (1982) states that cul-de-sac resonance can result from an anterior nasal obstruction and a posterior aperture (opening). Cul-de-sac resonance associated with tongue retraction often occurs on a functional basis, as well as in patients with deafness, flaccid and spastic dysarthria, athetoid cerebral palsy, or oral verbal apraxia (Boone & McFarlane, 1988; Prater & Swift, 1984).

Thin vocal resonance, also known as an *effeminate voice quality,* seems related to an anterior tongue posture. The habitually high and excessively anterior tongue position is almost always due to functional, not organic, reasons. Prater and Swift explain:

> [T]he voice sounds very weak and lacking in resonance, particularly for the back vowels . . . patients . . . articulate with a minimal oral opening and with little range of movement of the jaw. Because of . . . anterior tongue carriage and . . . restricted oral movement for articulation, the general impression . . . is that this type of speaker is using immature, baby-like, effeminate speech. Often, the speaker's vocal pitch is also elevated slightly, which aids in this perception of vocal immaturity and effeminacy. (1984, p. 241)

CASE HISTORY AND GENERAL VOICE ASSESSMENT

The evaluation of a resonance disorder is often an outgrowth of a general voice evaluation; the clinician may not know beforehand the specific nature of a patient's problem. Consequently, the evaluation session proceeds along the lines described in Chapter 10. Suffice it to say that, first, a case history interview is done. Routine information is gathered, but particular questions need to be asked concerning the patient's description of the voice problem and known or suspected causes of the disorder. Oronasopharyngeal injuries, structural defects, and surgeries need to be thoroughly discussed. Second, the oral peripheral examination is crucial to the evaluation of resonance disorders; and, third, all parameters of the voice must be assessed.

Any of the assessment instruments mentioned in Chapter 10 would be appropriate to use. *A Voice Assessment Protocol for Children and Adults* (Pindzola, 1987) is useful in assessing a multitude of vocal parameters. It evaluates the resonance of the patient's voice on a severity continuum. The patient may be scored as exhibiting normal resonance balance, cul-de-sac resonance, hyponasality (slight or intermittent versus moderate-to-severe), hypernasality on vocalic elements (slight, intermittent, or assimilative versus moderate versus severe), and nasal emission on pressure consonants (slight or intermittent versus moderate-to-severe).

After a thorough, overall voice assessment, emphasis is given to the appraisal of the resonance imbalance. Specific techniques can be employed by the speech-language pathologist.

ASSESSMENT TECHNIQUES AND PROBES
FOR RESONANCE IMBALANCE

In this section, we would like to discuss techniques requiring little or no instrumentation that the speech-language pathologist can and should do to assess the various resonance imbalances. Before concluding the evaluation, we feel very strongly that the clinician should experiment, or probe, to see what improvements, or changes in general, can be effected in the patient's voice. Some writers have discussed this as *stimulability*. Wilson (1987) maintains that the ability of a patient to produce a clear voice upon stimulation means that voice treatment has a good chance of being successful.

Hyponasality. Since denasality is often due to obstruction in the nasal cavity, an examination of the nasal region is in order during the oral peripheral part of the assessment. Additionally, during the case history intake, the patient may indicate knowledge of having a deviated septum, nasal polyp, enlarged adenoids, and the like. On the other hand, the basis of a patient's hyponasality may be neuromuscular in origin and reflect improper timing of velar movements. Case history questions should probe for trauma- or disease-related etiologies.

To evaluate a patient for hyponasal voice quality, speech-language pathologists rely on critical listening. While the patient is conversing or reading a standard paragraph, the clinician acutely listens for denasality shadowing the vowel portions of speech and, in particular, listens for the articulatory distortions or substitutions of b/m, d/n, and g/n. By using specially constructed phrases, sentences, or paragraphs that have a preponderance of nasal phonemes, the clinician has a heightened opportunity to perceive denasal resonance. Suggested stimuli include the following examples, some of which we have devised or borrowed from the literature (Bloomer & Wolski, 1968; Lippmann, 1981):

> Mama made some lemon jam.
> I know a man on the moon.
> Many a man knew my meaning.
> Mike needs more milk.
> My mom makes money.
> When may we know your name?
> I'm naming one man among many.

Having the patient count aloud from 90 to 100 is contextually appropriate, as well. Shupe (1968) provides word pairs useful in detecting hyponasality: bake/make, rib/rim, dine/nine, mad/man, wig/wing, bag/bang. In hyponasality, nasal resonance would be lacking and so, for example, the bake/make pair would sound like bake/bake.

Another clinical task that is helpful in revealing hyponasal speech is to have the patient read a list of words initiated with the /m/ phoneme. Bzoch (1979) suggests these 10 words: meat, moat, mit, moot, mate, mut, met, Mert, mat, and might. While the patient is reading, or repeating, each word from the list twice, the clinician alternately compresses and releases the patient's nostrils. In normal velopharyngeal function, the resonance becomes hypernasal when the nares are occluded, but no resonance change is heard in true hyponasality. Bzoch counts the number of words with no change in resonance and uses this figure as an index of hyponasality.

Operating on this same principle is the humming technique. The inability of a patient to hum or to hum clearly is suggestive of hyponasality (Prater & Swift, 1984).

> *Case Example.* Carmen Perez has fluctuating hyponasality. The severity of her hyponasality changes on a daily basis, but there is a more noticeable fluctuation with the seasons. Carmen's ear, nose, and throat doctor observed nasal cavity characteristics typical of allergic inflammation: tissue coloration changes and hypertrophy of the nasal turbinates secondary to edema. The planned course of treatment involved use of prescribed antihistamines and the option of undergoing a lengthy allergen tolerance program.

Hypernasality.   Judgments about resonance are truly judgments of a perceptual nature; a well-tuned clinical ear is essential—and adequate—for the speech-language pathologist. Critical listening by the clinician while the patient converses and/or reads a passage can be supplemented by rating the severity of the hypernasality on a rating scale. Several are available, including those by Subtelny, Van Hattum, and Myers (1972) and Van Demark (1974). Let us highlight a few others.

Fletcher (1978) rates the severity of hypernasality from mild to very severe. His descriptive categories are

- Normal nasality—speech has enough nasality to sound normal, but not so much as to call attention to it unless specifically listening for it.
- Mild nasality—nasality is apparent as the person speaks. It is somewhat greater than that of most speakers but would probably cause little or no distraction if not listening for it.
- Moderately nasal—nasality is obviously present and is moderately distracting to the listener.
- Severely nasal—nasality is prominent, is a highly distracting feature in the speech, and makes listening to the message difficult.
- Very severely nasal—nasality is so distracting that it dominates all aspects of speech and makes hearing the message extremely difficult.

Fletcher's rating system recognizes the perceptual nature of hypernasality and is based on listener impact.

The *Voice Profile System* (Wilson & Rice, 1977) includes a rating of resonance. Using a scale with one being a normal balance between nasality and orality, the following ratings are suggested:

    −2 = denasal voice
    +2 = assimilation nasality
    +3 = nasalization of some vowels and some shading of consonants
    +4 = nasalization with frequent consonant distortion by nasal emission.

The difficulty with such a scale is the "patient-fit" problem with dichotomous categories. Audiotaped samples, however, are available for reliability training.

The *Buffalo III Resonance Profile* (Wilson, 1987) is a 12-item supplement to Wilson's more general *Buffalo III Voice Profile* and is used when a patient has been rated two or higher on the nasal or oral resonance items of that voice profile. The profile for resonance uses a five-point rating scale where one is normal and five is very severe. Twelve parameters are then so rated: hypernasal resonance, hyponasal resonance, oral resonance, cul-de-sac resonance, nasal emission, facial grimaces, language level, articulation, speech intelligibility, speech acceptability, velopharyngeal competency, and overall resonance rating.

The speech-language pathologist can use a "listening tube" to heighten the perception of a patient's hypernasality, thus facilitating its recognition (Mason & Riski, 1982). We have used a make-shift listening tube fashioned from the plastic headsets provided by the airlines for in-flight movies. Prater and Swift explain an alternate construction and the use of a listening tube:

> The listening tube consists of a glass or plastic olive-shaped tip that is attached to a 2 to 3 foot piece of rubber tubing. Before beginning hypernasality assessment procedures, the nasal olive should be inserted into the patient's nostril and the free end of the tubing should be inserted into the clinician's ear. With

this device in place, even the slightest degrees of nasal emission or hypernasality can be easily detected in the patient's speech. (1984, pp. 55–56)

The speech-language pathologist may try a simple procedure sometimes known as the "nasal flutter test" (Hess, 1976; Weiss, 1974). Have the patient repeat in an alternate fashion the vowels /α/ and /i/ while the clinician alternately compresses and releases the patient's nostrils. It is presumed that if velopharyngeal closure is adequate, there will be no noticeable difference in vowel quality as the nostrils are pinched. Conversely, if the clinician hears an increase in the nasal resonance during the nose-occluded condition, velopharyngeal incompetence may be suspected. The resonance quality change has also been described as a flutterlike sound, hence the name of the test procedure.

Bzoch (1979) recommends a similar nose-occluded–unoccluded test procedure using plosive-vowel-plosive syllables. Ten vowels are tested in a /b——t/ context: beet, bit, bait, bet, bat, bought, boat, boot, but, Bert. In a person with normal velopharyngeal closure, the nose-occluded and unoccluded conditions sound the same.

Shelton, Brooks, and Youngstrom (1965) maintain that articulation tests are good measures of velopharyngeal closure and consequently are used for the clinical assessment of nasal emission and hypernasality. Most tests involve both consonants and vowels. Table 12.1 describes some commonly used articulation tests. Lintz and Sherman (1961) state that consonant environments influence the amount of nasality perceived on vowels. From least influential to most influential are /z, v, d, g, f, s, t, k/. It would seem, therefore, that nasality on vowels should be studied in these consonantal environments.

The perception of hypernasality can be heightened by using context-controlled stimuli. Mason and Grandstaff (1971) maintain that having the patient count aloud from 60 to 100 is an insightful, yet simple, assessment procedure. We offer the following summary of the counting task, which is a useful indicator of velopharyngeal incompetence and the symptoms of hypernasality, nasal emission, and hyponasality.

1. The 60 series of numbers may reveal velopharyngeal incompetence and nasal emission due to the frequent occurance of the /s/ pressure phoneme.
2. The 70 series may reveal assimilative hypernasality due to the embedded /n/ phoneme.
3. The 80 series should reveal normal or near-normal articulation and resonance.
4. The 90 series should sound normal when produced by a patient with hypernasality because of the frequent production of nasal consonants. The patient with hyponasality may display the articulatory substitution of d/n.

Shupe (1968) recommends testing for sound confusions in cases of suspected velopharyngeal incompetence. Have the patient read or repeat word pairs, such as bake/make, rib/rim, dine/nine, mad/man, wig/wing, bag/bang. In a patient with VPI, both sounds are hypernasal, making the bake/make pair, for example, sound like make/make.

Table 12.1 Articulation Tests Useful in Assessing Velopharyngeal Function

P-B Articulation Screening Test for Preschoolers
(Van Demark & Swickard, 1980)

A 25-item single-word test of two phonemes, /p/ and /b/. The authors claim that velopharyngeal inadequacy is indicated when errors occur on at least 50 percent of the sounds tested.

Error Pattern Screening Articulation Test
(Bzoch, 1979; Bzoch, Kemker, & Wood, 1984)

The 31 words are purported to be useful in identifying gross substitution errors in children aged 3 and 4. Plosives, fricatives, affricates, glides, nasals, and blends are tested. Scoring involves assigning an error value to each sound. Sounds are scored as correct, indistinct from nasal emission alone, distortion, simple substitution, gross substitution, or omission.

Bzoch Error Pattern Diagnostic Articulation Test
(Bzoch, 1979)

The diagnostic test has four forms, each with a different set of 100 words. Tested are 67 consonants and 33 blends in the initial, medial, final positions of the words. This is the full-length version of the screening test previously listed and is constructed with the same properties.

Iowa Pressure Articulation Test (IPAT)
(Templin & Darley, 1969)

Consists of 43 words containing pressure consonants. The percentage of correct responses is said to reflect the severity of velopharyngeal incompetence.

The reading passage "The Picnic"
(Wilson, 1987)

The 43 words from the IPAT are incorporated in the short paragraph called "The Picnic." Production of the test words therefore can be tested in reading, rather than the traditional single-word method.

Sentence articulation tests
(Fletcher, 1978; Van Demark, 1964, 1966)

These are two examples of informal tests at the sentence level, which may be more ecologically valid than single-word tests.

Articulation Protocol
(McCabe & Bradley, 1973)

The protocol, with a 10–15 minute administration time, compares accuracy of articulated words in automatic speech, single words, sentences, reading, and conversation.

Instrumentation is also available that purports to detect or measure hypernasality. Like Moll (1964), we maintain that hypernasality is a perceptual phenomenon and must be assessed perceptually. Attempts to measure hypernasality "objectively" are really attempts to measure velopharyngeal function, oral and nasal airflows, and the like. Although these data certainly relate to judgments of hypernasality, they are not measures of hypernasality per se. We will discuss instrumentation used to measure aspects of velopharyngeal function later in this chapter when we discuss the cleft palate population.

Once the speech-language pathologist has determined that the patient exhibits some degree of hypernasality, the evaluative session should turn to discovering what, if any, techniques and manipulations lessen the perception of nasality. Together, the patient and clinician should experiment to find "what works" and in doing so they are arriving at a prognosis for change and are mapping the direction of future treatment, if warranted.

The variability of the hypernasality as it relates to phonetic context should be explored. Does the perception of hypernasality diminish or worsen in sentences loaded with high vowels? With low vowels? With numerous nasal consonants? With many pressure consonants?

Does the degree of hypernasality improve when the patient speaks with "open-mouth articulation" where there is exaggerated mouth opening and speech sounds are enunciated with exaggerated movement? McDonald and Koepp-Baker (1951) discussed this technique as helpful in that air always takes the path of least resistance. By opening the anterior oral cavity wider, air will tend to flow outward rather than through the narrower, but opened velopharyngeal port.

The speech-language pathologist should also probe for possible improvements in hypernasality with changes in speaking rate, pitch, and loudness. These may be prime areas of manipulation in compensatory treatment programs. The literature reports that perceived hypernasality is lessened at higher pitch and intensity levels (Hess, 1959; Rampp & Counihan, 1970). The role of muscular fatigue can also be explored by having the patient determine whether there are times during the day that nasality is better or worse.

> *Case Example.* At the beginning of the second grade, Belinda Johnston was noticed by the speech-language pathologist during school-wide screenings. The child's voice was hypernasal and nasal emission occurred inconsistently on words starting with /s/, /f/, and /p/. Belinda was failed on this brief screening and the speech-language pathologist followed up on the case. In a telephone conversation with the mother, the clinician learned that Belinda had a tonsillectomy and adenoidectomy during the previous Easter break because of frequent ear infections and sore throats. The mother stated that Belinda's voice has sounded "unusual" only since the surgery, but she was told by the doctor that it would improve with time. The first grade teacher confirmed that Belinda's voice sounded normal the previous year. As six months had elapsed since the surgery, the speech-language pathologist and mother agreed to initiate appropriate school system procedures for a formal speech evaluation and subsequent intervention. In the evaluation, hypernasality was confirmed and its severity rated, as was the consistency and severity of nasal emission. The oral peripheral examination revealed several indicators of submucous clefting. There was a midline notching of the uvula (slight bifidity), an anteriorly placed velar dimple, midline translucency of the palate, and a highly vaulted hard palate. Velar movement occurred symmetrically but contact with the posterior pharyngeal wall could not be observed with certainty. Air came out the nose when the clinician used the modified tongue-anchor technique and Belinda was unable to blow up a balloon.
>
> The speech-language pathologist wondered whether adenoidectomy should have been done on this child—the oral exam revealed several factors that would contraindicate a routine removal. (The adenoid's bulk compensated for the child's VPI.) The school speech-language pathologist desired objective confirmation of the suspicions of VPI, available with sophisticated instrumentation, and expert opinions of the proper behavioral course of action, if any. Belinda was referred to the cleft palate team at a metropolitan hospital 100 miles away.
>
> *Case Example.* The speech-language pathologist at a rehabilitation hospital received Delondo Hayes as a transfer patient from an acute care facility. Mr. Hayes was a 22-year-old automobile crash victim who had sustained brain stem

and spinal cord injuries. The clinician noted in the initial speech consult that Mr. Hayes was partially paralyzed and wheelchair bound. His conversational speech was slow, slurred, and excessively hypernasal. In the oral examination, the speech pathologist also noted absence of the gag reflex and weak lingual muscles. The patient was diagnosed with the motor speech disorder of flaccid dysarthria. Early treatment efforts would be directed at oral muscle mobility and precision of articulation. Slow speech rates would be accepted, indeed, encouraged as a means of achieving target articulatory placements, including velar gestures. The hypernasality would be monitored for four to six weeks of rehabilitation before considering further alternatives.

Nasal Emission. Since nasal emission and hypernasality can both be due to inadequate velopharyngeal closure, it makes sense that they often co-occur; yet, we must keep in mind that the two problems are separate entities.

The assessment of nasal emission involves looking and listening. The expulsion of air through the nostrils may be so obvious as to flare the nares of the speaker. In contrast, in an attempt to decrease the outward flow of air, the person may constrict the nares. The clinician, then, looks for facial (nasal) grimaces.

Critical listening is crucial for the speech-language pathologist to accurately diagnose the presence of nasal emission. Sometimes the emitted air is obviously noisy; in fact, nasal snort is a descriptive term encountered in this body of literature. At other times, the nasal emission is barely audible or detectable only with special techniques, as we shall see.

A frequent way to assess the presence of nasal emission is by administering a single-word articulation test. Although any articulation test will do, a few commercially available tests are designed to more thoroughly tap production of pressure plosives, fricatives, and affricates. Table 12.1 described some of the more commonly used articulation tests. The results of the articulation test should answer the following questions posed by Morris and Smith (1962):

1. Does the speaker misarticulate fricatives, plosives, and affricates that have been demonstrated to require high intraoral breath pressure?
2. Do the misarticulations involve audible nasal emission?
3. Are there evidences of facial grimacing during the production of these consonants?
4. Does occluding the nostrils (preventing an air leakage) result in normal production of them?

We would add the following to this list of questions for clinicians:

1. Regarding nasal emission, are voiced consonants less defective than their voiceless cognates? Typically, the required amount of oral air pressure is greater for voiceless phonemes (Moll, 1968; Spriestersbach, 1955).
2. Are single consonants less affected than blends (Moll, 1968)?
3. Are consonants in the initial or final position in words articulated correctly more often than medial consonants (Moll, 1968)?
4. Does the patient use compensatory articulation patterns, such as glottal stop, pharyngeal stop, mid-dorsum palatal stop, pharyngeal fricative, posterior nasal fricative, and so forth (Trost, 1981)?

In addition to, or in place of, a formal articulation test, the clinician may listen for nasal emission in specially designed words and sentences. Have the patient read or repeat stimuli loaded with pressure consonants, such as the following (Bzoch, 1979; Hess, 1971; Lippmann, 1981; Warren, 1979):

> Pick the peas.
> Pappa piped up.
> Polish the shoes.
> Bessie stayed all summer.
> We'd better buy a bigger dog.
> Follow Sally, Charley.
> People, baby, paper, Bobby, puppy, bubble, pepper, B.B., piper, bye bye.

Likewise, the clinician can listen carefully as the patient counts aloud. The numbers between 60 and 79 are especially evocative of nasal emission (Mason & Grandstaff, 1971).

The speech-language pathologist can use simple items to enhance the detection and monitoring of nasal air emission. A small mirror held under the patient's nostrils will fog as air escapes. We have used a dental mirror with its convenient handle, a small lipstick mirror, and a special nonglass reflector manufactured by the Floxite Company (Niagara Falls, NY 14303). We prefer the latter for its sensitivity to fogging and its compact design with handle. Fog on the mirror during the patient's attempts at prolonging fricatives, repeating VCV syllables containing pressure consonants (such as /ipi ipi ipi/, /upu upu upu/), or saying the pressure-loaded sentences previously listed is strongly suggestive of velopharyngeal incompetence. These same procedures may be done with wisps of cotton on a wooden tongue depressor held beneath the nose when a mirror is not available. We find the cotton's sensitivity less reliable, though.

Bzoch (1979) describes an oral-nasal air paddle constructed from cardboard and Bloch (1979) suggests the use of an airline music headset or a stethoscope to detect air flow. The listening tube, described previously, is also useful for assessing nasal emission (Mason & Riski, 1982). A "scape-scope" (Shprintzen, McCall, & Skolnick, 1975) can be constructed with a clear plastic cylinder, styrofoam piston, and tubing with a nasal olive. The same type of device is available commercially as the See-Scape (PRO-ED, Austin, TX 78758). We would like to mention that all devices used to detect and visualize the nasal emission of air are useful in treatment as well as in assessment.

After determining that a patient has nasal emission, the clinician should probe for techniques that diminish air escape. If none is found, behavioral treatment may be contraindicated and physical management necessary. Here are some techniques the speech-language pathologist can try.

Have the patient use light articulatory contacts on pressure consonants—the plosives, fricatives, and affricates. McDonald and Koepp-Baker (1951) suggest explaining this concept to young children by teaching "fish-talking." A complementary technique that may diminish nasal emission is that of open-mouth articulation, as was suggested for hypernasality.

Perhaps having the patient extend the vowel portions of speech will lessen the emphasis placed on pressure consonant articulation and so improve nasal emission. The fluency-enhancing techniques that involve vowel/syllable prolongations, found in many stuttering approaches, may prove useful with some patients. Reduced rates of speech may also be useful, especially in patients who show velar movement potential but suffer from sluggish timing maneuvers.

Van Demark (1971) described a stimulability evaluation for children with resonance problems. Each item missed on the *Iowa Pressure Articulation Test* (Templin & Darley, 1969) is retested, using another picture. The speech-language pathologist repeats the item twice and the client responds immediately. Stimulation is then provided for the item in isolation, in nonsense syllables (all positions), and in words. Following this stimulation, the client is again shown the picture of the errored item and made aware that the word contains the stimulated sound. The child should then attempt the word correctly, read the word, and produce a sentence with it.

Wilson (1987) and Rampp, Pannbacker, and Kinnebrew (1984) advocate use of the *Miami Imitative Ability Test* (Jacobs, Philips, & Harrison, 1970) to determine the level of stimulability in patients with velopharyngeal incompetence. Twenty-four consonant sounds are used in the initial position, followed by a neutral vowel. The child is instructed to "watch and listen" as the clinician repeats each stimulus three times before attempting a production. The response is evaluated in two ways: the ability to imitate articulatory placement and the accuracy of the acoustic production. A three-point scoring system is used: 1 point if correct, $1/2$ point if questionable, and 0 if incorrect.

> *Case Example.* Philip Chang had a repaired cleft lip and palate. Due to persistent velopharyngeal incompetence, the surgeon established an inferiorly based pharyngeal flap. (The interested reader should consult Randall et al., 1978 for information about flaps.) After the appropriate recuperative period, the doctor was still concerned about Philip's speech and ordered further tests. As part of a thorough evaluation, the speech-language pathologist documented articulation errors of the type usually seen in cases of velopharyngeal incompetence. Stimulability probes, however, revealed some interesting changes. For example, Philip produced /t/ with nasal emission in place of /k/ on some test items, yet produced /k/ for /k/ on other items but did so with nasal emission. Glottal stops were noted in place of /g/ and sometimes for /k/. After stimulation, Philip was able to produce /k/ appropriately in phonetic contexts, without substituting. Furthermore, his /k/ productions were without nasal emission of air. A positive oral manometer ratio of 0.95 was obtained. The clinician interpreted Philip's stimulability as indication that velopharyngeal competence could be achieved, that old articulatory habits could be changed, and that phonetic placement training could be effective. Philip's prognosis for modifying his articulation toward normalcy was deemed good.

Cul-de-sac Resonance.   The hollow voice quality of this disorder is typically due to hyperfunction of the tongue. Speech is produced with the tongue posteriorly positioned in the oral cavity and oropharynx regions. The speech-language pathologist should try to observe this posterior retraction when possible; having the patient phonate an open vowel, such as /a/, may facilitate viewing of the posterior tongue placement.

De facto diagnosis may come from probing for improvements in the cul-de-sac resonance. Experiment by having the patient read sentences or word lists loaded with phonemes that promote anterior tongue placement and inhibit lingual retraction. Prater and Swift (1984) suggest the following phonemes for developing clinical stimuli:

> Tongue-tip: /t/, /d/, /s/, and /z/
> Front vowels: /i/, /I/, and /e/
> Front consonants: /w/, /hw/, /p/, /b/, /f/, /v/, /Θ/, and /l/.

It has been noted in the literature that hearing-impaired and deaf speakers often use too slow a rate of speech. The slow rate of speech seems attributable to altered syllable durations; this, in turn, adversely affects speech intelligibility and voice quality. Increasing the speaking rates of hearing-impaired persons may improve their perceived hypernasality of their cul-de-sac resonance and should be attempted by the speech-language pathologist.

Thin Vocal Resonance.   The thin, effeminate voice quality is usually related to anterior tongue carriage and thus the oral resonance of vowels and consonants is affected. By moving the place of the primary articulatory constriction more forward in the oral cavity, energy loci are shifted to higher frequencies and vocalic formants are likewise elevated (Minifie, 1973). The perception of effeminancy may be increased by the patient's use of an elevated fundamental frequency and/or exaggerated use of the upper range for pitch inflections. Pitch, as well as quality, should be evaluated in these patients. As suggested in Chapter 10, *A Voice Assessment Protocol for Children and Adults* (Pindzola, 1987), or a similar instrument, is a useful guide for appraising all parameters of a patient's voice. To assess thin resonance, have the patient read sentences or word lists containing many back vowels and back consonants (such as /k/ and /g/). Note whether there is an improvement in resonance with this probe technique.

ASSESSMENT ASSOCIATED WITH CLEFT PALATE

In addition to the information presented on assessing hypernasality and nasal emission, we would like to elaborate on the diagnostic process used with patients who have clefts of the hard or soft palate. In the diagnosis of communication problems associated with cleft palate, the speech-language pathologist is typically a member of a team. The "cleft palate team" is a well-accepted clinical entity, and in many communities it represents the ultimate in interdisciplinary cooperation between speech-language pathologists, audiologists, psychologists, surgeons, otolaryngologists, prosthedontists, orthodontists, pedodontists, and educational personnel (Bzoch, 1979; Wells, 1971). The speech-language pathologist is expected to inform the team members about the patient's communication abilities and disabilities, predict the effects of contemplated rehabilitative procedures, and serve as the primary agent for change in the patient's speech and language skills. The dramatic growth during the past three or four decades in the development of surgical and other rehabilitative procedures for the individual with a cleft has been encouraging.

The speech-language pathologist should endeavor to evaluate, or have evaluated at an appropriate facility, many aspects of velopharyngeal functioning. Table 12.2 lists areas and/or methods of appraisal. We will elaborate on many in the remainder of the chapter.

Case History. The routine case history data may need to be augmented for the cleft palate patient. Both general and special case history forms have been developed (Bloch, 1979; Darley, 1978; Peterson & Marquardt, 1981; Rampp, Pannbacker, & Kinnebrew, 1984; Saunders, 1972; Westlake, 1968).

Knowledge of the type and extent of cleft, as well as a description of the surgical, prosthodontic, orthodontic, and other rehabilitative procedures performed would be helpful. Some statement of the patient's current medical status and plans for future intervention procedures will also help direct the evaluative process. If the clinician is not a formal member of a cleft palate team, copies of reports from other professionals who have dealt with the patient should be obtained.

Critical Listening. Although the initial interaction between clinician and patient should be free and relatively unstructured, the clinician has a most demanding task. Once the patient is conversing in a spontaneous manner, the speech-language pathologist must apply critical listening skills to assess the individual's total communicative effectiveness. This involves systematically shifting perceptual sets from one aspect of the patient's speech to another. The speech-language pathologist should listen for the presence of a resonance imbalance (such as hypernasality, hyponasality, nasal emission, or a combination) and rate its severity. Although trained judges are able to identify nasality fairly adequately, the clinician may wish to tape-record the client and listen to several playbacks, or play the tape backwards to isolate the nasality from articulation (Sherman, 1954; Spriestersbach, 1955). After noting the degree of resonance imbalance on some scaling device, the clinician should listen to the general

Table 12.2 Areas Typically Appraised in Suspected Cases of Velopharyngeal Incompetence

Case History

Articulation and Intelligibility—formal tests, informal stimuli

Resonance—perceptual scales, listening tubes, various other devices

Intraoral Examination

Endoscopy—with rigid or fiberoptic scopes

Radiographic Studies—cephalometry (still, lateral x-rays), videofluoroscopy, cinefluorography, tomography (laminagraphy), and/or computerized tomography (CT) scanning

Pressure-Flow Studies—oral manometer, TONAR II (nasometer), PERCI, ZIPPO

Others—accelerometry, electromyography, ultrasound

Stimulability Testing (Probes)

articulatory pattern without recording actual errors. Is there an obvious preponderance of a particular type of error (such as glottal stops or pharyngeal fricatives)? Does the articulation appear to alter with differing communication situations, speech, or stress patterns? Next, listen to the language of the patient, particularly if it is a young child, and check for appropriate word choice, sentence complexity, and structure. The rate and rhythm of the patient's speech should be noted. Are there any other vocal quality differences (such as hoarseness)? Is there a facial grimace, constriction of the nares, or any other behavior that detracts from the individual's total communicative effectiveness?

Articulation Testing.   After formulating a general impression of the patient's speech patterns, detailed articulation testing should be done. Standard articulation tests may be satisfactory for cleft palate individuals, but there are several considerations that may be best examined by "specialized" articulation tests and context-controlled stimuli. Certainly, all of the functional, perceptual, and sensory factors that affect the normal person could be active, but in cleft palate individuals there are added possibilities. Most important are the degree of velopharyngeal closure and the resultant airflow and intraoral pressure. The deviant geography of the oral cavity may contribute to this problem, which is also complicated by the fact that the oral structure may well have undergone several architectural changes within the first few years of life. The speech-language pathologist must keep in mind that this individual has been trying to produce standard sounds with a nonstandard structure, and under these conditions, unique compensatory adjustments may have been made. The patient may have increased the airflow in order to build up adequate oral pressure, or minimized it to lessen nasal escape; in the latter case, we say that the patient is producing weak pressure consonants (McWilliams & Philips, 1979; Trost, 1981).

Many patients with VPI adopt compensatory articulations, including glottal stop substitutions, pharyngeal fricatives, velar fricatives, and aspirant productions of vowels and consonants; other, unusual compensations may also be used (Rampp, Pannbacker, & Kinnebrew, 1984; Trost, 1981).

Glottal stop substitutions are produced by approximation of the glottis; they are generally used in the place of plosives and sometimes in the place of fricatives. Glottal stop substitutions are a difficult habit to break even after management of the palate and seem to be especially persistent for sounds in the medial position (Bzoch, 1979; McWilliams & Philips, 1979). Pharyngeal and velar fricatives are also attempts by the patient to valve air at a point in the vocal tract that is nearer the source of air pressure than the velopharyngeal valve (Morris, 1979). The place of constriction is between the tongue and pharynx, or constriction of the pharynx, rather than more orally. Bzoch (1979) also reports that pharyngeal and velar fricatives persist longest for the /s/ and /z/ phonemes.

Trost (1981) described three types of compensatory articulation not typically reported in the literature: (1) The pharyngeal stop, used with /k/ and /g/, is produced with a posterior and inferior tongue placement. (2) The middorsum palatal stop is a stop consonant substitution for /t/, /d/, /k/, or /g/.

Posterior nasal fricatives are generally produced as substitutions for the /s/, /z/, /ʃ/, and /ʒ/ phonemes and may occur simultaneously with a fricative, affricate, or stop consonant.

The clinician should keep in mind that it is entirely possible for the compensatory habits that developed before the final surgical adjustments to persist after competence of the velopharyngeal mechanism is established and the patient can make the correct articulatory movements. Stimulability probes therefore are important in determining the patient's prognosis for change. Articulation errors may also be related to an existing or prior hearing loss.

In addition to providing an inventory of the patient's sound productions, articulation testing can indicate the adequacy of velopharyngeal closure (Shelton, Brooks, & Youngstrom, 1965). As we have said, certain sounds have a higher probability for error than others. The speech-language pathologist should obtain a thorough sample of these sounds in articulation testing. Since articulation involves dynamic and overlapping movements, the clinician should be certain to get samples of the patient producing isolated sounds, syllables, words, and connected speech. In certain cases of assimilation nasality, it is necessary to evaluate specific phonetic contexts containing nasal and non-nasal sounds to determine if the patient can make the rapid velopharyngeal alterations. There are several formal test instruments that have been traditionally associated with cleft palate articulatory assessment. These were described in Table 12.1. The context-controlled stimuli mentioned earlier in this chapter would be useful for the clinician, as well.

Nasal Resonance. Resonatory voice disorders are frequently heard in individuals with clefts. The assessment process described earlier in this chapter, then, certainly applies to the diagnostic workup of a cleft palate patient. Any quality aberration is possible in persons with clefts of the palate, but high probability disorders are hypernasality and nasal emission since both are related to inadequate velopharyngeal closure. It is worth mentioning that the clinician should attempt to determine to what extent the resonance imbalance is related to functional factors such as tension, fatigue, and learning or organic factors such as neurological dysfunction or the structural defect of the cleft itself. We would like to restate that listener evaluation of a speaking voice is the best way for the clinician to judge the resonance parameter.

The Oral Peripheral Examination. Although velopharyngeal closure cannot be visualized in an oral examination, it is important to examine the orofacial region of patients who manifest resonation disorders. The examination is an initial step in determining the general relationships among all structures in the vocal tract. For instance, the clinician can get a gross picture of palatal shape, total and effective velar lengths, movement ability and symmetry of movement of the velum, and dimensions of the pharynx and can determine if any defects, such as fistulas of the palate, are present. If the speech-language pathologist has any concerns regarding structure or function, the physician should be consulted.

Procedures for appraising the structure and function of the oral and peripheral regions are described in the literature (Bloch, 1979; Dworkin &

Culatta, 1980; Mason, 1969; Mason & Grandstaff, 1971; Mason & Simon, 1977; Rampp, Pannbacker, & Kinnebrew, 1984; St. Louis & Ruscello, 1981). General information on conducting an oral peripheral examination is provided in Chapter 9. We offer a few special comments here.

Perhaps the most important thing for the speech-language pathologist to do when VPI is suspected is to determine the effective length of the velum and the location of the velar dimple (Mason, 1969; Mason & Grandstaff, 1971). The effective velar length is that portion of the elevated velar tissue used in closure of the nasopharynx during phonation. The effected length can be estimated from intraoral inspection of the velar dimple during phonation relative to nasopharyngeal depth. The velar dimple on the oral surface of the velum is an indication of the point of maximum elevation on the nasal surface of the velum. It typically occurs at 80 percent of the total velar length. The more anteriorly the dimple is placed (say, at the 50 percent mark), the less the effective velar length, and the greater the degree of velopharyngeal incompetence.

Examination of the palate may reveal oronasal fistulas that are not always readily visible. What is the shape of the palatal vault? Is the coloration a healthy pink, or do there appear to be white or blue tinted regions? Is there a palatal translucency observed during the oral exam when, in a dark room, a flashlight is shined into a nostril? Upon palpation, does the bony substructure feel firm and have normal posterior edges? If there is a fistula, the degree to which it affects articulation or resonance may be determined by occluding the area with dental wax or chewing gum (Bloch, 1979; Colburn, 1982).

When overt clefting is present, the type and extent can be appraised. Many hospital-based cleft palate teams have devised specialized oral examination forms that contain diagrams of the lips and palate on which to mark the patient's features. Although many classification systems are still in use today (such as those proposed by Veau, 1931; Davis and Ritchie, 1922; Kernahan and Stark, 1958; and the American Cleft Palate Association as reported by Harkins, et al., 1962), the use of an individualized diagram not only documents the extent of the cleft but also facilitates communication among the team professionals.

Special Assessment Procedures for Velopharyngeal Function. As previously indicated, the oral peripheral examination does not allow definitive judgments of velopharyngeal adequacy to be made. Also, an articulation test, whether published or informal, is but an indirect measure of the client's velopharyngeal function (Shelton, Brooks & Youngstrom, 1965). Other techniques, many involving instrumentation, are available to directly or indirectly assess the velopharyngeal mechanism. We maintain that no single measure is adequate for appraisal of velopharyngeal function; and we also believe that articulation testing and resonance assessment *must* be part of any diagnostic process. Let us describe some of the other assessment procedures that are available for routine and/or sophisticated diagnostic sessions.

Fox and Johns (1970) describe a technique for measuring static closure whereby the patient is required to maintain intraoral pressure by puffing up the cheeks. If this is accomplished, the patient is then asked to protrude the tongue and puff up the cheeks (to prevent lingual valving). The clinician holds the patient's nostrils while this is done to aid in impounding pressure. If no air escapes when the nostrils are released, it is assumed that velopharyngeal closure is adequate.

As previously mentioned, informal and subjective measures of velopharyngeal leakage can be obtained by observing fog on a mirror held beneath the patient's nose, by seeing wisps of cotton move when so placed, by using listening tubes of various designs, and by critically listening to controlled stimuli spoken in nose-occluded–unoccluded conditions.

The oral manometer is an affordable piece of equipment helpful in discriminating between persons with good and poor velopharyngeal closure. Procedures for use of the manometer and advantages of using an open bleed valve have been described elsewhere (Hardy, 1965; Morris, 1966; Shelton, Hahn, & Morris, 1968). The patient either blows or sucks as forcefully as possible into/from a mouthpiece. The exhalation task yields a positive pressure reading from the manometer gauges, while the inhalation task gives a negative reading. A ratio is obtained by comparing pressures achieved in the nostrils-open and nostrils-occluded conditions. A normal ratio of 1.00 is suggestive of velopharyngeal closure adequacy, particularly if an open bleed valve was used to inhibit compensatory maneuvers, such as tongue-palate valving. Ratios less than 1.00 may be indicative of VPI, hypernasal speech, and reduced intelligibility in cleft palate patients; ratios less than 0.89 are particularly poor indicators (Subtelny & Subtelny, 1959; Van Demark, 1966).

Air pressure and air flow techniques are based on the fact that VPI results in a decrement of intraoral air pressure and an increase in airflow through the nose. Consequently, pressure and flow measurements can be part of the total diagnostic workup; they are often used for research purposes. Pressure transducers, such as strain gauge transducers, are used to measure air pressures while air flowmeters are used to measure volume rates of airflow. Types of flowmeters include warm-wire anemometers, pneumotachographs, and thermistors. The pneumotachograph is perhaps the most commonly used and requires the use of a face mask to collect the airflow and direct it through a sensing screen (Rampp, Pannbacker, & Kinnebrew, 1984). Air pressure and flow instrumentation is expensive and complex. McWilliams and Philips (1979) discuss the disadvantages of pressure-flow instrumentation and the limited information it actually provides about the velopharyngeal gap.

Warren (1979) designed an instrument called PERCI, which provides an oral and nasal air pressure ratio during the production of pressure (stop) consonants. A low oral/nasal pressure ratio is said to be indicative of velopharyngeal incompetence.

Fletcher (1970, 1976) developed the TONAR instrument, which measures the oral and nasal sound pressures. A ratio formed between the two measures, expressed as a percentage, is referred to as *nasalence*. Fletcher claims that nasalence is highly correlated with perceptual judgments of nasality. Normal oral/nasal ratios are said to be less than 10 percent, whereas patients with severe hypernasality have ratios in excess of 80 percent. The instrumentation has been simplified for use in clinician assessment; the modified version is TONAR II. Keuhn (1982) discusses limitations of this expensive instrumentation.

The Zemlin Index of Palatopharyngeal Opening, or ZIPPO, attempts to determine airflow leakage through the velopharyngeal port by measuring "vocal tract damping time" (Zemlin & Fant, 1972). Disadvantages of this instrumentation have been discussed by Keuhn (1982); its usefulness in the evaluation of VPI has yet to be determined.

Referral for direct visualization of the velopharyngeal closure mechanism is, perhaps, in order when articulation and nasal resonance have been determined to be abnormal. Direct visualization involves radiographic, ultrasonic, and/or endoscopic methods. Let us say a brief word about each.

Radiographic methods involve low doses of radiation to visualize the structures, including soft tissues. The speech-language pathologist should work closely with the radiologist in selecting the most appropriate radiographic method and conditions of study. Knowledge of the literature is important in selecting which speech and nonspeech tasks to have the patient perform (Shelton, Hahn, & Morris, 1968). Radiographic methods used in the assessment of velopharyngeal function were listed as part of Table 12.2. Several discussions of these methods are available in the literature (Bzoch, 1970; Pigott, 1980; Rampp, Pannbacker, & Kinnebrew, 1984; Spriestersbach et al., 1973).

Ultrasound offers a noninvasive means of visualizing lateral pharyngeal wall movement during speech. This technique has been described by Kuehn (1982) and involves placing an ultrasonic transducer against the neck. Soft tissues and air in the pharyngeal cavities transmit the pulse differently, thus creating an image on the display screen. A number of difficulties exist in using ultrasound to study velopharyngeal function; these may be resolved in future research.

Direct visualization is easily accomplished through an invasive technique that uses viewing devices called endoscopes. Rigid forms of endoscopy useful in observing velopharyngeal closure are the oral panendoscope and the nasal endoscope. Flexible endoscopes use fiberoptic bundles. We again remind the reader that closure, or lack of it, is best viewed from above and so the flexible fiberscope inserted through the nasal cavity is used quite often. Most, if not all, hospitals now have the necessary equipment. Cooperative patients can be examined while seated and performing speech and nonspeech tasks. Reviews of endoscopy can be found in the works of Osberg and Witzel (1981) and Karnell et al. (1983).

Other instrumental methods are available for research and clinician use. These include the use of accelerometers, or contact microphones, to measure the amplitude of nasal vibrations as an index of nasality in the patient's speech, electromyography to study muscle activity in velopharyngeal movement gestures, and photodetector assessment of velopharyngeal activity (Dalston, 1982). Rampp, Pannbacker, and Kinnebrew (1984) provide a review of these methods, which are used primarily in the research arena.

The speech-language pathologist may or may not have access to some of these instruments but should know that they are available. In this age of high technology, it can be expected that access to such equipment from universities, medical centers, and clinics will become easier and more widespread.

Auditory Acuity and Language Ability. The high incidence of auditory acuity problems among cleft palate children has been well documented (Heller, 1979; Prather & Kos, 1968). For this reason, it is absolutely essential that every cleft palate patient have a hearing examination. These examinations should include both air and bone conduction testing and should be a part of every speech diagnosis.

The speech-language pathologist will wish to see the cleft palate child or infant as soon as possible. Typically, in major hospitals, once an infant is born with an orofacial anomaly, the work of a multidisciplinary team is set into motion. The speech-language pathologist, as part of the team, will work closely with the parents—through counseling and training—to prevent future communication problems. During this early contact, the parents can be informed about the need for normal speech and language stimulation, what to expect from their child regarding speech and language production, and the need for frequent audiometric testing. Some speech clinicians use established language stimulation programs as a preventative measure with these children.

Several researchers have documented the existence of a language deficit among cleft palate children (Morris, 1962; Nation, 1970; Smith & McWilliams, 1968). Likewise, those children who received proper stimulation in the early years often do not have language problems that persist into the school years. To be sure, then, the clinician should examine the child's language abilities and pay particular attention to expressive skills. The procedures discussed in Chapters 4 and 5 should be sufficient for this evaluation.

PROGNOSIS ASSOCIATED WITH RESONANCE IMBALANCE

Let us now return to our general discussion of resonance imbalance and list some of the prognostic indicators for the treatment of resonatory disorders. We freely admit that much is speculation, opinion, or simply based on assumptions of etiology. Research documenting clinician effectiveness is sorely needed.

1. Prater and Swift (1984) state that voice treatment for cul-de-sac resonance is not usually successful in patients with neurologic involvement of the articulators. This includes conditions such as oral apraxia, athetoid cerebral palsy, flaccid dysarthria, and spastic dysarthria. Patients with functional cul-de-sac resonance and, to a lesser extent, deaf speakers can benefit from intervention directed toward anterior positioning of the tongue.

2. Thin resonance, with its assumed functional etiology, is remediated easily only in patients who are motivated to change. Treatment efforts should be directed toward correcting tongue carriage. The clinician may benefit from knowledge of male-female communication differences when assisting a patient

to reduce the effeminate aspects of speech. The emerging literature on communication treatment for transsexuals may be used as a resource, but applied in reverse for treating thin resonance. The works of Kline (1983) and Pryor and Scott (1983) can be consulted in this regard.

3. Hyponasality, when due to some nasal obstruction, necessitates physical management. Speech treatment alone is not likely to be beneficial.

4. The patient's motivation to change is paramount in predicting the outcome of voice treatment.

5. A favorable prognosis for treatment is indicated if the clinician was able to elicit a better voice from the patient during stimulability trials.

Pannbacker (1976) and Rampp, Pannbacker, and Kinnebrew (1984) reviewed the literature on indications and contraindications to speech treatment for individuals with cleft palate and concluded that there is much misunderstanding and a paucity of research evidence supporting its effectiveness. We will cite some of the treatment indicators here. Much of what is listed also applies to cases of hypernasality and nasal emission in the absence of clefting.

1. Speech treatment is contraindicated for patients with clearly inadequate velopharyngeal closure; physical management is warranted (Pannbacker, 1976). As discussed in this chapter, evidence of velopharyngeal inadequacy should come from a variety of sources, including articulation testing showing consistent hypernasality and nasal emission, observation of nasal grimacing, radiographic evidence, and oral examination findings of an anteriorly displaced velar dimple and/or excessive nasopharyngeal dimensions.

2. Since home programs are essential in most therapeutic approaches, motivated and cooperative patients and their parents are a requirement for enrollment in a speech intervention program (Shprintzen, McCall, & Skolnick, 1975).

3. Speech treatment is not warranted, or is low priority, when the patient needs language and communication improvement. Shelton, Hahn, and Morris (1968) stress the primacy of language treatment.

4. Pannbacker maintains that patients with borderline velopharyngeal closure "should not be subjected to the stress of speech therapy because of the chance that they may compensate laryngeally" (1976; p. 43). Speech treatment, then, is contraindicated if the patient presents with hoarseness. According to McWilliams, Bluestone, and Musgrave,

> [V]ocal cord nodules appear to be a danger signal and provide evidence that things are not quite as they should be higher in the tract; consideration should be given to secondary procedures designed to correct the velopharyngeal inadequacy which would appear to be related to the onset of vocal cord problems. (1969, p. 2076)

5. Patients who demonstrated improvement during the assessment probes are good candidates for speech treatment. Especially favorable are

reduced hypernasality when employing exaggerated, open-mouth articulation and a marked difference in velar activity when gagging and phonating (Mason & Grandstaff, 1971).

6. Some patients with inadequate velopharyngeal closure cannot benefit from further physical management. The speech-language pathologist may opt to provide compensatory treatment. The goal, then, is not normal-sounding speech, but the best speech of which the patient is capable. Tasks used in the assessment probes may be appropriate treatment techniques in that the perception of hypernasality is reduced by their use. These include increased mouth opening, low and forward placement of the tongue, auditory training, exaggerated articulation movements, light and quick articulatory contacts, overall slowed rate of speech, and altered pitch and/or loudness levels.

CONCLUSION

The evaluation of disorders of resonance is a challenge to the speech-language pathologist. The clinician must often work closely with medical personnel and other allied health workers, which necessitates knowing procedures and terminologies that are peripheral to speech-language pathology. The clinician must also remain abreast of current technological developments in electronics, surgery, and medical technology. Finally, the clinician must keep interpersonal clinical skills finely honed so that psychological aspects of vocal disorders can be detected and dealt with through treatment or referral.

BIBLIOGRAPHY

BLOCH, P. J. (1979). Clinical evaluation for the cleft palate team setting. In K. R. Bzoch (Ed.), *Communicative disorders related to cleft lip and palate.* Boston: Little, Brown.

BLOOMER, H. H., & WOLSKI, W. (1968). Office examination of palatopharyngeal function. *Clin. Pediatr., 7,* 611–618.

BOONE, D. R., & MCFARLANE, S. (1988). *The Voice and voice therapy* (3rd ed.). Englewood Cliffs, NJ: Prentice Hall.

BZOCH, K. (1970). Assessment: Radiographic techniques. *Asha Reports, 5,* 248–270.

BZOCH, K. (1979). *Communicative disorders related to cleft lip and palate.* Boston: Little, Brown.

BZOCH, K. R., KEMKER, F. J., & WOOD, V. L. D. (1984). The prevention of communicative disorders in cleft palate infants. In N. J. Lass (Ed.), *Speech and language: Advances in basic research and practice.* San Diego, CA: Academic Press.

COLBURN, N. (1982). Noninstrumental assessment of velopharyngeal adequacy in children. *Seminars in Speech, Language, Hearing, 3,* 212–221.

DALSTON, R. (1982). Photodector assessment of velopharyngeal activity. *Cleft Palate Journal, 19,* 1–8.

DARLEY, F. (1978). The case history. In F. Darley & D. Spriestersbach (Eds.), *Diagnostic methods in speech pathology.* New York: Harper & Row.

DAVIS, J. S. & RITCHIE, H. P. (1922). Classification of congenital clefts of lip and palate. *Journal of American Medical Association, 2,* 1323.

DWORKIN, J., & CULATTA, R. (1980). *Dworkin-Culatta oral mechanism examination.* Nicholasville, KY: Edgewood Press.

FLETCHER, S. (1970). Theory and instrumentation for quantitative measurement of nasality. *Journal of Speech and Hearing Disorders, 37,* 329–346.

FLETCHER, S. (1976). Nasalence vs. listener judgments of nasality. *Cleft Palate Journal, 13,* 31–44.

FLETCHER, S. (1978). *Diagnosing speech disorders from cleft palate.* New York Grune & Stratton.

FOX, D., & JOHNS, D. (1970). Predicting velopharyngeal closure with a modified tongue-anchor technique. *Journal of Speech and Hearing Disorders, 35,* 248–251.

HARDY, J. (1965). Airflow and air pressure studies. *Asha Reports, 1,* 141–152.

HARKINS, C. S., BERLIN, A., HARDING, R., LONGACRE, J., & SNODGRASSE, R. (1962). A classification of cleft lip and cleft palate. *Journal of Plastic and Reconstructive Surgery, 29,* 31.

HELLER, J. (1979). Hearing loss in patients with cleft palate. In K. R. Bzoch (Ed.), *Communicative disorders related to cleft lip and palate.* Boston: Little, Brown.

HESS, D. A. (1959). Pitch, intensity and cleft palate voice quality. *Journal of Speech and Hearing Research, 2,* 113–125.

HESS, D. A. (1971). Effects of certain variables on speech of cleft palate persons. *Cleft Palate Journal, 8,* 387–398.

HESS, D. A. (1976). A new experimental approach to assessment of velopharyngeal adequacy: Nasal manometric bleed testing. *Journal of Speech and Hearing Disorders, 41,* 427–443.

JACOBS, R. J., PHILIPS, B. J., & HARRISON, R. J. (1970). A stimulability test for cleft palate children. *Journal of Speech and Hearing Disorders, 35,* 354–360.

KARNELL, M., IBUKI, K., MORRIS, H., & VAN DEMARK, D. (1983). Reliability of the nasopharyngeal fiberscope (NPF) for assessing velopharyngeal function: Analysis by judgment. *Cleft Palate Journal, 20,* 200–208.

KERNAHAN, D. A., & STARK, M. D. (1958). A new classification for cleft tip and cleft palate. *Journal of Plastic and Reconstructive Surgery, 22,* 435–441.

KLINE, P. (1983). *Sex differences in communication: A therapy framework for the male to female transsexual client.* Paper presented at the annual convention of the American Speech-Language-Hearing Association, Cincinnati, OH.

KUEHN, D. (1982). Assessment of resonance disorders. In N. Lass, L. McReynolds, J. Northern, & D. Yoder (Eds.), *Speech, language and hearing (Vol. 11); Pathologies of speech and language.* Philadelphia, PA: W. B. Saunders.

LINTZ, L. B., & SHERMAN, D. (1961). Phonetic elements and perception of nasality. *Journal of Speech and Hearing Research, 4,* 381–396.

LIPPMANN, R. P. (1981). Detecting nasalization using a low-cost miniature accelerometer. *Journal of Speech and Hearing Research, 24,* 314–317.

MCCABE, R., & BRADLEY, D. (1973). Pre- and post-articulation therapy assessment. *Language, Speech and Hearing Services in Schools, 4,* 13–32.

MCDONALD, E. T., & KOEPP-BAKER, H. (1951). Cleft palate speech: An integration of research and clinical observation. *Journal of Speech and Hearing Disorders, 16,* 9–19.

MCWILLIAMS, B. J., BLUESTONE, C. D., & MUSGRAVE, R. D. (1969). Diagnostic implication of vocal cord nodules in children with cleft palate. *Laryngoscope, 79,* 2072–2080.

MCWILLIAMS, B. J., & PHILIPS, B. (1979). *Velopharyngeal incompetence: Audio seminars in speech pathology.* Philadelphia, PA: W. B. Saunders.

MASON, R. (1969). Improving the efficiency of the intra-oral examination. *Journal of the Tennessee Speech and Hearing Association, 14,* 4–10.

MASON, R. M., & GRANDSTAFF, H. L. (1971). Evaluating the velopharyngeal mechanism in hypernasal speakers. *Language, Speech and Hearing Services in Schools, 2,* 53–61.

MASON, R. M., & RISKI, J. E. (1982). The team approach in orofacial management. *Annals of Plastic Surgery, 8,* 71–78.

MASON, R., & SIMON, C. (1977). An orofacial examination checklist. *Language, Speech, and Hearing Services in Schools, 8,* 155–163.

MINIFIE, F. D. (1973). Speech acoustics. In F. D. Minifie, T. J. Hixon, & F. Williams (Eds.), *Normal aspects of speech, hearing, and language.* Englewood Cliffs, NJ: Prentice Hall.

MOLL, K. L. (1964). Objective measures of nasality. *Cleft Palate Journal, 1,* 371–374.

MOLL, K. (1968). Speech characteristics of individuals with cleft lip and palate. In D. Spriestersbach & D. Sherman (Eds.), *Cleft palate and communication.* New York: Academic Press.

MORRIS, H. (1962). Communication skills of children with cleft lips and palates. *Journal of Speech and Hearing Research, 5,* 79–90.

MORRIS, H. (1966). The oral manometer as a diagnostic tool in clinical speech pathology. *Journal of Speech and Hearing Disorders, 31,* 362–369.

MORRIS, H. (1979). Evaluation of abnormal articulation patterns. In K. Bzoch (Ed.), *Communicative disorders related to cleft lip and palate.* Boston: Little, Brown.

MORRIS, H. L., & SMITH, J. K. (1962). A multiple approach for evaluating velopharyngeal competency. *Journal of Speech and Hearing Disorders, 27,* 218–226.

NATION, J. (1970). Vocabulary comprehension and usage in preschool cleft palate and normal children. *Cleft Palate Journal, 7,* 639–644.

OSBERG, P., & WITZEL, M. A. (1981). The physiologic basis for hypernasality during connected speech in cleft palate patients: A nasoendoscopic study. *Plastic and Reconstructive Surgery, 67,* (1), 1–5.

PANNBACKER, M. (1976). Indications and contraindications for speech therapy in cleft palate. *Journal of National Student Speech and Hearing Association,* December, 4, pp. 40–47.

PETERSON, H., & MARQUARDT, T. (1981). *Appraisal and diagnosis of speech and language disorders.* Englewood Cliffs, NJ: Prentice Hall.

PETERSON, S. (1975). Nasal emission as a component of the misarticulation of sibilants and affricates. *Journal of Speech and Hearing Disorders. 40,* 106–114.

PETERSON-FALZONE, S. (1982). Resonance disorders in structural defects. In N. Lass, L. McReynolds, J. Northern, & D. Yoder (Eds.), *Speech, language and hearing (Vol. 2): Pathologies of speech and language.* Philadelphia, PA: W. B. Saunders.

PIGOTT, R. W. (1980). Assessment of velopharyngeal function. In M. Edwards & A. Watson (Eds.),

Advances in the management of cleft palate. New York: Churchill Livingstone, Inc.

PINDZOLA, R. H. (1987). *A voice assessment protocol for children and adults.* Austin, TX: PRO-ED.

PRATER, R. J., & SWIFT, R. W. (1984). *Manual of voice therapy.* Boston: Little, Brown.

PRATHER, W., & KOS, C. (1968). Audiological and otological considerations. In D. Spriestersbach & D. Sherman (Eds.), *Cleft palate and communication.* New York: Academic Press.

PRYOR, A. P., & SCOTT, C. S. (1983). *Communication therapy for the male transsexual.* Paper presented at the annual convention of the American Speech-Language-Hearing Association, Cincinnati, OH.

RAMPP, D., & COUNIHAN, D. (1970). Vocal pitch-intensity relationships in cleft palate speakers. *Cleft Palate Journal, 7,* 846–857.

RAMPP, D. L., PANNBACKER, M., & KINNEBREW, M. C. (1984). *VPI velopharyngeal incompetency: A practical guide for evaluation and management.* Austin, TX: PRO-ED.

RANDALL, P., WHITAKER, L. A., NOONE, R. B., & JONES, W. D. (1978). The case for the inferiorly based posterior pharyngeal flap. *Cleft Palate Journal, 15,* 262–265.

ST. LOUIS, K., & RUSCELLO, D. (1981). *The oral speech mechanism examination.* Baltimore: University Park Press.

SAUNDERS, L. (1972). *Procedure guides for evaluation of speech and language disorders in children.* Danville, IL: Interstate.

SHELTON, R. L., BROOKS, A. R., & YOUNGSTROM, K. A. (1965). Clinical assessment of palatopharyngeal closure. *Journal of Speech and Hearing Disorders, 30,* 37–43.

SHELTON, R. L., HAHN, E., & MORRIS, H. L. (1968). Diagnosis and therapy. In D. C. Spriestersbach & D. Sherman (Eds.), *Cleft palate and communication.* New York: Academic Press.

SHERMAN, D. (1954). The merits of backward playing of connected speech in the scaling of voice quality disorders. *Journal of Speech and Hearing Disorders, 19,* 312–321.

SHPRINTZEN, R. J., MCCALL, G. N., & SKOLNICK, M. L. (1975). A new therapeutic technique for the treatment of velopharyngeal incompetence. *Journal of Speech and Hearing Disorders, 40,* 69–83.

SHUPE, L. K. (1968). *Speech intelligibility measures of cleft palate speakers before and after pharyngeal flap surgery.* Unpublished doctoral dissertation, State University of New York at Buffalo.

SMITH, R., & MCWILLIAMS, B. (1968). Psycholinguistic abilities of children with clefts. *Cleft Palate Journal, 5,* 238–249.

SPRIESTERSBACH, D. (1955). Assessing nasal quality in cleft palate speech of children. *Journal of Speech and Hearing Disorders, 20,* 266–270.

SPRIESTERSBACH, D., DICKSON, D., FRASER, F., HOROWITZ, S., MCWILLIAMS, B., PARADISE, J., & RANDALL, P. (1973). Clinical research in cleft lip and cleft palate: The state of the art. *Cleft Palate Journal, 10,* 113–163.

SUBTELNY, J., & SUBTELNY, F. (1959). Intelligibility and associated factors of cleft palate speech. *Journal of Speech and Hearing Research, 2,* 353–360.

SUBTELNY, J., VAN HATTUM, R., & MYERS, B. (1972). Ratings and measures of cleft palate speech. *Cleft Palate Journal, 8,* 18–27.

TEMPLIN, M., & DARLEY, F. (1969). *The Templin-Darley Tests of Articulation* (2nd ed.). Iowa City, IA: University of Iowa Bureau of Educational Research and Service.

TROST, J. E. (1981). Articulatory additions to the classical description of the speech of persons with cleft palate. *Cleft Palate Journal, 18,* 193–203.

VAN DEMARK, D. (1964). Misarticulations and listener judgments of the speech of individuals with cleft palates. *Cleft Palate Journal, 1,* 232–245.

VAN DEMARK, D. (1966). A factor analysis of the speech of children with cleft palate. *Cleft Palate Journal, 3,* 159–170.

VAN DEMARK, D. (1971). Clinical research methodology in evaluating the therapeutic process. *Cleft Palate Journal, 8,* 26–35.

VAN DEMARK, D. (1974). Assessment of velopharyngeal competency for children with cleft palate. *Cleft Palate Journal, 11,* 310–316.

VAN DEMARK, D. R., & SWICKARD, S. L. (1980). A pre-school articulation test to assess velopharyngeal competency: Normative data. *Cleft Palate Journal, 17,* 175–181.

VEAU, V. (1931). *Division Palatine.* Paris: Masson et Cie.

WARREN, D. W. (1979). PERCI: A method for rating palatal efficiency. *Cleft Palate Journal, 16,* 279–285.

WEISS, C. (1974). The speech pathologist's role in dealing with obturator-wearing school children. *Journal of Speech and Hearing Disorders, 39,* 153–162.

WELLS, C. (1971). *Cleft palate and its associated speech disorders.* New York: McGraw-Hill.

WESTLAKE, H. (1968). Speech learning in cleft palate children. In R. Lencione (Ed.), *Cleft palate habilitation.* Syracuse, NY: Syracuse University Press.

WILSON, D. K. (1987). *Voice problems in children* (3rd ed.). Baltimore: Williams & Wilkins.

WILSON, F., & RICE, M. (1977). *A programmed approach to voice therapy.* Austin, TX: Learning Concepts, Inc.

ZEMLIN, W., & FANT, G. (1972). The effect of a velopharyngeal shunt upon vocal tract damping times: An analogue study. *Speech Transmission Laboratory Quarterly Report, 4,* 6–10.

13

THE DIAGNOSTIC REPORT

Only one very important phase of the evaluation remains to be considered: the preparation of the diagnostic report. Put the clinical situation, the interview, testing methods, results, and impressions in writing as soon as possible. Never trust a memory. Commit it to paper while the facial characteristics and voice inflections can still be remembered. Make the report "alive" so that others can experience what occurred just by reading about it. The raw data are of limited value to the clinician or other workers until they are assembled in a clear, precise, and orderly fashion.

A *diagnostic report* is a written record that summarizes the relevant information we have obtained—and how we have obtained it—in our professional interaction with a client. It serves the following functions: (1) It acts as a guide for further services to the client—providing a clear statement of how the person was functioning at a given point in time, so that we can document change or lack of change; (2) it communicates our findings to other professional workers; it provides answers to a number of clinical questions, including: Does the person have a problem? Will treatment be helpful? Will referrals be necessary?; and (3) it serves as a document for research purposes.

The importance of the first function should be obvious: Intelligent clinical plans evolve naturally from carefully prepared reports. The second purpose of diagnostic reports is to answer questions about clients so that other professionals can plan and provide appropriate services. In addition to transmitting necessary information, a carefully prepared examination report will also tend to establish the credibility of the speech-language pathologist in the eyes of other workers. To state it another way, a written document is an extension of the diagnostician, and even minor errors in spelling or grammar may cast doubt upon the accuracy and attention to detail with respect to substantive material. Although the clinician may be highly skilled in testing and interviewing, competence may be evaluated by the clinician's written communications. Clinical reports are the principal way we relate to other professionals.

FORMAT

There are several ways to organize a diagnostic report (Darley & Spriestersbach, 1978; Flower, 1984; Hollis & Dunn, 1979; Hutchinson, Hanson, & Mecham, 1979; Knepflar, 1976; Peterson & Marquardt, 1990). Because reports may vary, depending on the intended reader, no single schema is appropriate for all circumstances; in many instances, the format will be dictated by the agency the clinician serves. We will provide two examples: formats for reports in medical settings and in the public schools.

Clinicians in a medial setting may record their findings in a "problem-oriented" format (Kent & Chabon, 1980). Problem-oriented medical records (POMR) feature a carefully defined and "documented list of problems which encompass all the significant difficulties a patient is experiencing" (Enelow & Swisher, 1972, p. 69). The list includes the presenting complaint as well as those problems identified by the members of the treatment team. All available information about the person is then organized under the four headings shown in Figure 13.1 (Bouchard & Shane, 1977). The four headings of information form the acronym SOAP. Daily chart documentations can be written using the SOAP format, as well.

In recent years, there has been a growing trend in the health care industry toward the use of "functional outcome measures," in which the patient's behaviors are assessed categorically relative to levels of function. The Functional Communication Measures, a component of ASHA's Program Evaluation System, have a broad range of clinical applicability. A format for using the Functional Communication Measures in diagnostic reporting and treatment planning in speech-language pathology has been developed (Tonkovich, 1989).

Also, we would like to mention that technology has finally come to the aid of busy clinicians who are often inundated by clinical documentation. A large vocabulary voice recognition system with software specifically developed for generating diagnostic reports, treatment plans, progress notes, and discharge reports has been developed and field-tested at a large hospital (Tonkovich et al., 1990). This system allows clinicians to generate printed reports by speaking

Figure 13.1 The SOAP Format for Medical Reports

SUBJECTIVE	OBJECTIVE	ASSESSMENT	PLAN
Interview and case history	Test results	Collation of subjective and objective information	Additional testing Treatment options

aloud a set of words normally used in dictation. This practical application of voice recognition offers an attractive and cost-effective alternative to traditional reporting methods.

Public school clinicians report their diagnostic findings in a record called an Individualized Education Program. The IEP is a student-focused plan devised by a team—teachers, school administrators, special educators (including the speech-language pathologist), and others, particularly the parents. The plan is spelled out in response to very specific questions:

1. *What* is the problem(s)?
2. *Where* is the student now?
3. *Who* will do *what* with the student and *how often?*
4. *When* and *how* will progress be measured?

Figure 13.2 displays a portion of an IEP prepared for a child with a phonological disorder.

The speech-language pathologist in the schools will also be responsible for writing the Individualized Family Service Plan (IFSP). The assessment of infants and toddlers (birth to three) presents special considerations in terms of record keeping and evaluation procedures. Clearly, the family as well as the child become targets of assessment and possible intervention. Public Law 99-457 requires a multidisciplinary team approach to assessment of this population, since no single agency or discipline can meet the diverse needs of infants, toddlers, and their families. After assessment, the team is required by law to generate an IFSP that has the following components:

1. A statement of the child's present levels of development (cognitive, speech-language, hearing, motor, self-help, social)
2. A statement of the family's strengths and needs related to enhancing the child's development
3. A statement of major outcomes expected to be achieved for the child and family
4. The criteria, procedures, and timelines for determining progress
5. The specific early intervention services necessary to meet the unique needs of the child and family, including the method, frequency, and intensity of services
6. The projected dates for the initiation of service and the projected duration
7. The name of the case manager
8. The procedures for transition from early intervention into the preschool.

One can readily see that the format of the IFSP has clear implications for assessment. First, it mandates family assessment that forces the speech-language pathologist to focus on the child's total environmental system. Second, it requires that judgments be made in a variety of areas that require multidisciplinary cooperation (e.g., cognitive, social, language, motor, hearing). Third, it requires the practitioner to recommend evaluation procedures to be used to determine progress. We need to be prepared to address the issues included in the IFSP when we

Figure 13.2 Individualized Educational Program

Student: <u>David Grabowski</u>   Birthdate: <u>1/7/78</u>   Address: <u>224 Orchard</u>

Parents: <u>Gerard and Julie</u>   District/school: <u>Beaver Grove Schools</u>

Grade: <u>First</u>   District of residency: <u>Marquette County</u>

IEP conference date: <u>9/12/83</u>   Projected IEP review date: <u>9/10/84</u>

Eligibility Statement: (What decision/description requires this service?)

David has difficulty with frictional manner of articulation production resulting in several substitutional errors: th/s, th/z, s/sh, ts/ch, dz/dj.

Current Educational Level: (Where is child currently functioning?)

David is enrolled in a developmental first-grade classroom.

SPECIAL SERVICES		
GOALS	*OBJECTIVES*	*SERVICE DESCRIPTION*
1. David will produce *s, z* correctly at the word and sentence level. 2. David will produce *sh* correctly at the word and sentence level. 3. Progress reports will be sent to parents and teacher twice a year.	1. David will discriminate target sounds from other sounds with 90% accuracy. 2. David will produce target sounds at the beginning, middle, and end of single words with 90% accuracy. 3. David will correctly produce target sounds within sentences with 80% success.	Speech therapy
Dates of Services		Time in Programs	Responsible Individuals

Start	End	Daily	
9/19/83	6/1/84	Within small-group 20-minute sessions 2 times a week	Speech-language clinician

Evaluation Plan: (How is it planned to ascertain that goals have been reached?)

1. Goldman-Fristoe Test of Articulation
2. Pre- and postherapy word list containing target sounds
3. Five-minute sample of spontaneous speech

IEP Committee Members:

Name	Position
Ellen Mattson	Teacher
Roy Brown, Jr.	Principal
Rebecca Clark	Speech-language clinician
Gerard and Julie Grabowski	Parents

participate in staff meetings with other professionals subsequent to our evaluations of these children.

Regardless of the format employed, a diagnostic report should be organized for easy retrieval of information (Pannbacker, 1975) and prepared in a manner that reflects high professional standards. Here are additional criteria we use to judge a diagnostic report: Is it accurate? Is it complete? Is it efficiently written (clearly and with an economy of words)? Was it prepared promptly?

Figure 13.3 provides a generic format—one that we have found quite effective and recommend to the beginning clinician. It contains several major sections which we will discuss; these sections can be stored as a template in a word-processing program for ease of writing and editing. Of course, reports can continue to be written in longhand for later typing.

Routine Information

In this section, we present basic identifying information—client's name, sex, address, date of birth, telephone number, patient's name where relevant, and of course the date of the examination; an undated report is of very little use. In addition to these routine data, we generally identify the referral source (parent, teacher, physician) and the evaluator. If the client is a school-age child, we note the name and location of his/her school and the names of the teacher

Figure 13.3 Format for Diagnostic Report

I. Routine Information

Name:	File no.:
Sex:	Date:
Address:	Phone no.:
Birth date:	Age at Evaluation:
Parents:	Referred by:
Evaluated by:	Address:

II. Statement of the Problem
III. Historical Information
IV. Evaluation
V. Clinical Impressions
VI. Summary
VII. Recommendations

_____
                                Clinician

_____
                                Supervisor

and the principal. The keystone of this initial section of the report is meticulous attention to accuracy.

Statement of the Problem

In this section, we include a succinct statement of the presenting problem. What is the complaint and who is making it? Be sure to distinguish between the client's complaint and the problem stated by the referral source. In most instances, the reason for referral is stated in the client's (or parent's) own words— always indicated by quotation marks.

Historical Information

Before seeing a client for evaluation, many clinicians request that the individual fill out a brief case history form. Alternately, this information can be gathered in a face-to-face interview. Rather than present a generic example of a case history form, we refer the reader to the case history forms cited in all the preceding chapters. Different information needs to be collected with specific disorders.

Information obtained from referral letters, the case history, and the intake interview are included in this section of the diagnostic report. Material regarding the client's development (general and speech and language); medical, educational, and familial history; and estimates of psychosocial and behavioral adjustments are summarized. Only the most pertinent items are included in the diagnostic report. Because most of the historical information is obtained by questioning the client, a parent, or other informants, we suggest that the clinician briefly describe the interview situation—type of rapport established, the frankness and completeness of the respondent's answers, and any other pertinent observations.

Evaluation

The results of the various tests and examinations are delineated in this section. Before describing the assessment procedures and results, however, we include an opening statement that describes how the client approached the clinical setting and the tasks used to evaluate the communication abilities: Was the client apprehensive, bored, fatigued, cooperative? The name of each test, an explanation of what it does and how it was administered, and the results obtained should be included. Should the clinician include statements about communication skills that are within normal limits at the time of the evaluation? Knepflar (1976) believes that a complete diagnostic report should mention, even if briefly, all aspects of a client's speech, hearing, and language performance so that subsequent assessments can utilize the information as baseline observations. The information is simply presented, not interpreted, in this section of the report.

Clinical Impressions

In this section, we summarize our impressions of the individual and the communication impairment. What type of speech or language problem does the client have? How severe is it? What caused it? What factors seem to be perpetuating it? What impact has it had on the client and the client's family? How much does it interfere with everyday functioning? What are the prospects for treatment? Although we can offer interpretations here, we must still be able to support our impressions with information obtained during the interview or testing. Speculations based on previous clinical experience, such as similarity between the client and other cases the diagnostician has examined, should be clearly labeled as such.

Summary

The summary should be concise (not more than a short paragraph) statement abstracting the salient features of the whole report. What is the communication disorder? What are the primary features of the disorder? What is the probable cause of the disorder? What is the prognosis (and general estimate of the predicted time frame) for recovery?

Recommendations

This is perhaps the most crucial portion of the report. We must now translate our findings into appropriate suggestions or directions that will help the client solve communication and related problems. Do we recommend further speech and language evaluations? Is a medical referral necessary? Is treatment indicated? What direction should be taken? By whom, and when? The task, then, is to crystallize all the disparate interaction we have had with the individual, collate all the data, and then provide a flexible blueprint for further action. We must attempt to answer the question: What happens now—where do we go from here? Try to make the recommendations specific and brief. Suggestions for treatment or a more lengthy plan of therapy can be outlined in a letter or follow-up report. One final warning: Do not recommend *specific* evaluations or remediation procedures to workers in other professions. It is improper, for example, to recommend a client for electroencephalography to a neurologist, or for dental braces to an orthodontist; the speech clinician would be chagrined if a physician referred a child and recommended the administration of the ITPA. Be sure that your referrals for additional assessment are based on sound evidence; it is expensive, time-consuming, and stressful to the client to make recommendations for comprehensive medical or psychiatric evaluation without serious and compelling reasons:

> Early in the diagnostic session with five-year-old Mark we suspected the possibility of brain injury. Mindful of the family's limited finances, we wanted to document carefully all signs of apparent cerebral dysfunction before making a

referral for a complete pediatric neurological evaluation. Observation revealed a number of serious symptoms: difficulty with motor coordination; labile emotions; rapid and slurred speech; perseveration; and blanking out spells. The necessity for referral was then obvious.

CONFIDENTIALITY

In our view, confidentiality is basic to any helping profession. All reports and records should be kept secure so that no harm or embarrassment comes to the persons we serve. When a diagnostic report is released, we prefer to mail it to a specific person rather than to the agency itself. Before releasing any information about a client, however, we must secure the client's permission in writing; most speech and hearing centers have permission forms, which are completed prior to or during the diagnostic session.

Because clients and parents have a legal right (Public Law 93-380, Family Educational Rights and Privacy Act of 1974) to read any report containing information about them, we often find it useful to send them a copy of the diagnostic findings. Before mailing the report, however, we always review our findings and recommendations with them. By going over the report with the clients or parents, we can be sure that they understand its contents.

STYLE

An extended discussion of prose style for report writing is not possible within the scope of this text. The reader will want to consult several of the following sources for more definitive statements about common modes of report writing: Huber (1961), Jerger (1962), Moore (1969), Good (1970), Fishbein (1972), Haynes and Hartman (1975), Pannbacker (1975), Knepflar (1976), Hollis and Dunn (1979), and Tallent (1980). In the interest of brevity, then, we shall simply enumerate several principles of style that we have found useful.

1. Make your presentation straightforward and objective, using a topical outline. Use simple, brief but complete sentences. It is often helpful to write for a specific reader; picture the reader in your mind—the classroom teacher, physician, speech clinician—and then simply tell the story of what you observed and recommend regarding a particular client. When in doubt about a reader's level of understanding, it is better to err on the side of simplicity.

2. Use an impersonal style. Some clinicians use the first person when writing diagnostic reports, but in our view it is preferable to keep the "I" out of it; a reference to "the clinician" or "the examiner" is more in keeping with professional reports. We prefer to individualize the client described in the report, not the writer. Furthermore, we believe that not only does an impersonal style help to minimize the writer's verbal idiosyncrasies, but it also tends to encourage objectivity.

3. Edit the report carefully to make certain that spelling and use of tenses, grammar, and punctuation are accurate. Errors, even trivial ones, undermine the confidence of the reader in the diagnostician. Remember, competence is judged to a great extent by the precision of your reporting.

4. Watch your semantics. Be wary of overused or nebulous words such as "nice," "hopefully," "good," and the like. Avoid pet expressions or stereotyped ways of phrasing information. One clinician used the phrase "in terms of" 13 times in a two-page diagnostic report. Another laced his reports with currently popular words like "input," "interface," and "scenario." Some writers use the word "feel" inappropriately in statements like "The clinician felt the client understood the diagnostic task"; we believe (not feel!) that the word should be reserved for discussing emotions or tactile sensations. Use abbreviations sparingly. Avoid superlatives unless they are clearly indicated.

5. Avoid preparing an "Aunt Fanny" report (Sunberg & Tyler, 1962)— a bland written statement that could represent anyone or is so filled with qualifications ("perhaps," "apparently," "tends to") that it reveals nothing—nothing, that is, except a timid diagnostician.

6. Make the report "tight." Do not leave gaps or ambiguity where it is possible to read between the lines. If findings in certain areas are unremarkable, always state this explicitly. Do not leave the reader to guess whether you have investigated all possible aspects.

7. A diagnostic report is no place to display your learning or to parade a large vocabulary. Pedantic reports are misunderstood or unread.

8. Stay close to the data until you wish to draw the observations together and make some interpretations. For example, tell the reader which sounds were in error instead of simply stating that the child sounds infantile.

9. The very essence of good style is the willingness to take the time and energy to write and rewrite the report until it communicates what we did and what we found in the diagnostic session.

THE WRITING PROCESS

Many students have difficulty writing reports. Most of them have found the task onerous, and a few are threatened and overwhelmed by the prospect of a blank sheet of paper in the typewriter. It has been our experience, however, that rather than having a writing deficiency, most of these students have a writing bias—they do not think they can do it. There are, of course, no quick and simple solutions; but we offer the following suggestions that have proven helpful to more than one beginning report writer.

Write on a daily basis. Each night—before retiring, for example—sit down and write a descriptive paragraph concerning something that happened to you that day. It may be easier for you to tap into your own creative power by starting with material that arouses strong feelings (see Macrorie, 1968, 1970). At first it may be halting and difficult; as in any new task, your writing "muscles" will be sore. Do not wait for an inspiration, for that magic moment when, suddenly, it will come to you. Go to it. At the end of the week, review the writing you have done; edit, revise, ask yourself what you meant by each word or phrase. The best way to learn to write, in our opinion, is to write.

Get the message out and revise it later. It is especially important in writing reports to begin as soon as possible while the material is still fresh in your mind. A common error that some beginning writers make is to attempt to produce perfect writing in the initial draft. It does not matter how it looks at this point; you can always edit or have someone help you edit. When you meet barriers or mental blocks, do not linger; jump over them and go on with the rest of the report. When you come back later, you will find that your mind has filled in the blank spots.

It is helpful to have someone read and comment on the initial draft of your report. Although it is difficult to submit one's prose for dissection, ask the reader to be frank and honest in his/her editing. So many times, a phrase that seems clear to the writer who conceived it is vague or obscure to an objective reader. If writing continues to be a problem consult the work of Strunk and White (1959) and others (Berke, 1972; Ferguson, 1959; Jones & Faulkner, 1971; Kelly, Roth, & Altshuler, 1969; Leggett, Mead, & Charvat, 1974; Mayes, 1972; Wubben, 1971).

FOLLOW-UP

The clinician's responsibilities do not end when the diagnostic report is finished and filed. A complete evaluation includes one final important task: a careful follow-up. It is the examiner's professional obligation to determine that the diagnostic activities and recommendations are translated into action; it is useless, perhaps even harmful, to identify and describe problems unless the individual is seen for further testing or treatment as soon as possible. When the diagnostician is also the clinician, the follow-up can be handled directly and with a minimum of paperwork. In an agency such as ours (a university speech and hearing clinic), however, we regularly refer clients to other workers for further assessment or treatment. We use the following questions as guidelines in implementing a follow-up program:

1. Did the intended readers receive the report? The best of secretaries occasionally misfiles a document, so we generally call the referral source within a week after the diagnostic to determine if the report has arrived.
2. Does the reader understand the contents of the report? What questions did it raise, if any, about the client? We always log these phone calls in the client's folder.
3. What is the disposition of the client? Is the client being seen for further testing? Is the client on a waiting list or being seen for treatment?
4. How is the client responding to treatment? We call the local worker, usually on a monthly basis, to assess how the client is doing in treatment relative to our recommendations. Not only does this convey our interest and assistance, it also helps the diagnostic team evaluate the efficacy of its work.

BIBLIOGRAPHY

BERKE, J. (1972). *Twenty questions for the writer.* San Diego, CA: Harcourt Brace Jovanovich.

BOUCHARD, M., & SHANE, H. (1977). Use of the problem-oriented medical record in the speech and hearing profession. *Journal of the American Speech and Hearing Association, 19,* 157–159.

DARLEY, F., & SPRIESTERSBACH, D. (1978). *Diagnostic methods in speech pathology* (2nd ed.). New York: Harper & Row.

ENELOW, A., & SWISHER, S. (1972). *Interviewing and patient care.* New York: Oxford University Press.

FERGUSON, C. (1959). *Say it with words.* New York: Knopf.

FISHBEIN, M. (1972). *Medical writing.* Springfield, IL: Charles C Thomas.

FLOWER, R. (1984). *Delivery of speech-language pathology and audiology services.* Baltimore: Williams & Wilkins.

GOOD, R. (1970). The written language of rehabilitation medicine: Meaning and usages. *Archives of Physical Medicine and Rehabilitation, 51,* 29–36.

HAYNES, W. O., & HARTMAN, D. (1975). The agony of report writing. *Journal of the National Student Speech-Language-Hearing Association, 3,* 7–15.

HOLLIS, J., & DUNN, P. (1979). *Psychological report writing.* Muncie, IN: Accelerated Development.

HUBER, J. (1961). *Report writing in psychology and psychiatry.* New York: Harper & Row.

HUTCHINSON, B., HANSON, M., & MECHAM, M. (1979). *Diagnostic handbook of speech pathology.* Baltimore: Williams & Wilkins.

JERGER, J. (1962). Scientific writing can be readable. *Journal of the American Speech and Hearing Association, 4,* 101–104.

JONES, A., & FAULKNER, C. (1971). *Writing good prose.* New York: Scribner's.

KELLY, M., ROTH, A., & ALTSHULER, T. (1969). *Writing step by step.* Boston: Houghton Mifflin.

KENT, L., & CHABON, S. (1980). Problem-oriented records in a university speech and hearing clinic. *Journal of the American Speech and Hearing Association, 22,* 151–158.

KNEPFLAR, K. (1976). *Report writing.* Danville, IL: Interstate Printers and Publishers.

LEGGETT, G., MEAD, C., & CHARVAT, W. (1974). *Handbook for writers* (6th ed.). Englewood Cliffs, NJ: Prentice Hall.

MACRORIE, K. (1968). *Writing to be read.* Rochelle Park, NJ: Hayden.

MACRORIE, K. (1970). *Uptaught.* Rochelle Park, NJ: Hayden.

MAYES, J. (1972). *Writing and rewriting.* New York: Macmillan.

MOORE, M. (1969). Pathological writing. *Journal of the American Speech and Hearing Association, 11,* 535–538.

PANNBACKER, M. (1975). Diagnostic report writing. *Journal of Speech and Hearing Disorders, 40,* 367–379.

PETERSON, H., & MARQUARDT, T. (1990). *Appraisal and diagnosis of speech and language disorders* (2nd ed.). Englewood Cliffs: Prentice Hall.

STRUNK, W., & WHITE, E. B. (1959). *The elements of style.* New York: Macmillan.

SUNBERG, N., & TYLER, L. (1962). *Clinical psychology.* Englewood Cliffs, NJ: Prentice Hall.

TALLENT, N. (1980). *Psychological report writing.* Englewood Cliffs, NJ: Prentice Hall.

TONKOVICH, J. D. (1989). *Using functional outcome measures in diagnostic reporting and treatment planning.* Paper presented to the convention of the American Speech-Language-Hearing Association, St. Louis, MO.

TONKOVICH, J. D., HOROWITZ, D. M., GANS, B. M., & MATLOCK, M. C. (1990). *Automating speech-language pathology documentation with voice recognition.* Paper presented to the convention of the American Speech-Language-Hearing Association, Seattle, WA.

WUBBEN, J. (1971). *Guide writing.* New York: Random House.

CHILD LANGUAGE ASSESSMENT INTERVIEW PROTOCOL

GENERAL INFORMATION

Referral source:

Parent's statement of the problem:

History of prior assessments:

History of prior treatments:

Parent treatment attempts:

Preschool status (attendance at daycare/preschool):

Number and relationships of people living at home:

BIOLOGICAL PREREQUISITES

1.   Birth and general health:

Pregnancy:

Birth:

History of illnesses:

Present state of health:

2.   Auditory status

History of frequent colds:

History of earaches and ear infections:

Parent's estimation of hearing acuity:

3.   Neurological status

Concussions:

Unconsciousness:

Seizures:

Has the child been seen by a neurologist? For what?

Does the child evidence any motor difficulties?

SOCIAL PREREQUISITES

Approximate time spent in social interaction on typical day:

Who are the persons the child frequently interacts with?

What are the activities associated with social interactions?

Does the child exhibit any antisocial or socially inappropriate behaviors (avoiding interactions, consistent playing alone?, etc.):

Does the child exhibit any self-stimulating behaviors (e.g., rocking, flapping arms)?

Does the child maintain eye contact?

Does the child regulate your behavior nonverbally?

Does the child use objects or repeat actions to get your attention?

Does the child vocalize his/her social interactions?

Does the child joint reference with caretaker?

Describe the child's typical day in detail:

COGNITIVE PREREQUISITES

Does the child exhibit play routines and behavior which would indicate the following attainments (specify example activity):

Object permanence:

Means-end:

Immediate imitation:

Functional use of objects:

Deferred imitation:

Symbolic play with surrogate object:

Symbolic play with appropriate object:

What are the child's most frequent play activities?

LANGUAGE

Does the child exhibit phonetically consistent forms?

Parent estimation of the number of single words used expressively (follow up on word checklist):

Parent estimation of MLU:

Reports of presyntactic devices:

Parent's report of semantic relation types:

Parent's estimate of language comprehension:

Parent should provide anecdotal information on the following:

Phonetic inventory:

Phonological processes:

Intonation patterns:

Estimate of intelligibility:

B

EVALUATION CHECKLIST FOR CARETAKER-CHILD INTERACTION

William O. Haynes, Ph.D.
Auburn University

Child: _____   Date: _____   Age: _____

Nature of interaction in terms of toys, room, and interactants:

General Parameters

	No				Yes
1. Encourages communication by looking expectantly	1	2	3	4	5
2. Responds to communication by reinforcing it with action or utterance	1	2	3	4	5
3. Joint references with child	1	2	3	4	5
4. Alternates adult/child direction in joint referencing	1	2	3	4	5
5. Talks about present context (here and now)	1	2	3	4	5
6. Model is timed to coincide with joint referencing	1	2	3	4	5
7. Talks at child's eye level	1	2	3	4	5
8. Successful attempts at interpretation of child's utterances and communicative intents	1	2	3	4	5
9. Creates communicative opportunities by using sabotage or pause time	1	2	3	4	5
10. Does not anticipate child's needs ahead of time thus reducing communicative attempts	1	2	3	4	5

Language Model Parameters

1. Reduces sentence length	1	2	3	4	5
2. Reduces sentence complexity	1	2	3	4	5
3. Repeats utterances frequently (redundancy)	1	2	3	4	5
4. Paraphrases utterances ("throw the ball; throw it")	1	2	3	4	5
5. Uses exaggerated intonation patterns	1	2	3	4	5
6 Places stress on important words	1	2	3	4	5
7. Uses concrete, high frequency vocabulary	1	2	3	4	5
8. Does not talk too much and dominate conversation	1	2	3	4	5
9. Does not use excessive questions and commands	1	2	3	4	5
10. Uses slower speech rate	1	2	3	4	5

Use of Teaching Techniques

1. Self-talk	1	2	3	4	5
2. Parallel talk	1	2	3	4	5
3. Expansion	1	2	3	4	5
4. Expatiation (enlargement)	1	2	3	4	5
5. Buildup/breakdown sequences	1	2	3	4	5
6. Recast sentences	1	2	3	4	5

Average Score = _____

appendix
C

CODING SHEET FOR EARLY MULTIWORD ANALYSIS

CHILD UTTERANCE	SEMANTIC RELATION	FUNCTION	INITIATION	POST–STAGE 1 ELEMENT
Push car	Action + object	Regulation	CI	-ing
Push it	Action + object	Regulation	CI	
Car going	Instrument + action	Comment	CI	-ing
More car	Recurrence + X	Regulation	CI	
Car allgone?	X + disappearance	Questioning	CI	
Juice up there	Entity + locative	Elicited imitation	AI	
Gimme juice	Action + object	Regulation	CI	
That truck	Nomination + X	Answering	AI	

D

SUMMARY SHEET FOR EARLY MULTIWORD ANALYSIS

Summary Sheet for Early Multiword Analysis

Child: _____   Age: _____   Birth date: _____

Date of sample: _____   Context of sample (include people present): _____

Length of sample in time:

Activities performed during sample:

Mean length of utterance:

Total number of child utterances:

Longest utterance in morphemes:

Number of single-word responses:

Semantic relations evident in sample:

Functions evident in sample:

Syntactic constituents used most often:

Ratio of child-initiated to adult-initiated utterances:

Post–stage 1 elements noted:

Semantic relations missing from sample:

Functions missing from sample:

Recommendations for further sampling/treatment:

E

DATA CONSOLIDATION IN LIMITED-LANGUAGE EVALUATIONS

IDENTIFYING INFORMATION

Name:

Address:

Telephone:

Parents:

Date of Evaluation:

DATA OBTAINED (Check and Specify)

Case History _____

Reports from Professionals _____

Hearing Screening _____

Oral Peripheral _____

Behavioral Observation of Caretaker-Child _____

Behavioral Observation of Child _____

Parental Checklist (Lexicon) _____

Adaptive Behavior Scale _____

General Developmental Battery _____

Spontaneous Language Sample _____

Nonstandardized Tasks _____

Cognitive Scale _____

Comprehension Test _____

Imitation Test _____

Language Battery _____

Articulation Test _____

Other _____

ANALYSES PERFORMED (Check and Specify)

MLU _____

Distributional Analysis _____

Early Multiword Analysis (semantic relations/functions) _____

Sensorimotor Performative Analysis _____

Cognitive Analysis of Play _____

Vocalization Analysis _____

Phonetic Inventory _____

Phonological Analysis _____

Caretaker-Child Interaction Analysis _____

Scoring of Formal Procedures _____

Summarize Parent Checklist Information _____

Analysis of Social Behaviors _____

Scoring of Nonstandardized Procedures _____

Other(s) _____

REMARKS ON THE DATA

Remarkable Case History Information:

Remarkable Results from Prior Reports and Tests:

Remarkable Interview Information:

Remarkable Behavioral Observation Results:

Remarkable Informal Testing Results:

Remarkable Formal Test Results:

SYNTHESIS OF FINDINGS

A. Specific Areas of Interest (carry information forward from prior section and elaborate below).

    1. Prerequisites to Communication

        a. Biological

            (1) Hearing:

            (2) Neurological:

            (3) Medical:

            (4) Anatomical:

    b. Cognitive

        (1) Approximate Piagetian stage attainment and characteristic play/symbolic behaviors. List strengths and weaknesses.

    c. Social

        (1) Interpersonal manner (attachment, eye contact, reciprocity, affect, etc.):

        (2) Caretaker model of communication:

        (3) Nonverbal functions (include protoimperative/declarative):

        (4) Evidence of self-stimulation or abuse:

2. Communicative Effectiveness

    a. Nonverbal communication:

    b. Phonetically Consistent Form (PCF) vocalizations:

    c. Single-word forms and functions (describe):

    d. Presyntactic Device (PSD) vocalizations:

    e. Stage I forms and functions (describe):

    f. Phonetic inventory (describe):

    g. Phonological processes (describe):

    h. Intelligibility:

B. Areas of Strength and Concern

Child's age: MLU: Primary language stage: NV   SW   EMW   SYNT

Indicate areas of strength (+) and concern (−):

     biological prerequisites   _____

     cognitive prerequisites   _____

     social prerequisites   _____

     delayed language   _____

     adaptive behavior   _____

     phonology   _____

     communicative functions   _____

     phonetic inventory   _____

     caretaker model/cooperation   _____

RECOMMENDATIONS

A. Referrals:

B. Recommended Further Testing by SLP:

C. Prognosis and Treatment Directions/Suggestions:

E. Results of Parent Counseling and Recommendations for Further Interviews.

appendix

F

SELECTED LANGUAGE ASSESSMENT INSTRUMENTS FOR SYNTAX-LEVEL CHILDREN

INSTRUMENT/AUTHOR/SOURCE*	AGE RANGE
Analysis of the Language of Learning	
(Blodgett, E. & Cooper, E.; Linguisystems)	5–9
Adolescent Language Screening Test	
(Morgan, D. & Guilford, A.; Communication Skill Builders)	11–17
Assessment of Children's Language Comprehension	
(Foster, R., Giddan, J., & Stark, J.; Consulting Psychologists Press)	3–6.11
Assessing Semantic Skills through Everyday Themes	
(Barrett, N., Zachman, L., & Huisingh, R.; Linguisystems)	3–9
Auditory-Visual, Single Word Picture Vocabulary Test-Adolescent	
(Gardner, M.; Slosson)	12–17
Bankson Language Screening Test	
(Bankson, N.; PRO-ED)	4–7
Basic School Skills Inventory-Diagnostic	
(Hammill, D. & Leigh, J.; PRO-ED)	4–7.5
Basic School Skills Inventory-Screen	
(Hammill, D. & Leigh, J.; PRO-ED)	4–6.11
Bilingual Syntax Measure 1 and 2	
(Bkurt, M., Dulay, H., & Chavez, E.; Psychological Corp.)	5–12
Boehm Test of Basic Concepts — Preschool Version	
(Boehm, A.; Psychological Corp.)	3–5
Boehm Test of Basic Concepts — Revised	
(Boehm, A.; Psychological Corp.)	5–7
Bracken Basic Concept Scale	
(Bracken, B.; Psychological Corp.)	2.6–8
Carolina Picture Vocabulary Test	
(Layton, T. & Holmes, D.; United Educ. Services)	4–11.5

INSTRUMENT/AUTHOR/SOURCE*	AGE RANGE
Carrow Elicited Language Inventory (Carrow, E.; Learning Concepts)	3–7
Clark-Madison Test of Oral Language (Clark, J. & Madison, C.; PRO-ED)	4–8
Classroom Communication Screening Procedure for Early Assessment (Simon, C.; Interstate)	9–14
Clinical Evaluation of Language Fundamentals (Semel, E., Wiig, E., & Secord, W.; Psychological Corp.)	5–16
Clinical Evaluation of Language Functions (Semel, E., Wiig, E.; Merrill)	5–9
Cognitive Abilities Scale (Bradley-Johnson, S.; PRO-ED)	2–3
Del Rio Language Screening Test: English/Spanish (Toronto, A. et. al.; National Education Laboratory Pubs.)	3–6
Detroit Tests of Learning Aptitude —2 (Hammill, D.; PRO-ED)	6–17
Detroit Tests of Learning Aptitude —Primary (Hammill, D. & Bryant, B.; PRO-ED)	3–9
Diagnostic Achievement Battery (Newcomer, P. & Curtis, D.; PRO-ED)	6–14
Diagnostic Screening Test: Language (Gnagey, T. & Gnagey, P.; Slosson)	6–13
Dos Amigos Verbal Language Scales (Critchlow, D.; United Educ. Services)	5–13.5
Early School Inventory (Nurss, J. & McGauvran, M.; Psychological Corp.)	5–6
Evaluating Acquired Skills in Communication (Riley, A.; Communication Skill Builders)	<1–8
Early School Inventory —Preliteracy Nurss, J. & McGauvran, M.; Psychological Corp.)	5–6
Evaluating Communicative Competence: A Functional Pragmatic Procedure (Simon, C.; Communication Skill Builders)	9–17
Expressive One Word Picture Vocabulary Test: Upper Extension (Gardner, M.; Slosson)	12–15
Full Range Picture Vocabulary Test (Ammons, R. & Ammons, H.; Psychological Test Specialists)	2–21
Fullerton Language Test for Adolescents (Thorum, A.; Slosson)	11–18
Grammatical Analysis of Elicited Language (Moog, J., Kozak, V., & Geers, A.; Cent. Inst. Deaf)	3–6
Illinois Test of Psycholinguistic Abilities (Kirk, S., McCarthy, J., & Kirk, W.; Slosson)	2–10
Kindergarten Language Screening Test (Fauthier, S. & Madison, C.; PRO-ED)	4–5
Let's Talk Inventory for Adolescents (Wiig, E.; Psychological Corp.)	9–18
Let's Talk Inventory for Children (Bray, C. & Wiig, E.; Psychological Corp.)	4–8
Language Processing Test (Richard, G. & Hanner, M.; Linguisystems)	5–11
Language Inventory for Teachers (Cooper, A. & School, B.; United Educ. Services)	4–12

INSTRUMENT/AUTHOR/SOURCE*	AGE RANGE
Language Structured Auditory Retention Span Test	
(Carlson, L.; United Educ. Services)	3–21
MAP: The Miller Assessment for Preschoolers	
(Miller, L.; AGS)	3–6
Miller-Yoder Language Comprehension Test	
(Miller, J. & Yoder, D.; Slosson)	4–8
Northwestern Syntax Screening Test	
(Lee, L.; Northwestern University Press)	3–7
Oral Language Sentence Imitation Diagnostic Inventory	
(Zachman, L. et al.; Linguisystems)	none
Patterned Elicitation Syntax Test—Revised	
(Young, E. & Perachio, J.; United Educ. Services)	3–7
Peabody Picture Vocabulary Test—Revised	
(Dunn, L. & Dunn, L.; AGS)	2.5–21
Picture Story Language Test	
(Myklebust, H.; WPS)	7–12
Porch Index of Communicative Ability in Children	
(Porch, B.; Consulting Psychologists Press)	4–12
Pragmatics Screening Test	
(Prinz, P. & Weiner, F.; Psychological Corp.)	3–8
Preschool Language Assessment Instrument	
(Blank, M., Rose, S., & Berlin, L.; Linguisystems)	3–6
Preschool Language Scale	
(Zimmerman, I., Stiener, V., & Pond, R.; Merrill)	1.5–7
Psycholinguistic Rating Scale	
(Hobby, K.; WPS)	5–9
Rhode Island Test of Language Structure	
(Engen, E. & Engen, T.; United Educ. Services)	3–6
Receptive One Word Picture Vocabulary Test: Upper Extension	
(Brownell, R.; Slosson)	12–16
Reynell Developmental Language Scale	
(Reynell, J.; WPS)	1–7
Screening Test of Adolescent Language	
(Prather, E. et al.; United Educ. Services)	12–18
Screening Kit of Language Development	
(Bliss, L. & Allen, D.; Slosson)	2–5
Screening Children for Related Early Educational Needs	
(Hresko, W. et al.; PRO-ED)	3–7
Sequenced Inventory of Communication Development	
(Hedrick, E., Prather, E. & Tobin, A.; WPS)	<1–4
Slosson Articulation, Language Test with Phonology	
(Tade, W.; Slosson)	3–6
Spanish Language Assessment Procedures: A Communication Skills Inventory	
(Mattes, L.; Academic Communication Associates)	5–8
Test of Auditory Comprehension of Language—Revised	
(Carrow-Woolfolk, E.; DLM)	3–9
Test of Language Competence—Expanded Edition	
(Wiig, E. & Secord, W.; Psychological Corp.)	5–18
Test of Early Language Development	
(Hresko, W., Reid, K., & Hammill, D.; AGS)	3–7
Test of Adolescent Language 2	
(Hammill, D. et al.; AGS)	12–18

INSTRUMENT/AUTHOR/SOURCE*	AGE RANGE
Test of Language Development 2: Primary (Newcomer, P. & Hammill, D.; AGS)	4–8
Test of Language Development 2: Intermediate (Newcomer, P. & Hammill, D.; AGS)	8–12
Test de Vocabulario en Imagenes Peabody (Dunn, L. et al.; AGS)	2.5–18
Test of Relational Concepts (Edmonston, N. & Thane, N.; PRO-ED)	3–8
Test for Examining Expressive Morphology (Shipley, K., Stone, T., & Sue, M.; Communication Skill Builders)	3–8
Test of Pragmatic Skills (Shulman, B.; Communication Skill Builders)	3–8
Test of Problem Solving (Zachman et al.; Linguisystems)	6–11
Test of Word Finding (German, D.; DLM)	6–12
Test of Language Development 3 (Mecham, M. & Jones, D.; PRO-ED)	3–11
Thought and Language Inventory (Markoff, A.; Academic Communication Associates)	6
Token Test for Children (Disimoni, F.; Teaching Resources Corp.)	3–12
The Word Test (Barrett, M. et al.; Linguisystems)	7–11

*Addresses of major sources are included. In some cases, a general supplier (e.g., United Educational Services, Inc.) is listed because we did not have access to the original test instrument or specific catalogue.

Academic Communication Associates, Publications Division, Department 4, P.O. Box 6294, Oceanside, CA 92056

American Guidance Service (AGS), Publisher's Building, Circle Pines, MN 55014–1796

Central Institute for the Deaf, 818 South Euclid, St. Louis, MO 63110

Charles E. Merrill Publishing Co., 1300 Alum Creek Drive, Box 508, Columbus, OH 43216

Communication Skill Builders, 3830 E. Bellevue, P.O. Box 42050E, Tucson, AZ 85733

DLM Teaching Resources, One DLM Park, P.O. Box 4000, Allen, TX 75002

Interstate Printers and Publishers, Inc., P.O. Box 50, Danville, IL 61834

Linguisystems, Inc., Department ABCD, 3100 4th Avenue, P.O. Box 747, East Moline, IL 61244

PRO-ED, 8700 Shoal Creek, Austin, TX 78758–6897

Psychological Corporation, Harcourt Brace Jovanovich, P.O. Box 9954, San Antonio, TX 78204

Slosson Educational Publications, Inc., P.O. Box 280, East Aurora, NY 14052

United Educational Services, Inc., P.O. Box 605, East Aurora, NY 14052

Western Psychological Services, 12031 Wilshire Boulevard, Los Angeles, CA 90025

INDEX

Cultural groups, belief systems of regarding
    disabilities, 33
Cultural norms, 4
Curriculum, evaluation of school, 147–49
Curry, E.T., 329, 331
Czikszentmihalyi, M., 36

Dabul, B., 260, 328
Dale, P., 104
Damico, J., 146
Darley, F.L., 241, 246, 259, 263, 264, 270
Davis, S., 302
Deal, J., 256
Decision task, 136
Declarative, 103
Deferred initiation, 97
Definitions, ambiguous, 61–62
Degree of effort, 295
Delayed imitation, 97
Dementia, 242–43
Denasal voice, 339
DeRenzi, E., 259
Developmental apraxia, 263–66
Developmental Sentence Analysis, 140
Developmental stuttering, 200
Diadochokinesis, 216, 263, 270
Diagnosis, 1
    of adolescents, 19–20
    age groups in, 16–21
    of aphasic, 234–45
    of apraxia, 263–64
    arriving at, 3
    art of, 10–11
    and clinical management, 8–9
    defined, 2–3
    to determine etiology of problem, 6–8
    to determine reality of problem, 3–6
    differential, 199–205
    of dysarthrias, 267–69
    findings of, 14
    goal-oriented, 9
    through interview, 35–50
    precepts of, 88–90
    to provide clinical focus, 8
    of stuttering, 199–205
    synthesis of, 21–26
    of young children, 16–19
Diagnostician, as a factor, 11–14
Dialectal differences, 149
Dialectical variation, 159
Diaphragmatic breathing, 297
DiCarlo, L.M., 271, 272
Difference, 3–5
Differential diagnosis
    of aphasics, 239–45
    of developmental apraxia of speech, 263–64
    of dysarthrias, 267–69
Differentiating scales, 209
Dinnsen, D., 185
Diplophonia, 294
Direct visualization, 356
Discontinuous discourse, 145
Discourse analysis, 239
Discourse errors, specific, 146

Discursiveness, 137
Disfluencies
    assessing, 209
    characteristics of, 217
    distinguishing normal from stuttering, 203–05
    duration of child's, 204
    normal, 200
Disfluency Descriptor Digest, 220
Disfluent behaviors, frequency of, 204
Disorder, 3
    articulation, 154, 156, 165
    description of characteristics of, 7
    phonological, 128, 155, 156, 157–66
Disordered speech, detection of person with, 163
Distinctive feature acquisition, 158–59
Distinctive feature analysis, 172–75
Distortion, of sound, 156
Distractors, 333, 334
Distributional analysis, 112
Disturbance, 3, 5
Dore, J., 103, 107
Duchan, J., 98
Duguay, M.J., 311
Dunst, C., 101
Duration, 328
    of child's disfluency, 204
Dynamic assessment, 9
    of laryngectomee, 315–18
Dysarthria, 245, 261, 262
    adult, 255, 266–71
    appraisal of, 269–71
    ataxic, 268
    in children, 271–73
    flaccid, 267–68
    hyperkinetic, 269
    hypokinetic, 268
    mixed, 269
    prognosis of, 271
    spastic, 268
    testing for, 269
Dysphagia, 255

Early language cases, 102
Early utterance analysis, 106
Eckel, F., 299
Effeminate voice quality, 340, 350, 357
Egolf, D., 214
Elbert, M., 185
Elderly client, diagnosis of, 20–21
Electromyography, 300–301, 356
Elementary children
    evaluation of stuttering, 219
    screening later, 164
Elicited Articulatory System Evaluation, 178
Elicited imitation, 136–38
Emerick, L., 6
Emotion, responding appropriately to, 47
Emotional barriers, 34
Emotional release, 311
Empathy, 12, 50
Endoscopes, 356
Engmann, D., 173
Environmental reactions, 217
Environmental treatment, 216